369 0246815

O A O L
OXFORD AMERICAN ONCOLOGY LIBRARY

Lung Cancer

ONKLANDS HOSPITAL
LIBRARY
MONKSCOURT AVENUE
AIRDRIE ML60JS
☎ 01236712005

This material is not intended to be, and should not be considered, a substitute for medical or other professional advice. Treatment for the conditions described in this material is highly dependent on the individual circumstances. While this material is designed to offer accurate information with respect to the subject matter covered and to be current as of the time it was written, research and knowledge about medical and health issues are constantly evolving, and dose schedules for medications are being revised continually, with new side effects recognized and accounted for regularly. Readers must therefore always check the product information and clinical procedures with the most up-to-date published product information and data sheets provided by the manufacturers and the most recent codes of conduct and safety regulation. Oxford University Press and the authors make no representations or warranties to readers, express or implied, as to the accuracy or completeness of this material, including without limitation that they make no representations or warranties as to the accuracy or efficacy of the drug dosages mentioned in the material. The authors and the publishers do not accept, and expressly disclaim, any responsibility for any liability, loss, or risk that may be claimed or incurred as a consequence of the use and/or application of any of the contents of this material.

The Publisher is responsible for author selection and the Publisher and the Author(s) make all editorial decisions, including decisions regarding content. The Publisher and the Author(s) are not responsible for any product information added to this publication by companies purchasing copies of it for distribution to clinicians.

O A O L

OXFORD AMERICAN ONCOLOGY LIBRARY

Lung Cancer

Apar Kishor Ganti, MD, MS

Staff Physician
VA Nebraska Western Iowa Health Care System
Associate Professor
Division of Oncology-Hematology
Department of Internal Medicine
University of Nebraska Medical Center
Omaha, Nebraska

David E. Gerber, MD

Associate Professor
Division of Hematology-Oncology
Harold C. Simmons Cancer Center
University of Texas Southwestern Medical Center
Dallas, Texas

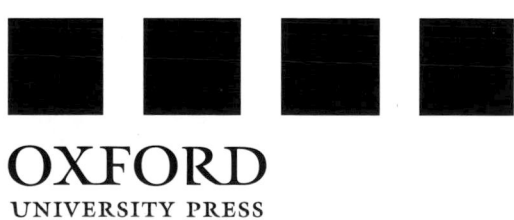

OXFORD
UNIVERSITY PRESS

BARCODE NO: 369024 6815.
CLASS NO: WF39 GAN
PRICE: 22.75
DATE: 20|11|13

OXFORD
UNIVERSITY PRESS

Oxford University Press is a department of the University of Oxford.
It furthers the University's objective of excellence in research, scholarship,
and education by publishing worldwide.

Oxford   New York
Auckland   Cape Town   Dar es Salaam   Hong Kong   Karachi
Kuala Lumpur   Madrid   Melbourne   Mexico City   Nairobi
New Delhi   Shanghai   Taipei   Toronto

With offices in
Argentina   Austria   Brazil   Chile   Czech Republic   France   Greece
Guatemala   Hungary   Italy   Japan   Poland   Portugal   Singapore
South Korea   Switzerland   Thailand   Turkey   Ukraine   Vietnam

Oxford is a registered trademark of Oxford University Press in the UK and certain
other countries.

Published in the United States of America by
Oxford University Press
198 Madison Avenue, New York, NY 10016

© Oxford University Press 2013

All rights reserved. No part of this publication may be reproduced, stored in a
retrieval system, or transmitted, in any form or by any means, without the prior
permission in writing of Oxford University Press, or as expressly permitted
by law, by license, or under terms agreed with the appropriate reproduction
rights organization. Inquiries concerning reproduction outside the scope of
the above should be sent to the Rights Department, Oxford University Press,
at the address above.

You must not circulate this work in any other form
and you must impose this same condition on any acquirer.

Library of Congress Cataloging-in-Publication Data
Lung cancer (2013)
Lung cancer / [edited by] Apar K. Ganti, David E. Gerber.
p. ; cm.—(Oxford American oncology library)
Includes bibliographical references and index.
ISBN 978–0–19–993593–2 (alk. paper)
I. Ganti, Apar K., editor of compilation.   II. Gerber, David E. (Professor of
Medicine), editor of compilation.   III. Title.   IV. Series: Oxford American
oncology library.
[DNLM: 1. Lung Neoplasms—Handbooks. WF 39]
RC280.L8
616.99'424—dc23
2013012325

JNKLANDS HOSPITAL
LIBRARY
MONKSCOURT AVENUE
AIRDRIE   ML60JS
230 06712005

9 8 7 6 5 4 3 2 1
Printed in the United States of America
on acid-free paper

To my wife Ketki and our children, Akhil and Anuraag. To my parents and mentors.

—Apar Kishor Ganti

To my wife Lara and our children, Jacob and Alexandra. To my mentors, colleagues, and students.

—David E. Gerber

We also dedicate this endeavor to lung cancer patients, as our goals are to improve patient care. If we are able in any way to help improve their care, we will consider our effort worthwhile.

Contents

Preface

Although lung cancer remains the leading cancer killer in the United States, recent years have seen major advances in the prevention, screening, diagnosis, staging, and treatment of this disease. Effective and well-tolerated pharmacologic agents are available for smoking cessation. For the first time in the history of the disease, there is evidence supporting radiographic screening for lung cancer, and low-dose computed tomography (CT) programs are being developed at centers around the world. With the advent of stereotactic radiation therapy, which features precise tumor targeting and high-potency beams, there now exist effective treatment options for patients with early-stage lung cancer who are not considered candidates for surgical resection. And finally, remarkable progress in the knowledge of the molecular underpinnings of the disease has resulted in a plethora of diagnostic studies and medical therapies not previously available to our patients.

Reading, processing, and implementing the barrage of new information related to lung cancer can overwhelm even those of us who focus on the disease, not to mention clinicians caring for patients with a wide range of diagnoses. Accordingly, we have written the volume *Lung Cancer* for the Oxford American Oncology Library with the practicing clinician in mind. We believe that medical oncologists, radiation oncologists, thoracic surgeons, pulmonologists, pathologists, and radiologists—whether in training or years into their career—will find the content highly applicable to questions and issues that arise in everyday patient management. We have provided specific guidance on ordering and interpreting molecular diagnostic studies; the selection and limitations of radiographic and invasive staging techniques; doses, schedules, and toxicities of medical and radiation treatments; management of numerous disease- and treatment-related complications; and the like. To support these recommendations, we present the available clinical data in concise yet comprehensive summaries.

To provide expertise on the increasingly nuanced and multidisciplinary approach to lung cancer, we invited numerous colleagues from the University of Nebraska Medical Center and the University of Texas Southwestern Medical Center to help us develop the content for this effort. The result is a volume covering the entire clinical course of the disease, from prevention, screening, and diagnosis to treatment and supportive care.

Apar Kishor Ganti, MD
VA Nebraska-Western Iowa Health Care System
University of Nebraska Medical Center

David E. Gerber, MD
University of Texas Southwestern Medical Center

Acknowledgments

We thank our editorial team of Rebecca Suzan, Andrea Zekus, and Andrea Seils at Oxford University Press; our copyeditor Aloysius Raj; and our administrative assistants, Carla Gaul, in the Division of Hematology-Oncology at the University of Nebraska Medical Center, and Cynthia Tingley in the Division of Hematology-Oncology at the University of Texas Southwestern Medical Center.

Contributors

I ONKLANDS HOSPITAL
LIBRARY
MONKSCOURT AVENUE
AIRDRIE ML60JS
250 1236712005

Daniel H. Ahn, DO
Department of Internal Medicine
University of Texas Southwestern
    Medical Center
Dallas, Texas

Matthew DeVries, MD
Assistant Professor of Radiology
Charles A. Dobry Professorship and
    Cardiothoracic Imaging Division
    Chief
Radiology Residency Program
    Director
Department of Radiology
University of Nebraska Medical
    Center
Omaha, Nebraska

Jonathan E. Dowell, MD
Program Director, Hematology
    Oncology Fellowship Program
Associate Professor
Division of Hematology-Oncology
Department of Internal Medicine
Harold C. Simmons Cancer
University of Texas Southwestern
    Medical Center
Dallas, Texas

**Apar Kishor Ganti, MD, MS,
FACP**
Staff Physician
VA Nebraska Western Iowa Health
    Care System
Associate Professor
Division of Oncology-Hematology
Department of Internal Medicine
University of Nebraska Medical
    Center
Omaha, Nebraska

David E. Gerber, MD
Associate Professor
Division of Hematology-Oncology
Department of Internal Medicine
Harold C. Simmons Cancer Center
University of Texas Southwestern
    Medical Center
Dallas, Texas

Puneeth Iyengar, MD, PhD
Assistant Professor
Department of Radiation Oncology
Harold C. Simmons Cancer Center
University of Texas Southwestern
    Medical Center
Dallas, Texas

Kemp H. Kernstine, MD, PhD
Professor
Division of Thoracic Surgery
Robert Tucker Hayes Foundation
    Distinguished Chair in
    Cardiothoracic Surgery
University of Texas Southwestern
    Medical Center
Dallas, Texas

Rudy P. Lackner, MD
Professor
Department of Surgery
Division of Surgical Oncology
Chief, Section of Thoracic Surgery
University of Nebraska Medical Center
Omaha, Nebraska

Raghav Murthy, MD
Resident
Department of Cardiovascular and
    Thoracic Surgery
University of Texas Southwestern
    Medical Center
Dallas, Texas

CONTRIBUTORS

Ameen A. Salahudeen, MD, PhD
Medical Scientist Training Program
    Fellow
Department of Biochemistry
University of Texas Southwestern
    Medical Center
Dallas, Texas

William W. West, MD
Associate Professor
Department of Pathology and
    Microbiology
University of Nebraska Medical
    Center
Omaha, Nebraska

Chapter 1

Lung Cancer Epidemiology, Etiology and Risk Factors

Daniel H. Ahn and David E. Gerber

Lung cancer is the second most common cancer in the United States and is the leading cause of cancer death in both men and women. Over 100,000 cases are diagnosed each year in both men and women with an estimated 87,750 deaths among men and 72,590 deaths in women (2008 estimates).[1] This exceeds the combined number of deaths from the other leading causes of cancer death (breast, prostate, and colon) and accounts for approximately 6% of all deaths in the United States.[1]

Worldwide, lung cancer is the leading cause of cancer death in men and the second leading cause of cancer death in women, with approximately 1.6 million new cases and 1.4 million deaths due to lung cancer in 2008.[1] International variations in the rates and trends in lung cancer are primarily due to the trends in the tobacco epidemic, as the majority of lung cancer–related deaths are due to smoking. In other Western countries, such as the United Kingdom and Canada, where the use of tobacco was established and has already peaked, lung cancer rates in men have been steadily decreasing.[2] In contrast, in countries where the tobacco epidemic has been established more recently and smoking rates continue to rise, including China, Korea, and numerous countries in Africa, lung cancer rates are increasing and will likely continue to increase, barring any interventions leading to smoking cessation.[3]

The median age at diagnosis of lung cancer is 71 years.[4] Due to cigarette smoking patterns, the epidemic of lung cancer started later in women than men. However, in contrast to men, rates in women have not begun to decrease consistently (Fig. 1.1). Far more men than women continue to die from lung cancer, but the gender gap in lung cancer mortality is narrowing and is anticipated to close. This trend is attributed to smoking patterns, with smoking prevalence having peaked approximately two decades earlier among men than women.

The highest incidence of lung cancer is found in African American men.[5] This racial disparity may be in part due to a greater susceptibility to carcinogens associated with smoking. In addition to a greater lung cancer incidence, African Americans also have worse survival outcomes in comparison with white individuals. The incidence of lung cancer–related deaths in the United States has been steadily decreasing. This trend appears to be attributable to the decrease in smoking prevalence.

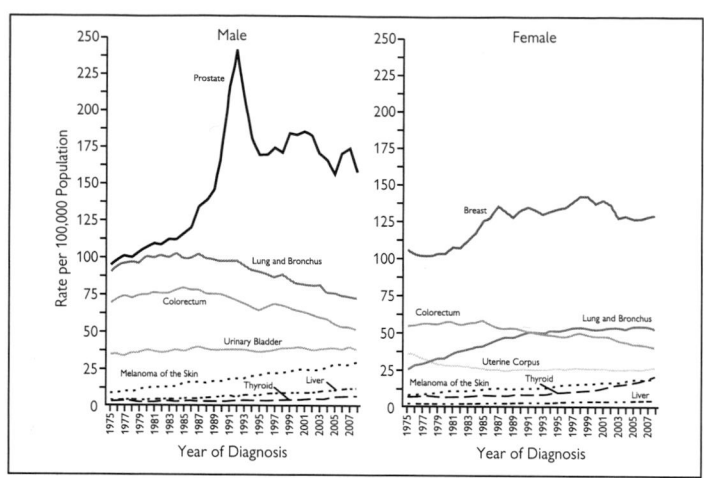

Figure 1.1 Cancer incidence by sex in the United States. (From Siegel R, Naishadham D, Jemal A. Cancer statistics, 2012. *CA Cancer J Clin.* 2012;62:10–29.)

Etiology and Risk Factors

Cigarette Smoking

Approximately 85% of all cases of lung cancer are related to cigarette smoking. There is a relatively strong dose–response relationship between cigarette smoking duration and intensity, and the development of lung cancer. The greater the number of cigarettes smoked on a daily basis and the greater the number of years of smoking, the greater the risk of cancer. Among smokers, the risk for lung cancer is on average 10-fold higher than in never smokers,[6] with individual estimated risk depending upon the duration and the amount smoked, shown in Table 1.1. There is also an association between cigar and pipe smoking and lung cancer risk, although it is not as strong as that for cigarette smoking.

Smoking cessation results in a decrease in precancerous lesions from 27% to 7%. For individuals who have quit smoking for 10 years, the risk for lung cancer may be 30% to 50% less than that of active smokers. Although smoking cessation decreases the risk of lung cancer, former smokers continue to have an elevated risk for lung cancer for years after quitting. Indeed, more lung cancer diagnoses occur in former smokers than in active smokers.

Tobacco cessation has been a major public health focus. Straightforward interventions such as brief physician counseling are associated with an increase in smoking cessation. Group therapy has also been shown to be effective. Additionally, pharmacologic therapy, such as all forms of nicotine replacement (nicotine gum, spray, patches), bupropion, and varenicline, improves smoking cessation rates. To date, complementary medicine approaches, such as acupuncture and hypnosis, have not been found to be effective.

Table 1.2 summarizes pharmacologic therapies available for smoking cessation.

Table 1.1 Ten-Year Risk (%) of Developing Lung Cancer

| Age (Years) | Duration of Smoking | | | | | |
| | 25 Years | | 40 Years | | 50 Years | |
	Quit (%)	Still Smoking (%)	Quit (%)	Still Smoking (%)	Quit (%)	Still Smoking (%)
One-pack-per-day smokers						
55	<1	1	3	5	NA	NA
65	<1	2	4	7	7	10
75	1	2	5	8	8	11
Two-packs-per-day smokers						
55	<1	2	4	7	NA	NA
65	1	3	6	9	10	14
75	2	3	7	10	11	15

Source: From Bach PB, Kattan MW, Thornquist MD, et al: Variations in lung cancer risk among smokers. J Natl Cancer Inst. 2003;95:470–478.

Table 1.2 Pharmacologic Treatment for Smoking Cessation

Medication	Dose	Side Effects	Comments
Nicotine replacement therapies			
Nicotrol NS inhaler	<40 mg/d	Local tissue irritation	Avoid in pregnant patients
Nicorette gum	18–24 mg/d	Sore throat, stomatitis, jaw ache	<20 pieces per day, decrease 1 piece every 4–7 days
Nicorette DS gum	36–48 mg/d		
Nicotine lozenges	40–80 mg/d	Local tissue irritation	Use for 12 weeks, <20 pieces per day
Habitrol nicotine patch	7–21 mg/d	Localized erythema, pruritis	Use for 6–12 weeks
NicoDerm CQ nicotine patch	7–21 mg/d		
Acetylcholine receptor partial agonist			
Varenicline	0.5 mg PO daily days 1–3, 0.5 mg PO bid days 4–7, then 1 mg PO bid through week 12	Nausea, insomnia, neuropsychiatric events	May repeat a second 12-week course in selected cases
Antidepressants			
Bupropion	150 mg PO daily x 3 days then increase to 300 mg PO daily x 12 weeks	Insomnia, dry mouth, dizziness	Do not take with other antidepressants, lowers seizure threshold
Fluoxetine	30–60 mg PO daily	Insomnia, dizziness, erectile dysfunction	

Randomized controlled trials have demonstrated efficacy of nicotine replacement and other pharmacologic therapies. For these interventions, odds ratios and 95% confidence intervals for smoking cessation (compared to placebo, with >1 favoring intervention) are as follows[7]:

- Bupropion 2.12 (1.76–2.56)
- Nicotine gum 1.65 (1.37–2.01)
- Nicotine inhaler 2.18 (1.38–3.45)
- Nicotine nasal spray 2.37 (1.57–3.60)
- Nicotine patch 1.88 (1.60–2.22)
- Nicotine tablet 2.06 (1.47–2.87)
- Varenicline 2.55 (1.99–3.24)

Environmental (Secondhand) Smoke

Exposure to smoke from those who are actively smoking poses a hazard to non-smokers. Non-smoking individuals who live in a household with a smoker have a 30% increased likelihood of developing lung cancer compared to those who live with nonsmokers. Estimates indicate that approximately 3000 lung cancer deaths per year in the United States are due to secondhand smoke exposure.[8]

Asbestos

Asbestos, a well-known occupational carcinogen, is another risk factor for lung cancer. It Is also a major risk factor for mesothelioma (covered in Chapter 13). Asbestos is a naturally occurring material that has been mined to use in a wide range of manufactured goods (see Table 1.3).

The term "asbestos" comprises six minerals divided into two classes. The serpentine class (which includes chrysotile) has curly fibers and is the most common type used in industry. The amphibole class (which includes amosite, crocidolite, tremolite, anthophyllite, and actinolyte) has straight, needle-like fibers. Amphibole (particularly amosite and crocidolite) is considered more hazardous and is more likely to cause cancer. However, exposure to serpentine asbestos has also been linked to lung cancer.

Table 1.3 Uses of Asbestos
Insulation (ceiling and pipe)
Fire retardant coatings
Concrete
Bricks
Pipes
Fireplace cement
Heat-, fire-, and acid-resistant gaskets
Fireproof drywalling
Flooring
Roofing
Lawn furniture
Drywall joint compound

The risk of asbestos exposure occurs via the inhalation of airborne friable asbestos particles. Continued exposure can increase the amount of fibers that remain in the lung, thus increasing the risk of malignancy. Studies have shown a 10-fold increase in the risk of developing lung cancer, primarily adenocarcinoma, in those exposed to asbestos. The latency period from asbestos exposure to diagnosis of lung cancer ranges between 10 and 40 years. In active smokers, the risk factors of smoking and asbestos act synergistically, resulting in a multiplicative effect.[9] The risk of lung cancer in smokers exposed to asbestos is 50 to 90 times greater than in smokers without asbestos exposure.

Radiation

Studies have demonstrated an association between lung cancer and exposure to ionizing radiation. However, the risk for low-dose radiation, such as that associated with X-rays and computed tomography (CT) scans, has been difficult to characterize. Although there have been no large epidemiologic studies examining the long-term risks of cancer from exposure to diagnostic ionizing radiation exposure, large cohort studies, particularly of Japanese atomic bomb survivors, have provided a greater understanding of the risks of low-dose radiation and the risk of cancer in patients exposed to higher doses of radiation.[10,11] A recent report estimated that the radiation organ doses corresponding to commonly performed CT studies could increase the risk of cancer, and that 0.4% of all cancers in the United States may be attributable to CT scans.

Radon

Radon, an inert gas produced naturally from uranium, is considered an occupational risk factor for lung cancer. Epidemiologic studies of uranium miners established exposure to radon as a cause of lung cancer in these populations.[12] Additionally, radon exists as an indoor air pollutant that enters buildings in soil gas. However, radon exposure in the general population is substantially less than the occupational exposure of uranium miners as the average home has less than 1% the radon concentration of a uranium mine.[12]

Nevertheless, residential radon exposure is estimated to account for up to 10% of lung cancer deaths in the United States each year.[13] Current risk estimates indicate an approximate increase in lifetime lung cancer risk of 12%–16% compared to the general population for every 2.7 pCi/L of radon exposure over a 20-year period of time, based on a ¾-day exposure period.[14,15]

High levels of radon have been found in every state within the United States, many of which have implemented programs that affect home buying and awareness. However, testing for radon is not mandatory unless specified by local jurisdiction.

Host Factors

Environmental agents, even cigarette smoking (1 in 13, or 7%), cause lung cancer in only a small proportion of exposed patients, leading to the hypothesis that genetic susceptibility plays a role in lung cancer risk. Epidemiologic studies have shown that a family history of lung cancer predicts an increased risk of the development of lung cancer.[16] Alterations in tumor suppressor genes and oncogenes have been associated with the development of lung cancer. Additionally, polymorphisms of certain genes, specifically those involved with carcinogen metabolism and DNA repair, are thought to alter DNA repair capacity and are associated with an increased cancer risk. Studies have shown significant interactions between these genetic variations and smoking in lung cancer risk.[17–21] Selected genes are listed in Table 1.4. To date, there is no established role for incorporating assessment of these genetic changes into lung cancer screening efforts.

Never Smokers

Although tobacco smoking accounts for the majority of lung cancer, 10%–15% of patients with lung cancer are lifelong never smokers.[22] Several molecular changes in never smokers have been identified that are unique in comparison to tobacco-related lung cancer. These include chromosomal abnormalities, activation of oncogenes, inactivation of tumor suppressor genes, and mutations of genes involved in DNA repair. Molecular aberrations in the epidermal growth factor receptor (EGFR) and anaplastic lymphoma kinase (ALK) genes occur more commonly in oligo-smokers and never smokers and predict response to EGFR- and ALK-directed therapy. By contrast, *KRAS* mutations are seen predominantly in current or former smokers.

Lung cancer in never smokers affects predominantly women, with up to 20% of women with lung cancer being lifelong never smokers.[22] Adenocarcinoma, particularly the subtype of adenocarcinoma *in situ* (previously known as bronchioloalveolar cancer [BAC]) is the most common histology among never smokers, accounting for approximately 60% of cases. In contrast, small cell lung cancer occurs almost exclusively in smokers.

Chemoprevention

To date, there is no proven role for chemoprevention in lung cancer. Early observational data suggested a potential benefit for prevention of lung cancer with beta-carotene and retinol (vitamin A). Laboratory research demonstrated that beta-carotene can decrease free radicals and/or deactivate oxygen

Table 1.4 Genetic Polymorphisms Associated with Lung Cancer
Genes involved in carcinogen metabolism
CYP1A1
GSTM1
GSTT1
GSTP1
Genes involved in DNA repair capacity
OGG1
ERCC1
XPD
XPF
XRCC3
XRCC1

Table 1.5 Phase III Trials of Chemoprevention for Lung Cancer

Study	Year	Intervention	End Point	Results
ATBC[23]	1994	Beta-carotene	Lung cancer	Increased risk of lung cancer. OR 1.19 (95% CI, 1.03–1.36); $P = 0.01$
ATBC[23]	1994	Vitamin E	Lung cancer	No difference in risk of lung cancer. OR 0.98 (95% CI, 0.86–1.12); $P = 0.8$
CARET[24]	1996	Beta-carotene and retinol	Lung cancer	Increased risk of lung cancer. OR 1.28 (95% CI, 1.04–1.57); $P = 0.02$
EUROSCAN[25]	2000	Retinol	Second primary lung cancer	No difference in risk of lung cancer. OR 1.008 (95% CI, 0.86–1.18); $P = 0.67$
EUROSCAN[25]	2000	N-Acetylcysteine	Second primary lung cancer	No difference in risk of lung cancer. OR 1.072, (95% CI, 0.92–1.25); $P = 0.93$

ATBC, Alpha-Tocopherol, Beta-Carotene Cancer Prevention Trial; CARET, Carotene and Retinol Efficacy Trial; CI, confidence interval; EUROSCAN, Randomized Trial of Vitamin A and N-Acetylcysteine; OR, odds ratio.

molecules, which may have an anticancer effect by preventing tissue damage; retinol, an antioxidant, was believed to reverse carcinogenesis. However, a protective association between beta-carotene and lung cancer was not found in randomized, double-blind, placebo-controlled trials. Indeed, a statistically significant increase in lung cancer incidence among high-risk populations of heavy smokers and asbestos-exposed workers using beta-carotene[23] and retinol[24] was noted in a number of trials. Additional studies, examining the use of aspirin, selenium, vitamin E, and N-acetylcysteine, have not shown statistically significant results in the prevention of lung cancer.[6] Table 1.5 summarizes the principal phase III trials that have been conducted in lung cancer chemoprevention.

References

1. Jemal A, Center MM, DeSantis C, Ward EM. Global patterns of cancer incidence and mortality rates and trends. *Cancer Epidemiol Biomarkers Prevent.* 2010;19:1893–1907.

2. Mortality from smoking in developed countries 1950–2000. 2006. [accessed February 22, 2013]. Available at http://www.ctsu.ox.ac.uk/~tobacco/SMK_All_PAGES.pdf.

3. Youlden DR, Cramb SM, Baade PD. The international epidemiology of lung cancer: geographical distribution and secular trends. *J Thorac Oncol.* 2008;3:819–31.

4. Hayat MJ, Howlader N, Reichman ME, Edwards BK. Cancer statistics, trends, and multiple primary cancer analyses from the Surveillance, Epidemiology, and End Results (SEER) Program. *Oncologist.* 2007;12:20–37.

5. Ries L, Eisner M, Kosary C, eds. *Cancer Statistics Review, 1975-2002.* Bethesda, MD: National Cancer Institute; 2005.

6. Gray J, Mao JT, Szabo E, Kelley M, Kurie J, Bepler G. Lung cancer chemo-prevention: ACCP evidence-based clinical practice guidelines. 2nd ed. *Chest* 2007;132:56S–68S.

7. Eisenberg MJ, Filion KB, Yavin D, et al. Pharmacotherapies for smok-ing cessation: a meta-analysis of randomized controlled trials. *CMAJ.* 2008;179:135–44.

8. United States Environmental Protection Agency. *Respiratory Health Effects of Passive Smoking: Lung Cancer and Other Disorders.* Washington, DC: US Government Printing Office; 1992.

9. Hammond EC, Selikoff IJ, Seidman H. Asbestos exposure, cigarette smoking and death rates. *Ann NY Acad Sci* 1979;330:473–90.

10. Pierce DA, Sharp GB, Mabuchi K. Joint effects of radiation and smoking on lung cancer risk among atomic bomb survivors. *Radiat Res.* 2003;159:511–20.

11. Brenner DJ, Hall EJ. Computed tomography—an increasing source of radiation exposure. *N Engl J Med.* 2007;357:2277–84.

12. Lubin JH, Boice JD, Jr., Edling C, et al. Lung cancer in radon-exposed miners and estimation of risk from indoor exposure. *J Natl Cancer Inst.* 1995;87:817–27.

13. United States Environmental Protection Agency. *EPA Assessment of Risks from Radon in Homes.* Washington, DC: US Government Printing Office; 2003.

14. Darby S, Hill D, Auvinen A, et al. Radon in homes and risk of lung cancer: collab-orative analysis of individual data from 13 European case-control studies. *BMJ.* 2005;330:223.

15. Krewski D, Lubin JH, Zielinski JM, et al. Residential radon and risk of lung cancer: a combined analysis of 7 North American case-control studies. *Epidemiology* 2005;16:137–45.

16. Matakidou A, Eisen T, Houlston RS. Systematic review of the relationship between family history and lung cancer risk. *Br J Cancer* 2005;93:825–33.

17. Kiyohara C, Takayama K, Nakanishi Y. Lung cancer risk and genetic poly-morphisms in DNA repair pathways: a meta-analysis. *J Nucleic Acids* 2010;2010:701–60.

18. Vineis P, Veglia F, Benhamou S, et al. CYP1A1 T3801 C polymorphism and lung cancer: a pooled analysis of 2451 cases and 3358 controls. *Intl J Cancer.* 2003;104:650–7.

19. Houlston RS. Glutathione S-transferase M1 status and lung cancer risk: a meta-analysis. *Cancer Epidemiol Biomarkers Prevent.* 1999;8:675–82.

20. Shen MR, Jones IM, Mohrenweiser H. Nonconservative amino acid substitution variants exist at polymorphic frequency in DNA repair genes in healthy humans. *Cancer Res.* 1998;58:604–8.

21. Goode EL, Ulrich CM, Potter JD. Polymorphisms in DNA repair genes and associations with cancer risk. *Cancer Epidemiol Biomarkers Prevent.* 2002;11:1513–30.

22. Subramanian J, Govindan R. Lung cancer in never smokers: a review. *J Clin Oncol* 2007;25:561–70.

23. Albanes D, Heinonen OP, Taylor PR, et al. Alpha-tocopherol and beta-carotene supplements and lung cancer incidence in the alpha-tocopherol, beta-carotene cancer prevention study: effects of base-line characteristics and study compli-ance. *J Natl Cancer Inst.* 1996;88:1560–70.

24. Omenn GS, Goodman GE, Thornquist MD, et al. Effects of a combination of beta carotene and vitamin A on lung cancer and cardiovascular disease. *N Engl J Med.* 1996;334:1150–5.

25. van Zandwijk N, Dalesio O, Pastorino U, et al. EUROSCAN, a randomized trial of vitamin A and N-acetylcysteine in patients with head and neck cancer or lung cancer. For the European Organization for Research and Treatment of Cancer Head and Neck and Lung Cancer Cooperative Groups. *J Natl Cancer Inst.* 2000;92:977–986.

Chapter 2

Biology of Lung Cancer

David E. Gerber, Ameen A. Salahudeen,
and William W. West

Over the course of several decades, therapies have emerged from research into the molecular biology of lung cancer. For example, certain lung cancers driven by specific growth pathways can be treated effectively by molecularly targeted agents. Despite such advances, however, the overall process of how normal lung parenchyma transforms and progresses into advanced or meta-static carcinoma remains poorly understood. Efforts to delineate these processes and characterize the underlying molecular changes are key not only to developing molecular approaches to therapy but also to identifying biomarkers for early detection, targets for prevention, and signatures predicting prognosis and response to specific treatments.

This chapter will review key molecular aberrations in lung cancer. Table 2.1 lists key terms and definitions related to lung cancer biology. Throughout the chapter, the name of a molecule refers to the gene when italicized (unless followed by the word "gene," in which case it is not italicized) and to the protein when not italicized.

Lung Carcinogenesis

As with many other malignancies, the development of lung cancer from normal pulmonary epithelium is a multistep process. Histologically, airway epithelium undergoes changes to atypical adenomatous hyperplasia, squamous dyaplasia/carcinoma *in situ*, or diffuse idiopathic pulmonary neuroendocrine cell hyperplasia—putative premalignant lesions for lung adenocarcinoma, squamous cell carcinoma, and neuroendocrine carcinoma, respectively. Multiple environmental and occupational carcinogens have been identified; however, those found in cigarette smoke statistically account for 85%–90% of lung cancers.[1] As reviewed in Chapter 1, the effects of multiple single nucleotide polymorphisms (SNPs) on the risk of developing lung cancer have been investigated. To date, most associations are modest and frequently inconsistent.

Carcinogenesis is a complex multistep process in the lung involving multiple genetic and epigenetic alterations and interactions between the involved molecular pathways. A framework for progression to carcinoma,

Table 2.1 Glossary of Commonly Used Terms in Lung Cancer Molecular Biology

Term	Explanation [and Lung Cancer Examples]
Actionable mutation	Mutation that guides clinical management [EGFR and KRAS mutations in adenocarcinoma]
Allele	One of two or more versions of a particular genetic sequence
Amplification	An increase in the amount of genomic material in a cell, ranging from regions within a gene to whole chromosomes [FGFR1 amplification in squamous cell carcinoma]
Angiogenesis	The production of vasculature mediated by growth factors during tissue repair or by tumors
Base pair (bp)	Two nitrogenous bases paired together in double-stranded DNA; refers to physical length of nucleotide sequence when quantified (eg, 100 bp)
Deletion mutation	Type of mutation entailing loss of genetic material from a single nucleotide to entire chromosomes [Deletion of P53, Rb, and CDKN2A in SCLC and NSCLC]
Driver mutation	Mutation that is essential, but not necessarily sufficient, for the uncontrolled proliferation of a cancer cell [EGFR L858R]
Epigenetic change	Increase or decrease in regulation of gene activity through chemical modification of nucleotides (e.g., methylation) or histones (eg, acetylation) without modification of the DNA sequence itself; in turn, these changes frequently modulate the binding of transcription factors [Methylation silencing of tumor suppressors PTEN and CDKN2A]
Exon	Portion of a gene that encodes amino acids
Fluorescence in situ hybridization (FISH)	Microscopy technique to analyze chromosomal DNA via fluorescent molecules covalently attached to antisense or complementary DNA strands to probe genomic DNA within a cell [Analysis of EGFR copy number or EML4-ALK rearrangement]
Gene	Sequence of nucleotides on a particular chromosome that encodes a specific protein or RNA molecule
Growth factor	Peptide or small molecule that upregulates growth of tissue or cells [EGF, VEGF, HGF]
Insertion mutation	Type of mutation entailing the introduction of a novel DNA sequence in a gene, resulting in disruption of gene expression or gene product function [EGFR exon 20 insertion mutation]
Kinase	An enzyme that catalyzes the transfer of phosphate groups from ATP or GTP to proteins or metabolites [AKT, EGFR]
Loss of heterozygosity (LOH)	Loss of normal function of one allele (either due to deletion or recombination event) of a gene in which the other allele was already inactivated [CDKN2A (p16), FHIT, p53]

Microarray	Technology for studying multiple genes simultaneously that entails placing thousands of gene sequences in specific locations on a glass slide, then placing a sample containing DNA or RNA on the slide; the binding of complementary base pairs from the sample and gene sequences on the chip is measured to determine the amount of specific sequences in sample
Microenvironment	The surrounding cells, vasculature, tissues, nutrients, and hormones that sustain a tumor's growth
microRNA (miRNA)	Short regulatory form of RNA that binds to target RNA and usually suppresses its translation to protein
Missense mutation	The erroneous substitution of one nucleotide(s) for another resulting in a change in the amino acid sequence of the gene product (e.g., AXXXB, where A is the original amino acid, XXX is the amino acid position number, and B is the mutated amino acid) [EGFR T790M mutation]
Monoclonal antibodies (mAbs)	Monospecific antibodies made by identical immune cells that are clones of unique parent cells [bevacizumab, cetuximab]
Mutation	Alteration in the sequence of DNA by deletion, insertion, rearrangement, or substitution of a nucleotide or a group of nucleotides [EGFR, KRAS, p53 gene mutations]
Nonsense mutation	Point mutation in DNA sequence resulting in premature stop codon and in a truncated, usually nonfunctional protein product
Oncogene	Gene that has the potential to cause cancer; in tumor cells, often mutated or overexpressed [KRAS]
Point mutation	Alteration in DNA sequence—often caused by chemicals or malfunction of DNA replication—that results in exchanging a single nucleotide for another
Polymerase chain reaction (PCR)	Biochemical technology employed to amplify DNA sequences; uses short, synthetic complementary DNA sequences (primers) to select portion of DNA to be amplified
Polyploidy	The number of chromosomes or genomes that exceeds the usual diploid (2n) in number
Predictive biomarker	Biomarker used to identify subpopulations of patients most likely to respond to a given therapy [EGFR mutations for EGFR inhibitors; EML4-ALK fusions for ALK inhibitors]
Prognostic biomarker	Biomarkers that provide information on the likely course of a disease in untreated individuals
Rearrangement	Chromosomal structural alteration that involves breakage and reattachment of chromosomal segment resulting in abnormal configuration; includes inversion and translocation [EML4-ALK fusion]

(continued)

Table 2.1 (Continued)

Term	Explanation [and Lung Cancer Examples]
Small molecule inhibitors	Synthetic or natural compounds of low molecular weight (i.e., not proteins or polysaccharides) that bind and downregulate a biological target's activity; also referred to as kinase inhibitors, tyrosine kinase inhibitors, and small molecules [erlotinib, crizotinib]
Stroma	The cellular and connective tissue network encompassing the functional cells of an organ or a tumor
Targeted therapy	Drugs designed to inhibit specific biological targets for treatment efficacy; typically refers to monoclonal antibodies and small molecule inhibitors [bevacizumab, erlotinib, crizotinib]
Telomere	Terminal part of a chromosome that contains a buffer of DNA repeats that are lost at the 3' end of the chromosome during the process of genomic replication during mitosis; the absence of telomeres results in cellular senescence and inability to replicate; telomere DNA is replenished on the 3' end of the chromosome through reverse transcription by telomerase
Tumor suppressor	Gene that protects a cell from one step in path to cancer development; when mutated to cause reduction or loss of function, may result in cancer [PTEN, p53]

referred to as the Hallmarks of Cancer, has been proposed by Hanahan and Weinberg[2]:

- Sustaining proliferative signaling
- Evading growth suppressors
- Avoiding immune destruction
- Enabling replicative immortality
- Tumor-promoting inflammation
- Invasion and metastasis
- Activation of angiogenesis
- Genomic instability mutations
- Resisting cell death
- Altering cell bioenergetics

Molecular Aberrations in Lung Cancer

In lung cancer and other malignancies, a number of molecular aberrations underlie tumor development and progression. These include the following:

- Oncogenic alterations (mutations, amplifications, overexpression)
- Tumor-suppressing alterations (mutations, deletions, loss of expression)
- Epigenetic changes
- Telomerase alterations
- Micro RNA modifications

Common Genetic Alterations

Early genomic analysis techniques, such as karyotyping, permitted the assessment of only large-scale chromosomal changes in lung cancer. Studies identified a number of chromosomal losses (most commonly 3p, 4q, 9p, 17p) and gains (most commonly 1q, 3q, 5p, 17q).[3] By contrast, recent technological advances have resulted in the ability to perform high-resolution microarray analyses and whole-genome and transcriptome sequencing of lung tumor (and adjacent normal tissue) samples. The nature and prevalence of specific molecular aberrations vary according to histologic subtype. Within a single histologic type (specifically adenocarcinomas), there may be further variation according to smoking status. The function and clinical relevance of many of these genetic aberrations remain under investigation.

Adenocarcinoma

In a study involving whole-genome sequencing of 188 lung adenocarcinomas,[4] over 1000 nonsynonymous somatic mutations were identified, of which the 10 most common were the following: TP53 (35%), KRAS (32%), STK11 (18%), EGFR (18%), LRP1B (10%), NF1 (9%), ATM (9%), APC (8%), EPHA3 (6%), and PTPRD (6%).

In a separate study of 1000 lung adenocarcinomas, "driver" mutations were identified in approximately 60% of tumors.[5] The majority were mutually exclusive. In contrast to whole-genome sequencing studies, this analysis included only preselected "driver" mutations. In the patient cohort, there was an overrepresentation of never smokers and oligo-smokers. The most common molecular aberrations were as follows:

- *KRAS* mutations (25%)
- *EGFR* mutations (23%)
- *ALK* rearrangements (6%)
- *BRAF* mutations (3%)
- *PIK3CA* mutations (3%)
- *MET* amplifications (2%)

Squamous Cell

The characterization and targeting of genetic alterations in squamous cell tumors have lagged behind developments in adenocarcinoma. Recently, however, The Cancer Genome Atlas (TCGA) profiled 178 lung squamous cell carcinomas to provide a comprehensive landscape of genetic and epigenetic alterations.[6] There were a mean of 360 exonic mutations, 165 genomic rearrangements, and 323 segments of copy number alteration per tumor. Frequent events included the following: *TP53* mutations (nearly all cases), *NFE2L2* and *KEAP1* mutations (34%), PI3K pathway alterations (47%), as well as alterations in genes within the *CDKN2A* locus (72%).

Small Cell Lung Cancer

Recent comprehensive and integrative genomic analyses of small cell lung cancer have revealed this malignancy to have one of the highest mutational rates of any cancer (7.4 mutations per million base pairs, compared to 6.3 for melanoma and 0.4–1.5 for various other solid and liquid tumors).[7] Among the more frequently detected molecular aberrations were the following[7,8]: *SOX2* amplifications, *MYC* fusions, *TP53* mutations, *RB1* mutations, *CREBBP* mutations, *EP300* mutations, *MLL* mutations, *PTEN* mutations, *EPHA* mutations, *FGFR1* amplifications, *RASSF8* mutations, *COL22A1* mutations, and *BCL-2* mutations.

Actionable/Druggable Molecular Targets

Currently, there are four molecular targets in lung cancer that guide treatment selection. These targets—KRAS, EGFR, ALK, and ROS1—are predominantly found in adenocarcinoma tumors and appear to be mutually exclusive. The FDA-approved targeted therapies erlotinib (for *EGFR* mutant tumors) and crizotinib (for *ALK* rearranged tumors) are associated with high response rate and prolonged disease control in these molecular subsets. While there are no specific KRAS-targeting drugs currently available, presence of a *KRAS* mutation precludes one of these other events and is associated with resistance to EGFR inhibitors.

In clinical practice, these and other molecular targets are inhibited by two classes of drugs: small-molecule tyrosine kinase inhibitors (TKIs) and monoclonal antibodies (mAbs), which are collectively referred to as targeted therapy. Table 2.2 lists features of mAbs and TKIs.

KRAS

Function

KRAS is a member of the Ras family of GTPases that promote cell growth and division through Ras/Raf signaling. These enzymes are activated by the binding

Table 2.2 Characteristics of Monoclonal Antibodies and Small Molecule Inhibitors

	Small Molecule Inhibitors	Monoclonal Antibodies (mAbs)
Nomenclature	"-ib"*	"-mab"
Examples in lung cancer	Erlotinib (Tarceva)	Bevacizumab (Avastin)
	Crizotinib (Xalkori)	Cetuximab (Erbitux)
Mechanism(s)	Inhibition of tyrosine kinase function	1. Antagonism of ligand-receptor binding
		2. Receptor internalization, degradation
		3. Recruitment of host immune functions (e.g., ADCC, CMC)
Target specificity	+++	+++++
Site of action	Intracellular	Extracellular
Molecular weight	~400–500 daltons	~150,000 daltons
Administration	Oral†	Intravenous
Half-life	Hours	Days
Hypersentitivity reactions	None	Yes
Drug interactions	Multiple (CYP450 substrates)	Minimal

*Exceptions: everolimus, temsirolimus.

†Exceptions: bortezomib, temsirolimus.

ADCC, antibody-dependent cellular cytotoxicity; CMC, complement-mediated cytotoxicity; CYP450, cytochrome P-450.

of guanosine triphosphate (GTP) and are able to phosphorylate proteins downstream in the signaling cascade until GTP is converted to guanosine diphosphate (GDP) through a GTPase activity instrinsic to the Ras family enzymes. The end effect is that KRAS kinase and signaling capacity is higher when the enzyme is bound to GTP instead of GDP.

Nomenclature

In lung cancer, *KRAS* is virtually the sole member of the Ras family (which also includes *HRAS* and *NRAS*) involved in tumorigenesis. The HRAS and KRAS genes were initially identified from studies of two cancer-causing viruses, the Harvey sarcoma virus and the Kirsten sarcoma virus. These viruses were originally discovered in rats by Jennifer Harvey and Werner Kirsten, hence the name Rat sarcoma (Ras).[9] *NRAS* is so named for its initial identification in human neuroblastoma cells.

Role in Tumorigenesis

KRAS acquires its tumorigenic ability when mutations (primarily in exons 12, 13, and 61) arise that decrease its intrinsic GTPase activity. As a result, an increased fraction of GTP- versus GDP-bound KRAS exists, causing marked upregulation of kinase activity and downstream growth and mitotic signaling. These mutations, which occur in approximately 15%–20% of non–small cell lung carcinoma (NSCLC), are associated with smoking and adenocarcinoma histology (30%–50%).[10] In Asian populations, *KRAS* mutations appear to be more common in males with poorly differentiated histology. Importantly, *KRAS* mutations are mutually exclusive of *EGFR* mutations and *ALK* and *ROS1* rearrangements, allowing clinicians to rule out these druggable aberrations if a *KRAS* mutation is present.

Clinical Significance

KRAS mutations have been shown to be prognostic (associated with worse overall survival) and predictive (associated with lack of benefit from adjuvant conventional chemotherapy in early disease and with resistance to EGFR TKIs in advanced disease).[11–13] In contrast to colorectal cancer, in NSCLC *KRAS* mutations are not clearly associated with resistance to the anti-EGFR mAb cetuximab.[14]

At the present time, there are no targeted therapies available for NSCLC patients with *KRAS* mutations. High-affinity binding to the GTP substrate has hindered the development of therapeutic agents that inhibit KRAS directly. However, agents are being developed to target downstream effector proteins in *KRAS* mutant NSCLCs, particularly in the PI3 kinases that interact with the Ras/Raf pathway.

Epidermal Growth Factor Receptor

Nomenclature

Epidermal growth factor receptor (EGFR) belongs to a four-member family of transmembrane receptor tyrosine kinases. These four receptors are known alternately as the HER (human epidermal growth factor receptor) and ErbB (so named for homology to a virus associated with erythroblastosis) family. Hence, EGFR is also referred to as HER1 or ErbB1.

Role in Tumorigenesis

Increased EGFR protein expression or EGFR gene amplification, mutation, or rearrangement has been demonstrated in multiple malignancies. EGFR is detectable in up to 90% of cases of NSCLC.[15,16] EGFR protein expression has been associated with more aggressive phenotype and worse prognosis in NSCLC, bladder, breast, and head and neck cancers.[17,18] EGFR is also expressed by normal epithelial cells, such as skin and gastrointestinal mucosa—a distribution that underlies the common toxicities of EGFR inhibitors. Anti-EGFR mAbs, which bind to the extracellular domain of EGFR and prevent ligand binding, are approved for colorectal and head and neck cancer treatment. EGFR TKIs, which bind directly to and inhibit the intracellular tyrosine kinase, are approved for NSCLC, pancreas cancer, and breast cancer treatment. For NSCLC, activating mutations in the *EGFR* kinase domain are associated with sensitivity to EGFR inhibitors and are used clinically as predictive biomarkers.

EGFR has an extracellular ligand-binding domain (621 amino acids), a transmembrane anchoring region (23 amino acids), and an intracellular tyrosine kinase (542 amino acids). After binding of the ligand, receptor subunits dimerize,

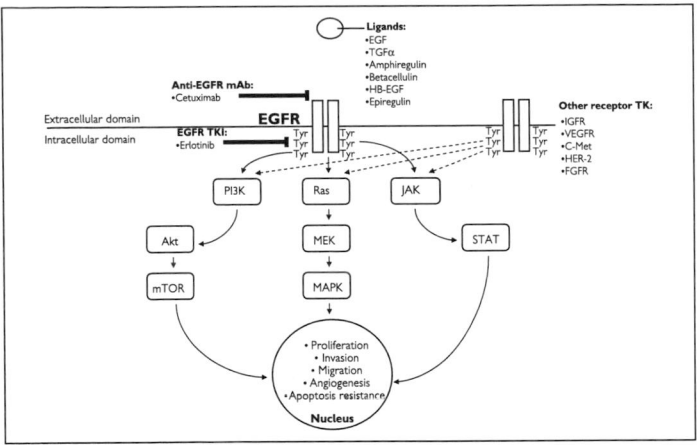

Figure 2.1 EGFR activation, inhibition, and signaling. EGF, epidermal growth factor; EGFR, epidermal growth factor receptor; FGFR, fibroblast growth factor receptor; HB-EGF, heparin-bound EGF; IGFR, insulin-like growth factor receptor; JAK, Janus kinase; mAb, monoclonal antibody; MAPK, mitogen-activated protein kinase; MEK, mitogen-activated and extracellular-signal regulated kinase kinase; mTOR, mammalian target of rapamycin; PI3K, phosphatidylinositol-3-kinase; STAT, signal transducer and activator of transcription; TGFα, transforming growth factor alpha; TK, tyrosine kinase; TKI, tyrosine kinase inhibitor; Tyr, tyrosine; VEGFR, vascular endothelial growth factor receptor.

resulting in autophosphorylation of intracellular tyrosine residues. This action creates docking sites for numerous intracellular effector proteins, thereby generating multiple signal transduction cascades. These include the Ras-Raf-MEK (mitogen-activated and extracellular-signal regulated kinase kinase), PI3K (phosphatidylinositol-3-kinase)-Akt, and STAT (signal transducer and activator of transcription) pathways (see Fig. 2.1).

These molecular signals ultimately result in cellular proliferation, resistance to apoptosis, cellular invasion, metastasis, and angiogenesis.[19-23] Independent of kinase-dependent signal-transduction pathways, the EGFR complex may also be internalized and translocated to the nucleus, where it modifies gene transcription and contributes to DNA repair mechanisms.[24,25]

EGFR Protein Expression

The relationship between EGFR protein expression (see Fig. 2.2) and tumor sensitivity to EGFR inhibition is unclear. Numerous retrospective analyses of NSCLC patients treated with EGFR TKIs have found no relationship between tumor EGFR protein expression (assessed by immunohistochemistry [IHC]) and objective response rate.[26-28] The association between EGFR protein expression and outcomes in studies of anti-EGFR mAbs is also unclear, as most of these studies mandated EGFR positivity for study entry.

EGFR Copy Number

As the case for EGFR protein expression, the association between the number of copies of the EGFR gene (most commonly assessed by fluorescence

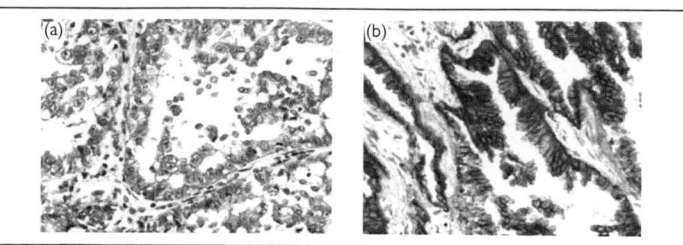

Figure 2.2 Weak (*a*) and strong (*b*) epidermal growth factor receptor (EGFR) staining by immunohistochemistry. (From Cappuzzo F, et al. *J Natl Cancer Inst* 2005;97:643–55.)

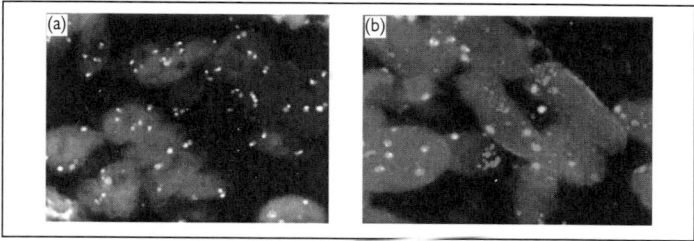

Figure 2.3 Epidermal growth factor receptor (EGFR) gene copy number by fluorescence *in situ* hybridization (FISH). Increased EGFR gene copy number due to high polysomy (*a*) and gene amplification (*b*). (From Cappuzzo F, et al. *J Natl Cancer Inst* 2005;97:643–55.)

in situ hybridization [FISH]) (see Fig. 2.3) and response to EGFR inhibitors is unclear. Increased *EGFR* copy number is highly correlated with the presence of *EGFR* mutations (see later), but, in Western populations, occurs more frequently.[27]

Increased *EGFR* copy number is usually due to chromosome 7 polysomy. True EGFR *gene amplification*—defined as the presence of tight gene clusters and an EGFR gene-to-chromosome 7 ratio of ≥2—occurs less commonly. There is no standardized scoring system for EGFR gene copy number. One definition of increased gene copy number, using FISH, is the presence of gene amplification (defined as tight gene clusters or an EGFR gene-to-chromosome ratio of ≥2 or ≥15 gene copies per cell) and/or chromosome polysomy (≥4 chromosomes in ≥40% of cells).[27] In this study, FISH positivity was associated with higher radiographic response rates (36% vs. 3%, $P < 0.001$) and longer median survival (18.7 months vs 7.0 months, $P = 0.03$).

EGFR Mutations

Of any biomarker, *EGFR* mutations have the clearest association with tumor sensitivity to EGFR inhibitors, particularly TKIs. In NSCLC, activating mutations in the EGFR tyrosine kinase domain, centered around exons 18–21, occur in 15%–20% of cases (see Fig. 2.4).[29–34] The current standard for *EGFR* mutational analysis is direct gene sequencing (see Fig. 2.5).

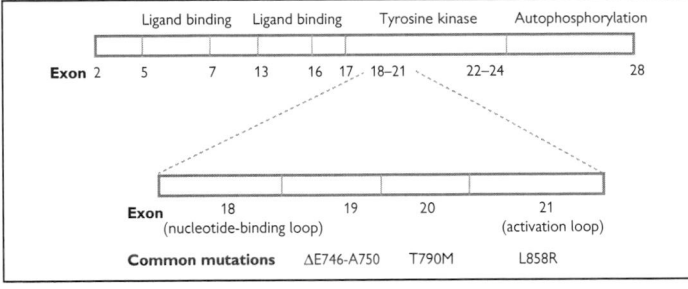

Figure 2.4 Epidermal growth factor receptor (EGFR) mutations in non–small cell lung carcinoma.

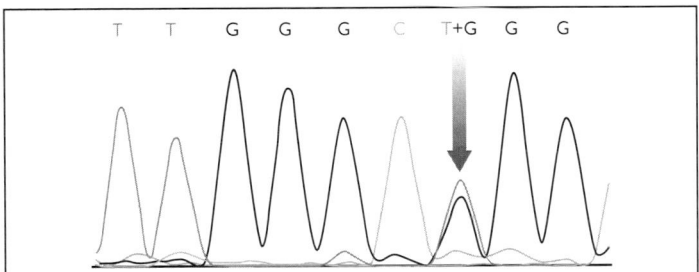

Figure 2.5 Epidermal growth factor receptor (EGFR) gene sequencing. Direct EGFR gene sequencing demonstrates point mutation in Exon 21. (Reprinted from Herbst RS, *The Lancet* 2009;373:1497–8, with permission from Elsevier.)

Mutations in exons 19 and 21 (termed classic *EGFR* mutations) each account for approximately 45% of *EGFR* mutations. These molecular alterations hyperactivate the EGFR tyrosine kinase, rendering cancer cells highly dependent on EGFR oncogenic pathways for survival (a concept known as oncogene addiction[35,36]) and thus highly sensitive to EGFR inhibition.

- Exon 19 mutations, most commonly in-frame deletions of amino acids 747–750, are clustered around the catalytic domain and flank the ATP-binding site. In addition to activating EGFR TK signaling, these structural changes enhance drug binding, resulting in complete blockade of mutated EGFR signaling at relatively low EGFR TKI doses.[37] Higher response rates are usually seen with exon 19 mutations than with exon 21 mutations.[38]

- Exon 21 mutations, which lie within the TK activation loop, are characteristically L858R substitutions.

- In NSCLC cases harboring classic *EGFR* mutations, EGFR TKIs yield response rates over 60%—compared with response rates of approximately 10% in wild-type *EGFR* cases—with progression-free survival exceeding 1 year, and overall survival exceeding 2 years.[38]

- *EGFR* mutations do not appear to predict response to anti-EGFR mAbs (e.g., cetuximab).[14,39]

- The impact of classic *EGFR* mutations is not limited to EGFR TKI therapy; response rates to conventional chemotherapy in this population may be up to twice those in *EGFR* wild-type patients.[40]
- Approximately 10% of NSCLC cases in North America and Western Europe harbor *EGFR* mutations, compared to 30%–50% of cases in East Asia.
- Classic *EGFR* mutations are associated with a number of clinicopathologic features[26,38,41–45]:
  - Female gender
  - East Asian ethnicity
  - Never-smoking status
  - Adenocarcinoma histology
  - Thyroid Transcription Factor-1 (TTF-1) positivity
  - Nonmucinous histology
  - Prominent lepidic, acinar, and/or papillary histologic patterns

The remaining 10% of *EGFR* TK mutations, in exons 18 and 20, generally do not confer sensitivity to EGFR TKIs and in some cases are associated with resistance (see section on "Acquired Resistance to EGFR Inhibition").

Any approach to testing tumor *EGFR* mutation status requires consideration of the following points:

- Even in highly clinically enriched populations (based on characteristics such as those listed earlier), *EGFR* mutations occur in only about 60% of patients.[40] Conversely, *EGFR* mutations may occur in patients lacking typical clinical predictors.[46]
- *EGFR* mutation status may change over the course of therapy or during progression.[47]
- Histologic designation (i.e., squamous cell versus adenocarcinoma) may not be sufficiently reliable to guide testing and treatment decision making.[48]

One common approach is to test all nonsquamous NSCLC cases for *EGFR* mutations. In squamous cases with less confident histologic designation (e.g., small specimens, patients with never-/oligo-smoking status), *EGFR* mutation profiling is also considered.

Acquired Resistance to EGFR Inhibition

On average, tumors harboring activating *EGFR* mutations develop resistance to EGFR inhibitors after 9–12 months. A number of mechanisms of this acquired resistance have been identified[49]:

- *EGFR* exon 20 T790M mutations (50% of acquired resistance cases): a threonine-to-methionine amino acid substitution at position 790 results in increased affinity of EGFR binding by ATP substrate as well as diminished binding by EGFR inhibitors. In such cases, it appears that a small population of cancer cells harboring T790M mutations is present at diagnosis and selected for during EGFR TKI therapy.
- *MET* amplifications (20% of acquired resistance cases): increased activity of this receptor tyrosine kinase results in bypass of EGFR signaling via molecular cross-talk, leading to activation of downstream mediators of signal transduction independent of EGFR inhibition

- *PIK3CA* mutations (5% of acquired resistance cases): result in increased activity of proto-oncogenic signaling molecule phosphatidylinositol 3-kinase (PI3K)
- Transition from epithelial cell morphology to mesenchymal cell-like appearance (epithelial-to-mesenchymal transition [EMT])
- Conversion from NSCLC histology to small cell lung cancer histology

Anaplastic Lymphoma Kinase

Nomenclature

The anaplastic lymphoma kinase (ALK) gene, which encodes a tyrosine kinase, was originally identified in a subset of anaplastic large cell lymphomas with a t(2;5)(p23;q35) translocation. In a rare subset of NSCLC, chromosome 2p inversion results in fusion of the protein encoded by the echinoderm (a phylum of sea animals, including sea stars, sea urchins, sand dollars, and sea cucumbers) microtubule-associated protein-like 4 (EML4) gene with the intracellular signaling portion of the ALK receptor tyrosine kinase (EML4-ALK). Unlike KRAS or EGFR, ALK is not expressed in normal lung tissue.

Role in Tumorigenesis

Analogous to *EGFR* mutations, *EML4-ALK* fusions result in constitutive tyrosine kinase activity, dependence of the cancer cell on activated downstream mitogenic pathways (including AKT, ERK, and STAT3), and sensitivity to ALK inhibition.[50] In contrast to *EGFR* mutations in NSCLC, *ALK* fusions do not appear to confer increased sensitivity to conventional, cytotoxic chemotherapy.[51] However, with the ALK inhibitor crizotinib, disease control rates approach 90% and 6 month progression-free survival rates exceed 70%.[52]

Other genetic aberrations involving the ALK gene have been identified in anaplastic large cell lymphomas, inflammatory myofibroblastic tumors, and neuroblastomas. Efficacy of the ALK inhibitor crizotinib for treatment of some of these other conditions highlights the increasing recognition that it is a tumor's molecular characteristics—and not anatomic site or histology—that may ultimately guide treatment selection in oncology.[53]

Clinical Significance

The selection of patients most likely to benefit from ALK inhibition has been a central tenet of the development and clinical use of ALK inhibitors. In contrast to EGFR inhibitors for NSCLC (which are approved regardless of *EGFR* mutation status), the use of ALK inhibitors is restricted to those patients with ALK-positive tumors.

The terms "ALK positivity," "ALK rearrangement," and "ALK fusion" are generally synonymous and refer to the presence of the *EML4-ALK* rearrangement. This molecular aberration is rare in NSCLC, occurring in 3%–5% of cases. Nevertheless, given the vast number of lung cancer cases worldwide, an estimated 40,000 such cases occur annually.[54] Similar to *EGFR* mutations, *EML4-ALK* translocations are associated with certain clinicopathologic features.[51,55] These include the following:

- Never or light smoking
- Younger age
- Mutual exclusivity with *EGFR* and *KRAS* mutations
- No clear association with patient sex or race/ethnicity (in contrast to *EGFR* mutations)
- Adenocarcinoma histology
- Solid to acinar histology
- Signet ring differentiation
- Prominent intracellular mucin
- Thyroid transcription factor-1 (TTF-1) positivity

Given the rarity of *ALK* translocations in NSCLC, the need for adequate tissue, and the time and expense of molecular profiling, prescreening patients for molecular testing may be appropriate. Restricting testing to never smokers with *EGFR* wild-type tumors yields the highest proportion of ALK-positive NSCLC (approximately 40% of such patients) but may not be sufficiently sensitive. Another approach is to perform ALK testing on patients with adenocarcinoma NSCLC with wild-type *EGFR* and *KRAS*, independent of smoking history.

ALK rearrangements can be identified by IHC, FISH, or polymerase chain reaction (PCR). Of these, FISH appears to be the most clinically applicable. However, dual IHC and FISH may increase the detection of these cases.[55]

ALK Immunohistochemistry

In NSCLC, ALK protein expression by IHC appears to be specific for ALK gene rearrangements. The widespread adoption of ALK IHC has been limited by technical and interpretive challenges. Amplification techniques improve the sensitivity of IHC substantially.

ALK Fluorescence *In Situ* Hybridization

EML4-ALK FISH employs differently labeled breakapart (split signal) probes on the 5' and 3' ends of the ALK gene. Normal *ALK* generates a fused (yellow) signal, while *ALK* rearrangements appear as separate red and green signals (see Fig. 2.6). The standard cutoff for a positive result is a split signal in >15% of cells examined.[56]

c-ros Oncogene 1

Rearrangements of the receptor tyrosine kinase c-ros oncogene 1 (ROS1) have recently been described in NSCLC. ROS1 is located on chromosome 6 and has a high degree of amino acid homology with ALK (49% within the kinase domain and 77% within the ATP-binding site).[57] *ROS1* fusions appear to occur in approximately 1%–2% of NSCLC and may be detected by FISH, PCR, and IHC.

Given the high homology in the kinase domains of ROS1 and ALK, ALK inhibitors have been tested in this population and have demonstrated efficacy. Among the 14 ROS1-positive patients in the phase I trial of crizotinib, preliminary response rate was 57% with a disease control rate of 79% at 8 weeks.[58]

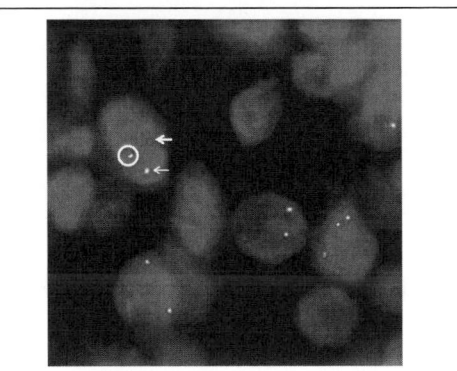

Figure 2.6 Anaplastic lymphoma kinase (ALK) fluorescence in situ hybridization (FISH). Non-small cell lung cancer with positive (rearranged) ALK FISH study. The FISH probe is designed to detect rearrangements of the ALK locus at 2p23. When the ALK locus is intact (nonrearranged), the signals are located close to each other resulting in a fused signal (circle). When rearrangement has occurred, the two signals are distant from each other (thick arrow: 3'-ALK probe signal; thin arrow: 5' ALK probe signal). (Vysis LSI ALK Break Apart Rearrangement Probe, Abbott Laboratories, Downer's Grove, IL). (Courtesy of Julia A. Bridge, MD, University of Nebraska Medical Center.)

Clinicopathologic features of ROS1-positive cases resemble those of ALK rearranged NSCLC and include the following[59]:

• Younger age
• Never smokers
• Adenocarcinoma histology

Additional Molecular Targets under Investigation

In addition to KRAS, EGFR, ALK, and ROS1, a number of other molecular changes in lung cancer are under investigation as potential therapeutic targets:

AKT: The serine-threonine kinase AKT is a downstream mediator of PI3K signaling (PI3K → AKT → mTOR → survival) and is inhibited by the tumor suppressor PTEN. Mutations in AKT1 (E17K) occur in approximately 1% of NSCLC (both adenocarcinoma and squamous) and appear nonoverlapping with other driver mutations. The role of AKT1 mutations in the selection of therapy is not established.

BRAF: BRAF is a serine-threonine kinase in the MAP kinase pathway (RAS → RAF → MEK → ERK → proliferation). BRAF mutations are found in 1%–3% of NSCLC. These cases are predominantly adenocarcinoma and occur in former/current smokers. In contrast to melanoma (in which almost all BRAF mutations are V600), a number of BRAF mutations have been identified in NSCLC: V600E (50%), G469A (40%), and D594G (11%).[60]

DDR2: DDR2 (discoidin death receptor 2) is a receptor tyrosine kinase activated by collagen that may signal via the SRC and STAT pathways. DDR2 mutations occur in 4% of squamous NSCLC and in <1% nonsquamous cases. The multitargeted kinase inhibitor dasatinib inhibits DDR2 in preclinical models.[61]

FGFR: The fibroblast growth factor receptor (FGFR) family includes four receptor tyrosine kinases (FGFR1, FGFR2, FGFR3, and FGFR4). *FGFR1* amplifications occur in approximately 20% of squamous NSCLC but in <2% of adenocarcinomas.[62] These amplifications appear to confer "oncogene addiction" to FGFR signaling. Studies of FGFR inhibitors for NSCLC therapy are underway.

HER2 (ErbB2): Human epidermal growth factor receptor 2 (HER2) is a tyrosine kinase in the HER (ErbB) family. It has no known ligand but is a dimerization partner for all other HER family members. In contrast to breast cancer, in lung cancer *HER2* amplification does not appear to have a prognostic or predictive role. Instead, *HER2* mutations appear more relevant. *HER2* mutations occur predominantly in exon 20, are detected in 2%–4% of NSCLC, most commonly in never smokers with adenocarcinoma but also in other populations and histologies.[63] These mutations are nonoverlapping with other oncogenic mutations. Responses to therapies with HER2 activity (e.g., trastuzumab, afatinib) have been reported in NSCLC.

MEK1: MEK1 (also called MAP2K1) is a serine-threonine kinase involved in transduction of proliferation signals (RAS → RAF → MEK → ERK → proliferation). *MEK1* mutations (K57N, Q56P, and D67N) occur in approximately 1% of NSCLC (adenocarcinoma > squamous).[64] In preclinical models, *MEK1* mutations result in constitutive signaling and sensitivity to MEK inhibitors, but clinical effects are not known.

MET: MET is a receptor tyrosine kinase activated by binding of its ligand hepatocyte growth factor (HGF), which is also known as scatter factor (SF). MET protein overexpression occurs in 25%–75% of NSCLC and is associated with poor prognosis. Increased MET protein expression by IHC is associated with improved response to an anti-MET antibody. Amplification of the MET gene occurs in 2%–4% of NSCLC (up to 20% of *EGFR* mutant NSCLC with acquired resistance to EGFR inhibitors), is associated with poor prognosis, and may confer sensitivity to MET inhibitors (including the dual ALK and MET inhibitor crizotinib).[65]

PIK3CA: The PIK3CA gene encodes a catalytic subunit of PI3K, a lipid kinase involved in cell growth and proliferation (PI3K → AKT → mTOR → proliferation). *PIK3CA* mutations (principally exons 9 and 20) occur in 1%–3% of NSCLC (squamous > nonsquamous; smokers and never smokers), may coexist with *EGFR* mutations, and account for up to 5% of *EGFR* mutant NSCLC acquired resistance to EGFR inhibitors.[66] The clinical effect of PI3K, AKT, and mTOR inhibitors in these cases is not known.

PTEN: PTEN (phosphatase and TENsin homolog deleted on chromosome 10) is a lipid/protein phosphatase that acts as a tumor suppressor by negatively regulating PI3K/AKT signaling. *PTEN* mutations occur in various exons in 4%–8% of NSCLC, more commonly in smokers and squamous histology.[67]

RET: An estimated 1% of lung cancers have rearrangements in the RET (rearranged during transfection) gene, which encodes the RET receptor tyrosine kinase.[68] Two specific gene fusions (*CCDC6-RET* and *KIF5B-RET*) have been described. *RET* rearrangements appear limited to adenocarcinoma histology and are not seen concurrently with *EGFR, ALK,* or *KRAS* mutations. A number of multitargeted kinase inhibitors have RET activity (vandetanib, sorafenib, sunitinib), but the efficacy of these agents in *RET* rearranged lung cancer has not been established.

Epigenetic Changes

Epigenetics refers to changes in gene expression caused by mechanisms other than changes in the underlying DNA sequence. These events are potentially reversible. The best described epigenetic changes in lung cancer and other malignances are DNA methylation and histone modification:

- *DNA methylation*: the addition of methyl groups to DNA, mostly at CpG sites. Highly methylated areas of DNA are less transcriptionally active. Promoter hypermethylation is a common method for the inactivation of tumor suppressor genes.
- *Histone modification*: changes, such as acetylation, to the amino acid structure of histones. Histone acetylation results in loosening of DNA from the histone complex, resulting in increased transcriptional activity. Conversely, histone deactylation inhibits gene expression.

In lung cancer, genes commonly affected by epigenetic changes include *APC, CDH1, CDH13, CDKN2A (p16), DAPK1, FHIT, PTEN, RAR*β, *RASSF1A, SEMA3B,* and *TIMP3*.[69,70] DNA hypomethylating agents and histone deacetylase inhibitors are currently under study for lung cancer therapy.

MicroRNA

MicroRNA (miRNA) are non-protein-encoding RNA ranging in size from 20 to 25 nucleotides. They function as posttranscriptional regulators that bind to complementary sequences of mRNA transcripts, resulting in translational repression or target degradation and gene silencing. There are estimated to be over 1000 miRNAs in the human genome.

These recently described molecules have a standardized nomenclature system. The prefix "mir-" indicates pre-miRNA, while "miR-" denotes the mature form. The number indicates the order in which the miRNA was discovered. If miRNA have nearly identical sequences, an additional lowercase letter is added after the number.

A number of miRNA have been identified as having tumor-suppressing and oncogenic effects in lung cancer[71,72]:

Tumor-Suppressing miRNAs

- *lethal-7 (let-7)* miRNA family: regulates KRAS; underexpressed in NSCLC compared with normal lung; decreased expression associated with poor prognosis; in preclinical models, induction of let-7 miRNA expression inhibits tumor growth *in vitro* and *in vivo*
- *miR-126*
- *miR-29a/b/c*
- *miR-1*
- *miR-128b:* regulator of EGFR; frequent LOH in NSCLC cell lines

Oncogenic miRNAs

- *miR-17-92* cluster: thought to target PTEN and RB
- *miR-205*
- *miR-21*
- *miR-155*

Other Abnormalities

Telomeres

In normal cells, progressive shortening of telomeres (regions of repetitive nucleotides at the ends of chromosomes) occurs with each cycle of replication. Eventually, when telomeres become too short, cells undergo senescence or apoptosis. Activation of telomerase, an enzyme that lengthens telomeres, is a requisite for cell immortality. Telomerase is activated in more than 80% of NSCLCs and in almost all SCLCs.[73,74] Telomerase inhibitors are currently being investigated for the treatment of lung cancer in clinical trials.

Stem Cells

Recently published work has raised the possibility that solid tumors possess a niche of specialized stem cells that replicate and propagate cancer cells (perhaps ad infinitum). These stem cells are thought to resist the effect of current chemotherapeutic agents due to the fact that they do not divide rapidly and do not rely on the same growth pathways to survive as do their progeny. Despite this potential treatment breakthrough, no lung cancer stem cell has been identified thus far. Hedgehog (HH), Wnt, and Notch signaling are involved in stem cell self-renewal pathways. In lung cancer, these pathways are often deregulated or aberrantly activated, suggesting they may serve as therapeutic targets.[75]

Tumor Microenvironment and Angiogenesis

At the cellular level, lung and other cancers exist in a milieu of stroma, microvasculature, and inflammatory cells that together make up the tumor microenvironment. Overall, it is thought that the microenvironment is mainly driven by signaling molecules originating from tumor cells as a means to promote nutrient flow and suppress antitumor immune responses. These signaling molecules include tumor growth factor beta (TGF-β), nitric oxide (NO), and vascular endothelial growth factor (VEGF).[76]

VEGF is the principal mediator of angiogenesis, the growth of new blood vessels from preexisting vasculature. Specifically, the VEGF-VEGFR axis regulates endothelial cell survival, mitogenesis, migration, mobilization of endothelial progenitor cells from the bone marrow, and vascular permeability. Similar to normal cells, tumor cells require oxygen and nutrients for survival, placing angiogenesis among the many targets for cancer therapy.

The VEGF-related gene family of growth factors includes VEGF-A, VEGF-B, VEGF-C, VEGF-D, VEGF-E, and placental growth factor (PlGF)-1 and PlGF-2. VEGF-A, commonly referred to as VEGF, binds to three receptors: VEGFR1 (also known as Flt-1 [fms-like tyrosine kinase-1]), VEGFR2 (also known as Flk-1/KDR [fetal liver kinase-1/kinase domain region]), and VEGFR3 (also known as Flt-4). VEGFR2 is the principal mediator of malignant angiogenesis. VEGFR3 has been found to be primarily associated with lymphangiogenesis. VEGFRs are receptor tyrosine kinases. Similar to EGFR, they convey proliferation signals via intracellular mediators.

In advanced nonsquamous NSCLC, the anti-VEGF monoclonal antibody bevacizumab is approved for first-line therapy in combination with carboplatin-paclitaxel. Reflecting the importance of angiogenesis across tumor types, bevacizumab is also approved for the treatment of colorectal, kidney, and brain cancers.

In NSCLC, no biomarkers consistently predict response to anti-angiogenic agents. Tumor and plasma VEGF levels are prognostic, but not reliably predictive.[77] VEGF and VEGFR polymorphisms, which have been characterized in breast cancer patients treated with bevacizumab,[78] are under study in NSCLC. Other candidate pharmacodynamic markers include multiple plasma cytokines and angiogenic factors, among them intracellular adhesion molecule-1 (ICAM-1), E-selectin, soluble VEGFRs, matrix metalloproteinases, and interleukins.

Biomarkers Predictive of Sensitivity to Cytotoxic Chemotherapy in Lung Cancer

Conventional cytotoxic chemotherapy remains the backbone of medical therapy for most patients with lung cancer. In contrast to molecular targeted agents such erlotinib and crizotinib, these drugs do not have established biomarkers predicting efficacy. Nevertheless, a number of candidate biomarkers are under investigation.

Predictive biomarkers to chemotherapy can be categorized as DNA synthesis/repair genes, cell cycle regulators, class III beta-tubulin, signal transduction pathways, and gene expression profiling.[79]

DNA Synthesis/Repair Genes

Excision Repair Cross-Complementation Group 1
Excision repair cross-complementation group 1 (ERCC1) is a protein involved in DNA repair after platinum damage that is associated with platinum resistance. ERCC1 is specifically involved in nucleotide excision repair and interstrand cross-link repair. Generally, ERCC1 expression is assessed by IHC or PCR. In a retrospective analysis of the International Adjuvant Lung Cancer Trial (IALT), cisplatin-based chemotherapy significantly prolonged survival for patients with ERCC1-negative tumors (HR 0.65; 95% CI, 0.50–0.86; $P = 0.002$) but not for patients with ERCC1-positive tumors (HR 1.14; 95% CI, 0.84–1.55; $P = 0.40$). In this analysis, approximately 45% of tumors were ERCC1 positive and 55% were ERCC1 negative.[80] Prospective validation studies are ongoing.

Ribonucleotide Reductase Messenger 1
Ribonucleotide reductase messenger 1 (RRM1) is a regulator of ribonucleotide reductase (an enzyme involved in ribonucleotide synthesis and DNA repair) that is associated with resistance to gemcitabine-based chemotherapy.[81]

Thymidylate Synthase
Thymidylate synthase (TS) is the main target of the antifolate pemetrexed. TS is involved in DNA replication and repair mechanisms. Elevated levels of TS in squamous tumors are postulated to underlie the histology-specific effects of pemetrexed.[82,83] In a retrospective analysis of 285 cases of nonsquamous NSCLC treated with pemetrexed-based chemotherapy, TS-negative tumors had significantly higher response rate (33.7% vs 14.1%; $P = 0.002$) and progression-free survival (4.1 months vs. 2.0 months; $P = 0.001$).[84]

MutS Homologue 2

MutS homologue 2 (MSH2) is a protein involved in repair of platinum-induced DNA damage. In IALT, adjuvant cisplatin-based chemotherapy resulted in improved overall survival in the low-MSH2 group (38% of cases) (HR 0.76; 95% CI, 0.59–0.97; P = 0.03) but not in the high-MSH2 group (62% of cases) (HR 1.12; 95% CI, 0.81–1.55; P = 0.48).[85]

Cell Cycle Regulators

Expression levels of p27 (a member of the cyclin-dependent kinase inhibitory family that regulates G1 to S phase cell cycle progression), P53 (a tumor suppressor involved in genome stability and cell cycle regulation), and Bax (a proapoptotic factor activated by P53) have demonstrated associations with benefit from adjuvant chemotherapy.[86,87]

Class III Beta-Tubulin

Class III beta-tubulin (TUBB3) is a microtubule element that reduces microtubule stability and has been associated with resistance to antitubulin therapy. In a meta-analysis of over 550 patients in 10 studies of paclitaxel- or vinorelbine-containing chemotherapy, patients with low/negative class III beta-tubulin expression (assessed by mRNA) (50% of cases) had higher radiographic response rates and longer overall survival than patients with high-positive class III beta-tubulin.[88]

Signal Transduction Pathways

KRAS mutations may predict lack of benefit from adjuvant chemotherapy.[87] *EGFR* mutations are associated with improved response to conventional chemotherapy as well as to EGFR inhibitors.[40]

Gene Expression Profiling

Numerous gene signatures have been derived for the prediction of chemosensitivity, as well as for prognostication.[89] Issues of standardization and reproducibility have hindered the incorporation of these techniques into routine clinical practice.

Molecular Diagnostic Techniques

In both research and clinical practice, molecular diagnostic techniques play a central role in elucidating lung cancer biology. Selected techniques are discussed here.

Immunohistochemistry

IHC uses primary and secondary antibodies to stain for a molecular marker (usually a protein) of interest (see Fig. 2.2). The intensity, prevalence, and location of staining may be reported semiquantitatively. While IHC may be performed on small samples, such as bronchial brushings or fine needle aspirates, tissue blocks are preferred.

Because IHC is used for routine clinical testing (see Chapter 3), it has the advantage of availability in most medical centers. However, several factors influence the reproducibility and quantitative value of IHC, including tissue collection and handling techniques, time between slide preparation and staining, antibody detection protocols, and the size and quality of tissue sections used.[90] IHC of phosphorylated (activated) proteins is particularly fraught with challenges.

As seen in other malignancies, lung cancer biomarker expression may display substantial heterogeneity. For instance, there is variation in EGFR expression between primary and metastatic tumors, as well as within a single tumor.[91,92] Furthermore, in contrast to HER2 IHC in breast cancer, IHC scoring for lung cancer biomarkers, such as EGFR, is not standardized.

Fluorescence *In Situ* Hybridization

FISH uses fluorescence-tagged DNA probes corresponding to the gene(s) of interest (see Figs. 2.3 and 2.6). These probes may demonstrate changes in gene number (e.g., *EGFR* amplification/copy number) or gene rearrangements (e.g., *EML4-ALK*).

While more readily standardized than IHC, FISH is less widely available. FISH may be performed on small samples, including cytology specimens such as bronchial brushings and FNAs. However, tumor blocks, which provide more assessable tumor cell nuclei, are preferred.

Gene Expression Profiling

Microarray technology has provided the potential to interrogate thousands of genes simultaneously. A microarray is a two-dimensional array on a solid substrate (usually a glass slide or silicon thin-film cell) that employs specifically synthesized DNA probes to hybridize and immobilize fluorescently labeled genomic DNA or cDNA sequences from a biological sample.

Probe-target hybridization is quantified by fluorophore, silver, or chemiluminescence labeling and is visualized as a "heat map" (see Fig. 2.7). While promising, this technology introduces a number of technical issues, including standardization between platforms and data format, low throughput and accuracy, and low precision.

Gene Sequencing

Gene sequencing is the current standard for determining the mutation status of *EGFR* and *KRAS* (see Fig. 2.5). Rapid advances in sequencing technologies have markedly reduced the cost and time required. A traditional sequencing reaction (also known as first-generation or Sanger sequencing) yields approximately 1 kb (1000 bp) of high-quality DNA sequencing data using specific DNA primers upstream and downstream of the target gene. Currently, the cost and capacity of first-generation sequencing is well suited for sequencing of a candidate region <1 kb in length.

In contrast, next-generation sequencing platforms have emerged as a rapid and cost-effective means of sequencing entire genomes of individuals as well as cancers. The basic technologic premise in next-generation sequencing platforms involves fragmenting sample DNA into small (<100 bp) fragments and sequencing each fragment during polymerase chain reaction (PCR) amplification in real time. This so-called sequence by synthesis allows for millions of fragments to be sequenced in parallel, yielding more than 100 Gb (100 billion bp) per "run." To put things into perspective, an entire cancer genome can be sequenced within

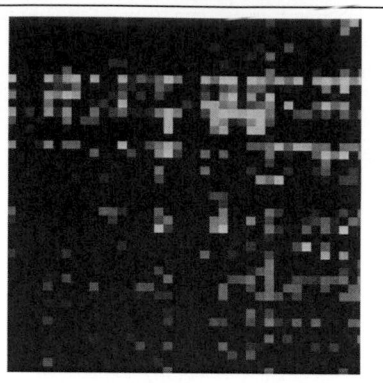

Figure 2.7 Data from microarray or other genomic data sets are often arranged in clusters on a heat map, a two-dimensional representation of either frequency or signal intensity (e.g., higher values are represented by brighter squares) versus sample number on one axis and gene on the other axis. Heat maps are often arranged to where genes are clustered by frequency or signal intensity (i.e., similarly colored squares are adjacent to one another). (Courtesy of Ameen Salahudeen, MD, PhD.)

days. Recently, using this technology, several groups have reported comprehensive genomic sequencing of NSCLCs.[6,8]

Because high tumor cell content (50%–70% tumor cells) is required for gene sequencing, tissue macro- or microdissection may be needed. Most techniques employ PCR to amplify (i.e., create multiple copies) the DNA segment of interest. Fresh tissue is preferred to formalin-fixed paraffin-embedded tissue because formalin fixation can cause nucleic acid degradation.

References

1. Dela Cruz CS, Tanoue LT, Matthay RA. Lung cancer: epidemiology, etiology, and prevention. *Clin Chest Med* 2011;32:605–44.

2. Hanahan D, Weinberg RA. The hallmarks of cancer. *Cell* 2000;100:57–70.

3. Fong KM, Sekido Y, Minna JD. Molecular pathogenesis of lung cancer. *J Thorac Cardiovasc Surg* 1999;118:1136–52.

4. Ding L, Getz G, Wheeler DA, et al. Somatic mutations affect key pathways in lung adenocarcinoma. *Nature* 2008;455:1069–75.

5. Kris MG, Johnson BE, Kwiatkowski DJ, et al. Identification of driver mutations in tumor specimens from 1,000 patients with lung adenocarcinoma: The NCI's Lung Cancer Mutation Consortium (LCMC). *J Clin Oncol* 2011;29 (suppl; abstr CRA7506).

6. Cancer Genome Atlas Research Network. Comprehensive genomic characterization of squamous cell lung cancers. *Nature* 2012;489:519–25.

7. Peifer M, Fernandez-Cuesta L, Sos ML, et al. Integrative genome analyses identify key somatic driver mutations of small-cell lung cancer. *Nat Genet* 2012;44:1104–10.

8. Rudin CM, Durinck S, Stawiski EW, et al. Comprehensive genomic analysis identifies SOX2 as a frequently amplified gene in small-cell lung cancer. *Nat Genet* 2012;44:1111–6.

9. Kranenburg O. The KRAS oncogene: past, present, and future. *Biochim Biophys Acta* 2005;1756:81–2.

10. Rodenhuis S, Slebos RJ. Clinical significance of ras oncogene activation in human lung cancer. *Cancer Res* 1992;52:2665s–9s.

11. Coate LE, John T, Tsao MS, et al. Molecular predictive and prognostic markers in non-small-cell lung cancer. *Lancet Oncol* 2009;10:1001–10.

12. Miller VA, Riely GJ, Zakowski MF, et al. Molecular characteristics of bronchioloalveolar carcinoma and adenocarcinoma, bronchioloalveolar carcinoma subtype, predict response to erlotinib. *J Clin Oncol* 2008;26:1472–8.

13. Shepherd FA, Rodrigues Pereira J, Ciuleanu T, et al. Erlotinib in previously treated non-small-cell lung cancer. *N Engl J Med* 2005;353:123–32.

14. Gatzemeier U, Paz-Ares L, Rodrigues Pereira J, et al. Molecular and clinical biomarkers of cetuximab efficacy: data from the phase III FLEX study in non-small cell lung cancer (NSCLC). *J Thorac Oncol* 2009;4:S324 (abstract B2.3).

15. Rusch V, Baselga J, Cordon-Cardo C, et al. Differential expression of the epidermal growth factor receptor and its ligands in primary non-small cell lung cancers and adjacent benign lung. *Cancer Res* 1993;53:2379–85.

16. Dutu T, Michiels S, Fouret P, et al. Differential expression of biomarkers in lung adenocarcinoma: a comparative study between smokers and never-smokers. *Ann Oncol* 2005;16:1906–14.

17 Hirsch FR, Varella-Garcia M, Bunn PA, Jr., et al. Epidermal growth factor receptor In non small-cell lung carcinomas: correlation between gene copy number and protein expression and impact on prognosis. *J Clin Oncol* 2003;21:3798–807.

18. Nicholson RI, Gee JM, Harper ME. EGFR and cancer prognosis. *Eur J Cancer* 2001;37(Suppl 4):S9–S15.

19. Schreiber AB, Winkler ME, Derynck R. Transforming growth factor alpha: a more potent angiogenic mediator than epidermal growth factor. *Science* 1986;232:1250–3.

20. Petit AM, Rak J, Hung MC, et al. Neutralizing antibodies against epidermal growth factor and ErbB-2/neu receptor tyrosine kinases down-regulate vascular endothelial growth factor production by tumor cells in vitro and in vivo: angiogenic implications for signal transduction therapy of solid tumors. *Am J Pathol* 1997;151:1523–30.

21. Gibson S, Tu S, Oyer R, et al. Epidermal growth factor protects epithelial cells against Fas-induced apoptosis. Requirement for Akt activation. *J Biol Chem* 1999;274:17612–8.

22. O-charoenrat P, Modjtahedi H, Rhys-Evans P, et al. Epidermal growth factor-like ligands differentially up-regulate matrix metalloproteinase 9 in head and neck squamous carcinoma cells. *Cancer Res* 2000;60:1121–8.

23. Harari PM, Allen GW, Bonner JA. Biology of interactions: antiepidermal growth factor receptor agents. *J Clin Oncol* 2007;25:4057–65.

24. Lin SY, Makino K, Xia W, et al. Nuclear localization of EGF receptor and its potential new role as a transcription factor. *Nat Cell Biol* 2001;3:802–8.

25. Dittmann K, Mayer C, Fehrenbacher B, et al. Radiation-induced epidermal growth factor receptor nuclear import is linked to activation of DNA-dependent protein kinase. *J Biol Chem* 2005;280:31182–9.

26. Perez-Soler R, Chachoua A, Hammond LA, et al. Determinants of tumor response and survival with erlotinib in patients with non-small-cell lung cancer. *J Clin Oncol* 2004;22:3238–47.

27. Cappuzzo F, Hirsch FR, Rossi E, et al. Epidermal growth factor receptor gene and protein and gefitinib sensitivity in non-small-cell lung cancer. *J Natl Cancer Inst* 2005;97:643–55.

28. Tsao MS, Sakurada A, Cutz JC, et al. Erlotinib in lung cancer—molecular and clinical predictors of outcome. *N Engl J Med* 2005;353:133–44.

29. Kosaka T, Yatabe Y, Endoh H, et al. Mutations of the epidermal growth factor receptor gene in lung cancer: biological and clinical implications. *Cancer Res* 2004;64:8919–23.

30. Lynch TJ, Bell DW, Sordella R, et al. Activating mutations in the epidermal growth factor receptor underlying responsiveness of non-small-cell lung cancer to gefitinib. *N Engl J Med* 2004;350:2129–39.

31. Pao W, Miller V, Zakowski M, et al. EGF receptor gene mutations are common in lung cancers from "never smokers" and are associated with sensitivity of tumors to gefitinib and erlotinib. *Proc Natl Acad Sci USA* 2004;101:13306–11.

32. Kobayashi S, Boggon TJ, Dayaram T, et al. EGFR mutation and resistance of non-small-cell lung cancer to gefitinib. *N Engl J Med* 2005;352:786–92.

33. Pao W, Miller VA, Politi KA, et al. Acquired resistance of lung adenocarcinomas to gefitinib or erlotinib is associated with a second mutation in the EGFR kinase domain. *PLoS Med* 2005;2:e73.

34. Kwak EL, Sordella R, Bell DW, et al. Irreversible inhibitors of the EGF receptor may circumvent acquired resistance to gefitinib. *Proc Natl Acad Sci USA* 2005;102:7665–70.

35. Weinstein IB, Joe AK. Mechanisms of disease: Oncogene addiction—a rationale for molecular targeting in cancer therapy. *Nat Clin Pract Oncol* 2006;3:448–57.

36. Weinstein IB. Cancer. Addiction to oncogenes—the Achilles heal of cancer. *Science* 2002;297:63–4.

37. Yun CH, Boggon TJ, Li Y, et al. Structures of lung cancer-derived EGFR mutants and inhibitor complexes: mechanism of activation and insights into differential inhibitor sensitivity. *Cancer Cell* 2007;11:217–27.

38. Rosell R, Moran T, Queralt C, et al. Screening for epidermal growth factor receptor mutations in lung cancer. *N Engl J Med* 2009;361:958–67.

39. Hanna N, Lilenbaum R, Ansari R, et al. Phase II trial of cetuximab in patients with previously treated non-small-cell lung cancer. *J Clin Oncol* 2006;24:5253–8.

40. Mok TS, Wu YL, Thongprasert S, et al. Gefitinib or carboplatin-paclitaxel in pulmonary adenocarcinoma. *N Engl J Med* 2009;361:947–57.

41. Fukuoka M, Yano S, Giaccone G, et al. Multi-institutional randomized phase II trial of gefitinib for previously treated patients with advanced non-small-cell lung cancer (The IDEAL 1 Trial). *J Clin Oncol* 2003;21:2237–46.

42. Kris MG, Natale RB, Herbst RS, et al. Efficacy of gefitinib, an inhibitor of the epidermal growth factor receptor tyrosine kinase, in symptomatic patients with non-small cell lung cancer: a randomized trial. *JAMA* 2003;290:2149–58.

43. Janne PA, Gurubhagavatula S, Yeap BY, et al. Outcomes of patients with advanced non-small cell lung cancer treated with gefitinib (ZD1839, "Iressa") on an expanded access study. *Lung Cancer* 2004;44:221–30.

44. Kim KS, Jeong JY, Kim YC, et al. Predictors of the response to gefitinib in refractory non-small cell lung cancer. *Clin Cancer Res* 2005;11:2244–51.

45. Veronese ML, Algazy K, Bearn L, et al. Gefitinib in patients with advanced non-small cell lung cancer (NSCLC): the expanded access protocol experience at the University of Pennsylvania. *Cancer Invest* 2005;23:296–302.

46. D'Angelo SP, Pietanza MC, Johnson ML, et al. Incidence of EGFR exon 19 deletions and L858R in tumor specimens from men and cigarette smokers with lung adenocarcinomas. *J Clin Oncol* 2011;29:2066–70.

47. Maheswaran S, Sequist LV, Nagrath S, et al. Detection of mutations in EGFR in circulating lung-cancer cells. *N Engl J Med* 2008;359:366–77.

48. Grilley-Olson JE, Hayes DN, Qaqish BF, et al. Diagnostic reproducibility of squamous cell carcinoma in the era of histology-directed non-small cell lung cancer (NSCLC) chemotherapy: a large prospective study. *J Clin Oncol* 2009;27(suppl);abstract 8008.

49. Sequist LV, Waltman BA, Dias-Santagata D, et al. Genotypic and histological evolution of lung cancers acquiring resistance to EGFR inhibitors. *Sci Transl Med* 2011;3:75ra26.

50. Gerber DE, Minna JD. ALK inhibition for non-small cell lung cancer: from discovery to therapy in record time. *Cancer Cell* 2010;18:548–51.

51. Shaw AT, Yeap BY, Mino-Kenudson M, et al. Clinical features and outcome of patients with non-small-cell lung cancer who harbor EML4-ALK. *J Clin Oncol* 2009;27:4247–53.

52. Kwak EL, Bang YJ, Camidge DR, et al. Anaplastic lymphoma kinase inhibition in non-small-cell lung cancer. *N Engl J Med* 2010;363:1693–703.

53. Butrynski JE, D'Adamo DR, Hornick JL, et al. Crizotinib in ALK-rearranged inflammatory myofibroblastic tumor. *N Engl J Med* 2010;363:1727–33.

54. Palmer RH, Vernersson E, Grabbe C, et al. Anaplastic lymphoma kinase: signalling in development and disease. *Biochem J* 2009;420:345–61.

55. Rodig SJ, Mino-Kenudson M, Dacic S, et al. Unique clinicopathologic features characterize ALK-rearranged lung adenocarcinoma in the western population. *Clin Cancer Res* 2009;15:5216–23.

56. Camidge DR, Kono SA, Flacco A, et al. Optimizing the detection of lung cancer patients harboring anaplastic lymphoma kinase (ALK) gene rearrangements potentially suitable for ALK inhibitor treatment. *Clin Cancer Res* 2010;16(22):5581–90.

57. Chin LP, Soo RA, Soong R, et al. Targeting ROS1 with anaplastic lymphoma kinase inhibitors: a promising therapeutic strategy for a newly defined molecular subset of non-small-cell lung cancer. *J Thorac Oncol* 2012;7:1625–30.

58. Shaw AT, Camidge DR, Engelman JA. Clinical activity of crizotinib in advanced non-small cell lung cancer (NSCLC) harboring ROS1 gene rearrangement. *J Clin Oncol* 2012;30 (suppl; abstr7508).

59. Bergethon K, Shaw AT, Ou SH, et al. ROS1 rearrangements define a unique molecular class of lung cancers. *J Clin Oncol* 2012;30:863–70.

60. Paik PK, Arcila ME, Fara M, et al. Clinical characteristics of patients with lung adenocarcinomas harboring BRAF mutations. *J Clin Oncol* 2011;29:2046–51.

61. Hammerman PS, Sos ML, Ramos AH, et al. Mutations in the DDR2 kinase gene identify a novel therapeutic target in squamous cell lung cancer. *Cancer Discov* 2011;1:78–89.

62. Dutt A, Ramos AH, Hammerman PS, et al. Inhibitor-sensitive FGFR1 amplification in human non-small cell lung cancer. *PLoS One* 2011;6:e20351.

63. Buttitta F, Barassi F, Fresu G, et al. Mutational analysis of the HER2 gene in lung tumors from Caucasian patients: mutations are mainly present in adenocarcinomas with bronchioloalveolar features. *Int J Cancer* 2006;119:2586–91.

64. Marks JL, Gong Y, Chitale D, et al. Novel MEK1 mutation identified by mutational analysis of epidermal growth factor receptor signaling pathway genes in lung adenocarcinoma. *Cancer Res* 2008;68:5524–8.

65. Cappuzzo F, Marchetti A, Skokan M, et al. Increased MET gene copy number negatively affects survival of surgically resected non-small-cell lung cancer patients. *J Clin Oncol* 2009;27:1667–74.

66. Kawano O, Sasaki H, Endo K, et al. PIK3CA mutation status in Japanese lung cancer patients. *Lung Cancer* 2006;54:209–15.

67. Jin G, Kim MJ, Jeon HS, et al. PTEN mutations and relationship to EGFR, ERBB2, KRAS, and TP53 mutations in non-small cell lung cancers. *Lung Cancer* 2010;69:279–83.

68. Ju YS, Lee WC, Shin JY, et al. A transforming KIF5B and RET gene fusion in lung adenocarcinoma revealed from whole-genome and transcriptome sequencing. *Genome Res* 2012;22:436–45.

69. Ito M, Ito G, Kondo M, et al. Frequent inactivation of RASSF1A, BLU, and SEMA3B on 3p21.3 by promoter hypermethylation and allele loss in non-small cell lung cancer. *Cancer Lett* 2005;225:131–9.

70. Zochbauer-Muller S, Minna JD, Gazdar AF. Aberrant DNA methylation in lung cancer: biological and clinical implications. *Oncologist* 2002;7:451–7.

71. Yu SL, Chen HY, Chang GC, et al. MicroRNA signature predicts survival and relapse in lung cancer. *Cancer Cell* 2008;13:48–57.

72. Yanaihara N, Caplen N, Bowman E, et al. Unique microRNA molecular profiles in lung cancer diagnosis and prognosis. *Cancer Cell* 2006;9:189–98.

73. Albanell J, Lonardo F, Rusch V, et al. High telomerase activity in primary lung cancers: association with increased cell proliferation rates and advanced pathologic stage. *J Natl Cancer Inst* 1997;89:1609–15.

74. Hiyama K, Hiyama E, Ishioka S, et al. Telomerase activity in small-cell and non-small-cell lung cancers. *J Natl Cancer Inst* 1995;87:895–902.

75. Daniel VC, Peacock CD, Watkins DN. Developmental signalling pathways in lung cancer. *Respirology* 2006;11:234–40.

76. Whiteside TL. The tumor microenvironment and its role in promoting tumor growth. *Oncogene* 2008;27:5904–12.

77. Longo R, Gasparini G. Challenges for patient selection with VEGF inhibitors. *Cancer Chemother Pharmacol* 2007;60:151–70.

78. Schneider BP, Wang M, Radovich M, et al. Association of vascular endothelial growth factor and vascular endothelial growth factor receptor-2 genetic polymorphisms with outcome in a trial of paclitaxel compared with paclitaxel plus bevacizumab in advanced breast cancer: ECOG 2100. *J Clin Oncol* 2008;26:4672–78.

79. Felip E, Martinez P. Can sensitivity to cytotoxic chemotherapy be predicted by biomarkers? *Ann Oncol* 2012;23(Suppl 10):x189–92.

80. Olaussen KA, Dunant A, Fouret P, et al. DNA repair by ERCC1 in non-small-cell lung cancer and cisplatin-based adjuvant chemotherapy. *N Engl J Med* 2006;355:983–91.

81. Bepler G, Kusmartseva I, Sharma S, et al. RRM1 modulated in vitro and in vivo efficacy of gemcitabine and platinum in non-small-cell lung cancer. *J Clin Oncol* 2006;24:4731–7.

82. Ceppi P, Volante M, Saviozzi S, et al. Squamous cell carcinoma of the lung compared with other histotypes shows higher messenger RNA and protein levels for thymidylate synthase. *Cancer* 2006;107:1589–96.

83. Scagliotti GV, Parikh P, von Pawel J, et al. Phase III study comparing cisplatin plus gemcitabine with cisplatin plus pemetrexed in chemotherapy-naive patients with advanced-stage non-small-cell lung cancer. *J Clin Oncol* 2008;26:3543–51.

84. Sun JM, Han J, Ahn JS, et al. Significance of thymidylate synthase and thyroid transcription factor 1 expression in patients with nonsquamous non-small cell lung cancer treated with pemetrexed-based chemotherapy. *J Thorac Oncol* 2011;6:1392–9.

85. Kamal NS, Soria JC, Mendiboure J, et al. MutS homologue 2 and the long-term benefit of adjuvant chemotherapy in lung cancer. *Clin Cancer Res* 2010;16:1206–15.

86. Filipits M, Pirker R, Dunant A, et al. Cell cycle regulators and outcome of adjuvant cisplatin-based chemotherapy in completely resected non-small-cell lung cancer: the International Adjuvant Lung Cancer Trial Biologic Program. *J Clin Oncol* 2007;25:2735–40.

87. Tsao MS, Aviel-Ronen S, Ding K, et al. Prognostic and predictive importance of p53 and RAS for adjuvant chemotherapy in non small-cell lung cancer. *J Clin Oncol* 2007;25:5240–7.

88. Zhang HL, Ruan L, Zheng LM, et al. Association between class III beta-tubulin expression and response to paclitaxel/vinorebine-based chemotherapy for non-small cell lung cancer: a meta analysis. *Lung Cancer* 2012;77:9–15.

89. Zhu CQ, Ding K, Strumpf D, et al. Prognostic and predictive gene signature for adjuvant chemotherapy in resected non-small-cell lung cancer. *J Clin Oncol* 2010;28:4417–24.

90. Eberhard DA, Giaccone G, Johnson BE. Biomarkers of response to epidermal growth factor receptor inhibitors in Non-Small-Cell Lung Cancer Working Group. standardization for use in the clinical trial setting. *J Clin Oncol* 2008;26:983–94.

91. Italiano A, Vandenbos FB, Otto J, et al. Comparison of the epidermal growth factor receptor gene and protein in primary non-small-cell-lung cancer and metastatic sites: implications for treatment with EGFR-inhibitors. *Ann Oncol* 2005;17:981–5.

92. Suzuki S, Dobashi Y, Sakurai H, et al. Protein overexpression and gene amplification of epidermal growth factor receptor in nonsmall cell lung carcinomas. An immunohistochemical and fluorescence in situ hybridization study. *Cancer* 2005;103:1265–73.

Chapter 3

Pathology of Lung Cancer

William W. West

In the adult lung, carcinomas comprise 95% of primary tumors, carcinoids account for 2%–3% and a wide variety of benign and malignant lesions make up the remaining 1%–2%. This chapter will discuss lung carcinomas in the adult. Tumors seen in the pediatric population vary significantly from the adult tumors and the reader should refer to a pediatric pathology reference for information regarding pediatric tumors.

Anatomy

Lungs

The lungs are bilateral, but asymmetric, intrathoracic air-exchange organs encased by the musculoskeletal chest wall, mediastinum, and diaphragm. The right lung is subdivided into three lobes (upper, middle, and lower). The left lung consists of two lobes (upper and lower) with the lingula, part of the upper lobe. The right lung is larger than the left due to the leftward location of the heart within the mediastinum. Combined lung weights vary from 750 to 850 grams and vary with sex and height.

While each lung is relatively mobile within the thoracic cavity, it is attached at the hilum to the mediastinal structures. The lungs are located adjacent to multiple significant anatomic structures that lie within the mediastinum— heart, great vessels, trachea, esophagus, thymus, nerves, and mediastinal nodes. Lymphatics, nerves, major airways, and blood vessels traverse the hilum, which is located along the mediastinal surface at the medial aspect of each lung.

Pleura

The lung, including the surfaces of the major and minor fissures, is covered by a thin translucent serosal surface lined by mesothelial cells (visceral pleura). This pleural surface reflects off the medial aspect of the lung at the hilum and pulmonary ligament to form the parietal pleura, which covers the mediastinum, diaphragm, and inner aspect of the chest wall. The potential space between the visceral lining and the parietal lining constitutes the pleural space.

Under normal circumstances the pleural space, lubricated by a minimal amount of pleural fluid, allows mobility of the lung surface to accommodate respiration. The visceral pleural space is lined by a layer of flattened mesothelial cells, which overlie a basal lamina, a connective tissue layer, and 1–2 layers of thickened elastic fibers (visceral pleura elastica). The submesothelium then gives way to looser connective tissue that includes collagen, fine elastic fibers, small vessels, and lymphatics. The pleural elastica is important in staging small peripheral lung cancers and may require special histochemical stains (elastic stain) to evaluate for evidence of visceral pleural invasion.

Airways

Much of the lung anatomy is characterized by continuous asymmetric dichotomous branching of the airways starting at the trachea and continuing peripherally to the level of the acinus. Lung cancer can originate in the mucosa of the conducting airway system (tracheobronchial tree) or in the lung periphery from acinar/alveolar lining cells. The source of the tumor may affect the morphology and the immunoprofile.

The conducting airways consist of the trachea, bronchi, and conducting bronchioles. The trachea asymmetrically branches to form the right and left mainstem bronchi within the mediastinum. The mainstem bronchus on each side enters the lung and subsequently branches and directly forms the lobar bronchi on the left and the bronchus intermedius and upper lobe bronchus on the right. Within the lungs, the lobar bronchi continue to branch forming segmental, subsegmental, and subsequent generations of smaller airways.

Bronchi are larger airways with mural cartilage and/or submucosal seromucinous glands, while *bronchioles* are the smaller airways that lack cartilage and glands. The last conducting airway is the terminal bronchiole. Lung parenchyma distal to one terminal bronchiole is known as the pulmonary *acinus* (approximately 0.5–0.7 cm), the functional air exchange portion of the lung. The pulmonary *lobule* (1–2 cm) is the portion of lung parenchyma delimited by interlobular septa. Each lobule consists of 4–8 acini.

Lymphatics

Lymphatics extend throughout the bronchoarterial connective tissue sheath to anastomose with visceral pleural lymphatics and the septal, perivenous lymphatics. These lymphatics drain to ipsilateral intrapulmonary, subsegmental, segmental, lobar, interlobar, and hilar lymph nodes (N1 nodes). N1 nodes potentially drain to ipsilateral N2 nodes (mediastinal, subcarinal) and/or supraclavicular and scalene lymph nodes (N3 nodes).

Pathologic Diagnosis

The pathologic diagnosis of lung cancer is based upon the light microscopic evaluation of cytology specimens (fine-needle aspiration, brushing, washing, endobronchial ultrasound, effusion), biopsies (core needle, bronchoscopic), and/or resection specimens. Since most (70%) lung cancers have spread beyond the lung at the time of initial presentation, the diagnosis of lung cancer is frequently based upon small samples of larger lesions with the inherent potential for sampling bias.

Diagnosis requires proper sampling of the tumor, careful tissue handling, adequate fixation, processing, cutting and staining in the laboratory, and careful examination by a trained pathologist. While numerous ancillary studies are available to assist in the evaluation of the tissue sample, a properly prepared, well-stained hematoxylin and eosin (H&E) stained slide or cytology preparation remains the cornerstone for the diagnosis and classification of lung cancer.[1]

The 2004 World Health Organization (WHO) classification of lung tumors serves as the basis for the current nomenclature for lung cancers.[2] A more recent multidisciplinary consensus classification from the International Association for the Study of Lung Cancer, the American Thoracic Society, and the European Respiratory Society (IASLC/ATS/ERS) has recommended important updates for the classification of lung adenocarcinoma and the diagnostic terminology for small biopsy specimens and resection specimens.[3] The WHO classification of lung carcinomas as modified by the IASLC/ATS/ERS proposal is shown in Table 3.1.

Four histologic types account for the majority of lung carcinomas:

- Adenocarcinoma (ADC) (approximately 40% of cases)
- Squamous cell carcinoma (SCC) (30%)
- Large cell carcinoma (LCC) (9%)
- Small cell carcinoma (SCLC) (14%)

Each histologic type includes one or more subtypes as listed in Table 3.1.

Table 3.1 Pathologic Classification of Lung Carcinomas in Resection Specimens

Adenocarcinoma
- Minimally invasive adenocarcinoma (MIA) (≤3 cm lepidic predominant tumor with ≤5 mm invasion)
- Invasive adenocarcinoma
  - Lepidic predominant (nonmucinous with >5 mm invasion)
  - Acinar predominant
  - Papillary predominant
  - Micropapillary predominant
  - Solid predominant with mucin

Variants
- Invasive mucinous adenocarcinoma
- Colloid
- Fetal
- Enteric

Squamous cell carcinoma
Variants
- Papillary
- Clear cell
- Small cell
- Basaloid

Small cell carcinoma
Variant
- Combined small cell carcinoma

Large cell carcinoma
Variants
- Large cell neuroendocrine carcinoma

(continued)

Table 3.1 (Continued)
• Basaloid carcinoma
• Lymphoepithelioma-like carcinoma
• Clear cell carcinoma
• Large cell carcinoma with rhabdoid phenotype
Adenosquamous carcinoma
Sarcomatoid carcinoma
• Pleomorphic carcinoma
• Spindle cell carcinoma
• Giant cell carcinoma
• Carcinosarcoma
• Pulmonary blastoma
Carcinoid tumor
• Typical carcinoid
• Atypical carcinoid
Salivary gland tumors
• Mucoepidermoid carcinoma
• Adenoid cystic carcinoma
• Epithelial-myoepithelial carcinoma

2004 WHO Classification[2] as modified by IASLC/ATS/ERS Classification of Lung Adenocarcinoma.[4] The table includes only lung carcinomas and does not include nonepithelial tumors (mesenchymal, lymphoid, etc.).

All four major types of lung cancer are associated with cigarette smoking. SCC and SCLC have the strongest association; adenocarcinoma has the weakest.

While a resection specimen allows ample histologic evaluation of a lung tumor, small biopsies and/or cytology specimens by their nature are only limited samples of a larger lesion. For several decades small samples of lung tumors were divided into two broad categories by the pathologist: non–small cell lung cancer (NSCLC) and small cell lung cancer (SCLC). Recent changes in molecular biology, oncology, radiology, and pathology have driven the need for further subclassification of the NSCLC group, even on small biopsy/cytology specimens.[4]

The IASLC/ATS/ERS recommendations suggest revised terminology for the pathologic reporting of small nonresection biopsy/cytology specimens. This revised terminology is included in the algorithm for the evaluation of small biopsy/cytology specimens in Figure 3.1. The purpose is to minimize use of the term *NSCLC* for small biopsy or cytology specimens by utilizing more standardized terminology for morphologic findings on H&E stained slides as well as a panel of immunohistochemical studies (thyroid transcription factor-1 [TTF-1], napsin, p63, cytokeratin 5/6 [CK5/6]) for some cases in an attempt to classify the tumor further. Most important, the recommendations attempt to standardize the discrimination of adenocarcinoma from squamous cell carcinoma in small biopsies of unresectable cases.

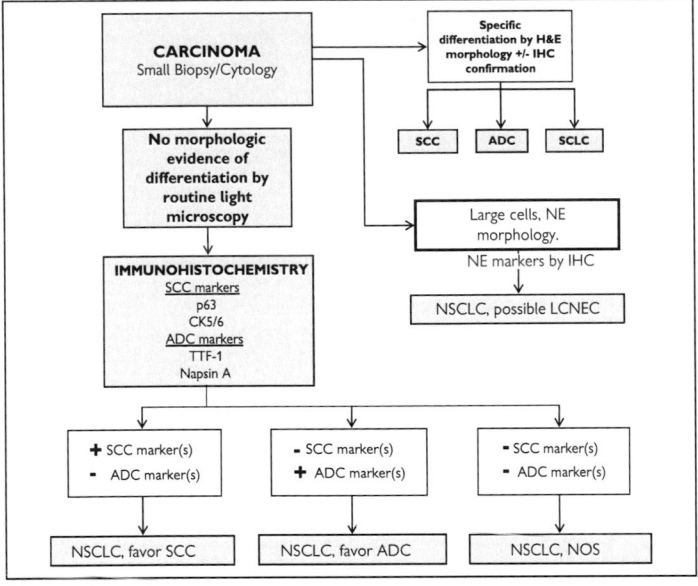

Figure 3.1 Outline for the pathologic evaluation of lung carcinoma in a small biopsy and/or cytology specimen. If there is clear morphologic evidence of differentiation by routine light microscopy, the diagnosis of squamous cell carcinoma (SCC), adenocarcinoma (ADC), or small cell lung cancer (SCLC) can be rendered, although immunohistochemistry (IHC) may be utilized for confirmation in some cases. Tumors of large cells with a neuroendocrine (NE) morphology should be evaluated by IHC for neuroendocrine markers (synaptophysin, chromogranin, CD56) as large cell neuroendocrine carcinoma (LCNEC) is a consideration. If the tumor is composed of large cells without evidence of differention by routine microscopy, IHC may be helpful. In addition, histochemical stains for mucin (PAS with diastase, mucicarmine) can be evaluated for evidence of glandular differentiation (i.e., adenocarcinoma). If the IHC staining is positive for both the squamous markers and the adenocarcinoma markers but in different cell populations, the possibility of adenosquamous carcinoma should be considered. The algorithm listed does not exclude the possibility of metastatic tumor; thus, the evaluation must be viewed in light of the clinical and radiologic data. (Based on Travis WD, Rekhtman N, Riley GJ, Geisinger KR, Asamura H, Brambilla E, et al. Pathologic diagnosis of advanced lung cancer based on small biopsies and cytology: a paradigm shift. *J Thorac Oncol.* 2010;5:411–4.)

To maximize the diagnostic accuracy of cytology and small biopsy specimens, the IASLC/ATS/ERS recommendations also include the following:

- Collection of cytology specimens whenever feasible in addition to small biopsies, as cytology is often a powerful tool in the morphologic separation of squamous cell carcinoma from adenocarcinoma as well as small cell carcinoma

- Concomitant review of cytology specimens with the corresponding biopsy to optimize the accurate separation of adenocarcinoma from squamous carcinoma and to minimize discrepancies in the classification of tumors

• Preparation of cell blocks whenever possible (aspirations, effusions), as cell blocks are often useful for subsequent immunohistochemical and/or molecular studies

Pathologic Classification of Lung Cancer

Preinvasive Lesions

Based on the 2004 WHO classification of lung tumors and the 2011 IASLC/ATS/ERS proposal, there are four categories of preinvasive lesions (see Figs. 3.2a–3.2d)[2,3,5]:

• Bronchial squamous dysplasia/carcinoma *in situ* (CIS)

• Atypical adenomatous hyperplasia (AAH)

• Adenocarcinoma *in situ* (AIS)

• Diffuse idiopathic pulmonary neuroendocrine cell hyperplasia (DIPNECH)

Squamous Dysplasia/Carcinoma *In Situ*

Squamous dysplasia/carcinoma *in situ* represents a spectrum of atypical histologic changes found in the bronchial mucosa that, analogous to intramucosal

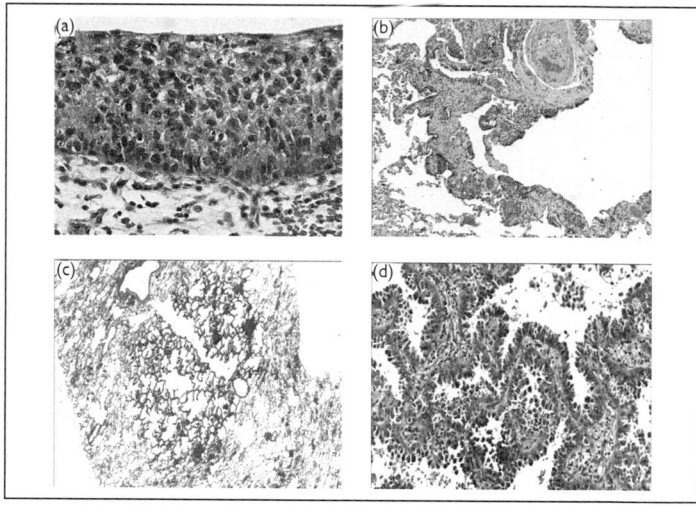

Figure 3.2 Preinvasive epithelial lesions. (*a*) Squamous dysplasia/carcinoma *in situ* (CIS). There is squamous metaplasia with virtual full thickness dysplasia of the bronchial epithelium (H&E stain, 400× original magnification). (*b*) Diffuse idiopathic pulmonary neuroendocrine cell hyperplasia (DIPNECH). Bronchiole with neuroendocrine hyperplasia and fibrotic thickening of airway wall (H&E stain, 400× original magnification). (*c*) Atypical adenomatous hyperplasia (AAH). Rounded central area approximating 3 mm of slight alveolar wall thickening lined by an increased number of mildly atypical alveolar epithelial cells (H&E stain, 10× original magnification). (*d*) Adenocarcinoma *in situ* (AIS). Thickened alveolar walls lined by crowded cytologically atypical epithelial cells (H&E stain, 400× original magnification). (Images courtesy of William W. West, MD.)

dysplastic lesions of the uterine cervix, are graded from mild squamous dysplasia to carcinoma in situ.[6,7] This lesion is considered a nonobligate precursor of invasive squamous cell carcinoma of the lung. The intramucosal change of dysplasia/carcinoma in situ (CIS) may be focal, but more often it is multifocal and predominantly involves the mucosa of larger airways (main bronchi to subsegmental bronchi) frequently at bifurcation points. The spectrum of squamous dysplasia/CIS is frequently seen in resected invasive carcinoma specimens, in which the changes involve the mucosa of bronchial airways in the surrounding lung.

Increasing degrees of squamous dysplasia are associated with more frequent invasive carcinomas, although the predictive significance of dysplasia in isolation is not well established. Squamous dysplasia may also serve as a pitfall for pathologists when it extends into the ducts of seromucinous glands and superficially mimics an invasive SCC or when a superficial biopsy of a lung tumor yields only dysplastic squamous mucosa and the underlying malignancy is not sampled, resulting in a misclassification of the tumor as squamous cell carcinoma.

Squamous dysplasia/CIS is highly associated with cigarette smoking and some forms of chronic obstructive airways disease. In addition to the histologically visible mucosal atypia seen in the bronchi, additional investigation has revealed a variety of genetic and molecular aberrations that increase in number and complexity as the degree of squamous dysplasia progresses. These findings add further support to the concept that squamous dysplasia/CIS is a progenitor in the multistep carcinogenesis of invasive squamous cell carcinoma.

Changes of dysplasia/CIS may be detected by cytology, fluorescence bronchoscopy (less autofluorescence than adjacent normal mucosa), biopsy of the bronchial mucosa, or in resection specimens. Although many of these intramucosal lesions are not grossly visible, some may produce leukoplakia, erythroplakia, or exophytic/polypoid lesions of the bronchial mucosa. The intramucosal lesions of squamous metaplasia, goblet cell metaplasia, and basal cell/reserve cell hyperplasia, while often seen in association with squamous dysplasia/CIS, are considered reversible non-neoplastic mucosal changes, often reactive in nature, and should not be considered true dysplastic processes.

Squamous dysplastic change of the mucosa in the central airways is often heterogeneous, multifocal, and migratory, confounding efforts to diminish the risk of subsequent invasive lung cancer by treating high-grade dysplastic lesions (moderate/severe dysplasia, CIS). As many of these patients suffer from the carcinogenic "field effect" of smoking, metachronous lung cancers may occur not only in the central airways, where the squamous dysplastic lesions are located, but also in the lung periphery, where there is an increased incidence of other lung cancers, including adenocarcinoma, not detectable by bronchoscopy.

Despite these limitations, the 2007 American College of Chest Physicians Clinical Practice Guidelines suggest bronchoscopic follow-up for patients with high-grade squamous dysplastic lesions (moderate/severe dysplasia, CIS) but no localizing abnormality on chest imaging. No specific follow-up is suggested for isolated low-grade dysplastic lesions as many regress and the risk of invasive cancer is low.[8–10]

Atypical Adenomatous Hyperplasia

Atypical adenomatous hyperplasia (AAH) is a bronchioloalveolar epithelial proliferation of mild to moderately atypical nonmucinous cells that form local-ized lesions, often in centriacinar areas of the peripheral lung.[6,7,11] The atypical epithelial cells resemble the nonciliated secretory cells of the distal bronchi-oles (Clara cells) and/or type II pneumocytes and grow along the surface of the alveolar parenchyma and/or respiratory bronchiole to create a localized lesion that is usually less than 5 mm in diameter. The atypical cells of AAH grow along the alveolar framework in a lepidic fashion similar to adenocar-cinoma *in situ* (AIS; formerly termed bronchioloalveolar carcinoma [BAC]); however, the cells of AAH are generally cuboidal to low columnar nonmuci-nous cells with less nuclear atypia and less confluent growth than AIS. AAH may be isolated or multifocal.[12]

AAH is most frequently seen by the pathologist as an incidental observation in resection specimens for lung cancer, where the incidence of AAH varies from 5% to 20%. Although these lesions may be found in association with a variety of smoking-related lung cancers, the association is most prevalent with peripheral adenocarcinomas. The lesions of AAH are small (1–5 mm). Although AAH is microscopically discrete, it is often difficult to detect grossly because it is only slightly elevated against the background uninvolved lung parenchyma. Inflated lung parenchyma is helpful in localizing these small lesions. Furthermore, the atypical cells of AAH must be differentiated from the reactive atypia of pneu-mocytes and Clara cells associated with inflammatory conditions.

Morphologic, cytofluorometric, molecular, immunoperoxidase, and epide-miologic studies support the hypothesis that AAH is part of the spectrum of putative precursors of a subset of peripheral lung adenocarcinoma and that AAH is often a smoking-related change. The current hypothesis is that AAH and AIS represent a spectrum of peripheral *in situ* lesions (pulmonary alveolar intraepithelial neoplasia) that may lead to peripheral invasive lung adenocarci-nomas. While lesions of AAH are generally not detectable on routine chest X-rays, high-resolution computed tomography (CT) scans in screening pro-grams not infrequently detect AAH as small (2–5 mm) pure ground glass opaci-ties. Longitudinal imaging studies lend further credence to the probability that AAH is a precursor lesion for invasive adenocarcinoma. Several studies have failed to show a prognostic difference between lung cancer resection patients with associated AAH and those without AAH. The incidental finding of AAH in isolation without evidence of cancer does not warrant surgical therapy, although clinical follow-up may be appropriate in some cases.

Even though AAH is a putative precursor of certain peripheral adenocarci-nomas, there is evidence that progression is distinctly uncommon and extends over a prolonged time frame. As most incidentally discovered AAH detected by high-resolution CT are <5 mm and do not progress, there is currently no recommendation for routine CT follow-up, especially in the elderly. However, pure ground glass opacities measuring >5 mm or expanding lesions include a sufficient number of higher grade lesions (AIS, minimally invasive adenocarci-noma [MIA], invasive adenocarcinoma) that surveillance and/or resection may be indicated. Individual clinical histories and imaging data may substantially alter these preliminary guidelines.[12–14]

Adenocarcinoma *In Situ*

Adenocarcinoma *in situ* (AIS), formerly termed bronchioloalveolar carcinoma (BAC), may be nonmucinous or mucinous. AIS consists of a localized peripheral lung lesion characterized by a pure lepidic growth pattern of atypical glandular epithelial cells.[15] By definition, the lesion is <3 cm and lacks stromal, vascular, or pleural invasion. Intra-alveolar papillary growth or a micropapillary pattern excludes AIS.

The proliferating epithelial cells in AIS are most often nonmucinous with evidence of differentiation toward Clara cells or type II pneumocytes (similar to atypical adenomatous hyperplasia). There are also rare cases of *mucinous* AIS. Before making a diagnosis of mucinous AIS, an *invasive* mucinous adenocarcinoma must be carefully excluded. Nonmucinous AIS differs from atypical adenomatous hyperplasia in that the cellular proliferation is more confluent, often columnar, with more cytologic atypia and the tumors are generally larger (1–3 cm in greatest dimension). Similar to AAH, the proliferation in AIS does not destroy the background alveolar architecture; thus, AIS is also difficult to identify grossly in noninflated specimens.

Nonmucinous AIS is often seen as a pure ground glass opacity on high-resolution CT scan. The uncommon case of mucinous AIS may present a more solid appearance by CT. The entire lesion should be no more than 3 cm in greatest dimension and the entire tumor should be submitted for histologic evaluation before rendering a diagnosis of AIS.

Nonmucinous AIS conveys an excellent prognosis with disease-free survival rates approaching 100%. Like AAH, AIS is considered a smoking-related precursor of some forms of invasive peripheral adenocarcinoma of the lung.

Diffuse Idiopathic Pulmonary Neuroendocrine Cell Hyperplasia

Diffuse idiopathic pulmonary neuroendocrine cell hyperplasia (DIPNECH) consists of a diffuse intramucosal proliferation of bland neuroendocrine cells within the confines of the bronchial and bronchiolar basement membranes, often accompanied by varying numbers of carcinoid tumorlets (<5 mm) and sometimes carcinoid tumor(s) (≥5 mm).[6,7,16] The intramucosal neuroendocrine hyperplasia is many times associated with varying degrees of airway fibrosis thought to be the etiology of many of the pulmonary symptoms and the functional deficits (obstructive, mixed obstructive/restrictive, decreased diffusion capacity) noted on pulmonary function testing. Most diffuse cases are idiopathic, although rare associations with multiple endocrine neoplasia I (MEN I) and other hormonal syndromes have been reported.

The diffuse neuroendocrine hyperplasia of DIPNECH must be clinically and pathologically distinguished from secondary forms of neuroendocrine hyperplasia that may be seen in association with chronic fibrotic and/or inflammatory conditions of the lung (e.g., abscess, diffuse fibrosis, bronchiectasis). In contrast to DIPNECH, secondary cases of neuroendocrine hyperplasia are not thought to predispose to the development of carcinoid tumors.

Although once thought to be rare, DIPNECH is now recognized more often due to the increased use of high-resolution CT scans for follow-up of other unrelated disorders. DIPNECH has a wide age spectrum, occurs in both males and females, but most commonly presents in middle-age females often 40–50 years of age.[17] Symptomatic individuals frequently present with slowly worsening dry cough, shortness of breath, and asthma-like symptoms. DIPNECH is not considered a smoking-related disorder.

Although the diagnosis of DIPNECH once required biopsy confirmation *and* evidence of pulmonary functional deficits, it is now recognized that only about half of cases currently present in the classic symptomatic fashion (cough/dyspnea, obstructive pulmonary function tests). The other half are largely asymptomatic and most often discovered by high-resolution CT performed for other disorders.[18] High-resolution CT scans in cases of DIPNECH often mimic diffuse interstitial lung disease and/or metastatic tumor, as the scans most often demonstrate bilateral mosaic attenuation, thickened airway walls, and small (<5 mm) centrilobular nodules. If carcinoid tumors are present, larger tumor nodules or masses may be noted.

DIPNECH is thought to be the precursor for some carcinoid tumors, which can be found in up to 55% of cases of DIPNECH. The carcinoid tumors may be single or multiple and often have a spindle cell histologic pattern. Although most associated carcinoid tumors behave in the typical low-grade fashion, a few cases of atypical carcinoid tumors have been reported in association with DIPNECH. DIPNECH is not associated with large cell neuroendocrine carcinoma (LCNEC).

Patients with DIPNECH generally have a stable to slowly progressive pulmonary course spanning multiple years with reported 5-year survival of >80%; however, a few (5%–10%) may suffer a more rapid decline in pulmonary function.

Invasive Lung Carcinoma

Adenocarcinoma

Lung adenocarcinoma is a malignant epithelial tumor characterized by glandular differentiation and/or the production of mucin (Fig. 3.3).[2] These tumors are

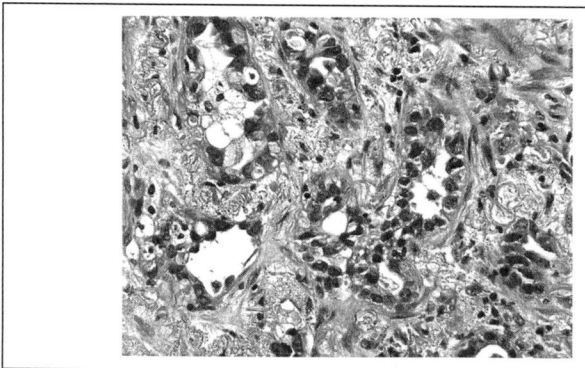

Figure 3.3 Invasive adenocarcinoma, acinar pattern, demonstrating irregular poorly formed glands infiltrating desmoplastic stroma (H&E stain, 400×). (Image courtesy of William W. West, MD.)

often histologically heterogeneous. Recognized histologic patterns, which are often mixed, include the following[3]:

- Acinar
- Papillary
- Lepidic
- Micropapillary
- Solid with mucin

Variants of adenocarcinoma include the following:

- Invasive mucinous
- Colloid
- Fetal
- Enteric

Adenocarcinoma is now the most frequent histologic type of lung cancer, accounting for approximately 40% of cases and replacing squamous cell carcinoma as the most frequent type in many countries. The incidence of lung adenocarcinoma is related to cigarette smoking, but more weakly than squamous cell carcinoma and small cell carcinoma. Adenocarcinoma is the most common subtype of lung cancer in nonsmokers.

Clinical Presentation

Although many lung adenocarcinomas present as a peripheral nodule or mass, they not infrequently produce other gross patterns with the corresponding spectrum of radiologic changes. The most common presentation is a subpleural peripheral nodule that may involve the overlying pleura. Central or endobronchial tumors are less common. Pneumonic consolidation may be seen in adenocarcinomas with a prominent lepidic and/or papillary pattern. A multifocal pneumonic pattern may be seen in mucinous adenocarcinomas with a lepidic predominant pattern. Peripheral adenocarcinomas that penetrate the visceral pleura and seed the pleural space may result in diffuse pleural thickening, producing a "pseudomesotheliomatous" pattern. Although many adenocarcinomas are isolated lesions, some individuals may present with multiple nodules or infiltrates, sometimes with bilateral distribution.

Lung cancer screening programs frequently identify small peripheral adenocarcinomas with a spectrum of ground glass opacities, solid or mixed radiologic densities. For small peripheral adenocarcinomas, ground glass opacities often represent the lepidic component of the tumor. The larger the solid component by CT, the more likely there is an associated invasive component.

The prognosis in lung adenocarcinoma is highly dependent upon the presence or absence of invasion, stage of tumor, and to a lesser extent the histologic type and grade of tumor. There is evidence that micropapillary predominant, solid predominant, colloid predominant, and invasive mucinous subtypes act more aggressively than other subtypes for small tumors.[19,20] Overall 5-year survival for invasive adenocarcinoma approaches 15%–20% based upon SEER data; however, early-stage resectable small tumors may yield 70%–80% 5-year survival, and AIS/MIA survival reports approach 100% in several studies. Invasive adenocarcinomas often spread to distant sites as well as regional lymph nodes. Distant metastatic disease most often involves brain, bone, adrenals, and/or liver.

Pathologic Diagnosis

The pathologic diagnosis of adenocarcinoma can often be rendered by cytology (bronchial brushings/washings, aspiration); however, the predominant pattern of tumor and assessment of invasion usually require biopsy or resection specimens. Most adenocarcinomas display a mixture of histologic patterns, although one or more may predominate.

A pure lepidic pattern requires growth of tumor cells along preexisting alveolar walls without significant destruction of the parenchymal architecture and without invasion (stromal, vascular, or pleural). Pure lepidic adenocarcinoma <3 cm in greatest dimension represents adenocarcinoma *in situ* (AIS). The great majority of AIS is nonmucinous. Malignant mucinous lepidic tumors most often represent multifocal mucinous adenocarcinoma and have a poor prognosis; these lesions rarely represent mucinous AIS.

The recent IASLC/ATS/ERS recommendations significantly affect the histologic classification of small (<3 cm) adenocarcinomas of the lung.[3]

- Use of the term bronchioloalveolar carcinoma (BAC) is no longer recommended.

- Tumor spread along preexisting alveolar structures without destruction of the architecture is now referred to as a *lepidic* pattern (formerly BAC pattern).

- The concept of adenocarcinoma *in situ* (AIS) is introduced as a preinvasive pure lepidic form of adenocarcinoma associated with a near 100% 5-year survival.

- The term *minimally invasive adenocarcinoma* (MIA) is utilized for lepidic predominant tumors with focal invasion measuring ≤5 mm. Some studies report that MIA 5-year survival also approaches 100%.[15]

- Nonmucinous tumors with invasive components >5 mm but a dominant lepidic pattern are now called *lepidic predominant adenocarcinoma* (LPA).

Almost all AIS and minimally invasive adenocarcinoma cases are nonmucinous tumors; only rarely do mucinous adenocarcinomas fulfill the diagnostic criteria. Most mucinous tumors formerly called "mucinous BAC" are now reclassified as invasive mucinous adenocarcinoma. Micropapillary carcinoma is now recognized by the IASLC/ATS/ERS proposal as a pattern of adenocarcinoma with a poor prognosis.

For invasive adenocarcinomas, the term "mixed" subtype has been replaced by itemization of the histologic subtypes present in each adenocarcinoma with classification according to the predominant subtype. Clear cell and signet ring cell carcinomas are no longer recognized as distinct histologic subtypes, as these are morphologic changes that may be a component of multiple other subtypes.

Comparison of the comprehensive histologic subtyping between tumors can be useful in determining whether a separate tumor nodule represents intrapulmonary metastasis or an independent primary. Preliminary studies suggest this comparative histologic approach correlates well with molecular studies and clinical outcome in patients with more than one lung lesion.

By immunohistochemistry, lung adenocarcinomas are positive for pankeratin cocktails, usually positive for cytokeratin 7 (CK7), and uncommonly positive for

CK20. Thyroid transcription factor-1 (TTF-1) positivity is found in 75% of lung adenocarcinomas with a similar proportion staining for napsin A. Less differentiated tumors have a lower rate of staining for TTF-1 and napsin A. Mucinous adenocarcinomas are often positive for CK20 and CK7 but negative for TTF-1.

Squamous Cell Carcinoma

Squamous cell carcinoma (SCC) of the lung is a malignant epithelial tumor with evidence of squamous differentiation (i.e., intercellular bridges and/or keratinization) (Fig. 3.4). Squamous dysplastic lesions/CIS are thought to be the precursor for invasive squamous cell carcinoma.

Histologic variants of squamous cell carcinoma include the following:

- Papillary
- Clear cell
- Small cell
- Basaloid

Clinical Presentation

Approximately 60% of cases of SCC arise from the more central bronchi (segmental, lobar, main), while the remainder arise as more peripheral lesions with a tendency to cavitate. As SCC arises from the bronchial mucosa and is frequently associated with adjacent squamous dysplastic changes, there is a higher diagnostic yield on bronchoscopic sampling and cytology evaluation.

Better differentiated lesions have a tendency for direct local extension and intrathoracic nodal metastasis before developing distant metastases. Poorly differentiated lesions often metastasize distantly as well as spread locally. SCC may produce a parathyroid hormone-like substance with resultant hypercalcemia. Superior sulcus SCC (Pancoast tumor) may cause Horner's syndrome (ipsilateral ptosis, miosis, anhidrosis).

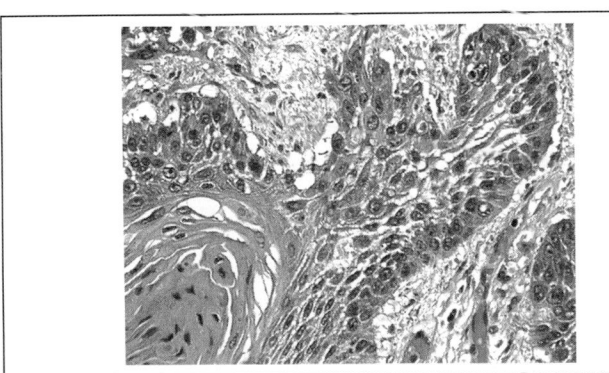

Figure 3.4 Invasive squamous cell carcinoma with intercellular bridges between tumor cells and keratinization in the lower left portion of the photo (H&E stain, 400×). (Image courtesy of William W. West, MD.)

Pathologic Diagnosis

The histologic diagnosis of squamous cell carcinoma requires identification of intercellular bridges and keratinization (individual cells and/or squamous pearls). By electron microscopy, squamous cell carcinoma demonstrates numerous desmosomes and abundant cytokeratin filaments.

Well-differentiated lesions are readily identified by H&E stained slides as well as by cytology, while moderately to poorly differentiated lesions may require additional studies. SCC is usually positive for p63, high molecular weight keratins, and CK5/6 by immunohistochemistry. Most SCC are TTF-1 negative and CK7 negative.

Small Cell Lung Cancer

Small cell carcinoma of the lung (SCLC) (Fig. 3.5) is an aggressive carcinoma of the lung characterized by the following:

- Small tumor cells with scant cytoplasm
- High nuclear/cytoplasmic (N/C) ratio
- Finely granular chromatin pattern
- Nuclear molding
- Necrosis
- Absent to inconspicuous nucleoli
- High mitotic rate (average >60 mitoses/2 mm^2)

(For mitotic counts, 2 mm^2 is approximately 10 high-power fields [hpf] on a standard microscope with a 40× objective. Eyepiece field of view may vary significantly between models of microscopes; thus, each microscope should be calibrated to cover 2 mm^2.)

Clinical Presentation

SCLC accounts for 14% of US lung cancers and is the most common neuroendocrine tumor of the lung. Like squamous cell carcinoma, SCLC is

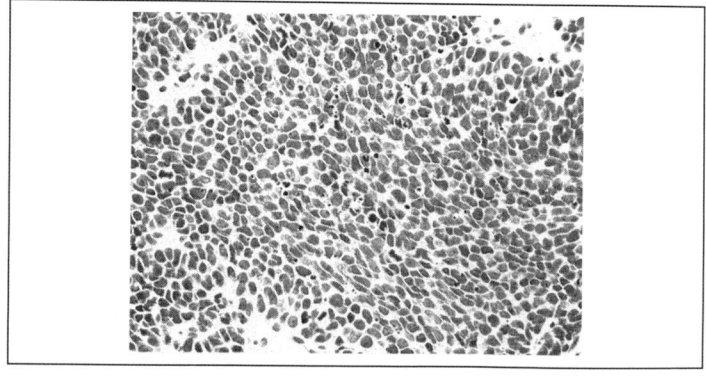

Figure 3.5 Small cell carcinoma composed of anaplastic small epithelial cells with prominent nuclear molding, apoptotic bodies, and mitotic figures (H&E stain, 400×). (Image courtesy of William W. West, MD.)

highly associated with cigarette smoking. SCLC characteristically presents as a poorly defined central mass/infiltrate extensively involving the bronchial submucosa and surrounding structures, commonly with hilar and mediastinal adenopathy.[2,21]

The tumor deceptively infiltrates the submucosa of the bronchi without producing a significant endobronchial component. SCLC presenting as an isolated peripheral nodule occurs, but it is distinctly uncommon and other diagnoses should be carefully considered. Although small cell cancers may arise in other primary sites (cervix, prostate, bladder, etc.), lung accounts for the great majority (95%) of these tumors.

Pathologic Diagnosis

By microscopy, SCLC consists of sheets of high-grade small cells with foci of nesting, palisading, and rosette formation as seen in other neuroendocrine tumors. The tumor cells are relatively small (≤3x the size of a resting lymphocyte), have a finely granular chromatin pattern, scant cytoplasm, high mitotic rate, prominent apoptosis, and often extensive necrosis. The tumor cell size varies with the size of the biopsy and the degree of preservation. Nuclei vary from round to oval or spindled. In combination with the characteristic nuclear chromatin of SCLC, these features make the diagnosis on H&E stains acceptable. Basophilic DNA encrustation of blood vessels (Azzopardi effect) is frequently seen in these tumors near zones of necrosis.

Despite the nomenclature ("small cell" carcinoma and "non–small cell" carcinoma), cell size alone is not sufficient to classify these tumors accurately because there is considerable overlap between the two groups and the degree of tumor cell preservation significantly affects the tumor cell size as assessed under the microscope. Due to the size overlap, other histologic features must also be considered. In general, when compared to SCLC, biopsies of NSCLC often have more vesicular chromatin pattern, prominent nucleoli, lower nuclear to cytoplasmic ratio, evidence of cytoplasmic differentiation, and less nuclear molding. It is the composite microscopic assessment of all of the morphologic features based upon a well-prepared H&E stained slide and/or cytologic preparation that allows the accurate identification of SCLC.

Immunohistochemical studies are most often weakly positive for one or more neuroendocrine markers (synaptophysin, chromogranin, CD56). Most (90%) are positive for TTF-1 and pankeratin. Ki-67 index is high, often 70%–90%.[1,21] Electron microscopy shows occasional cytoplasmic neuroendocrine granules in more than half of the cases.

The diagnosis of SCLC requires well-preserved tumor in a well-prepared cytologic or histologic sample. As crush artifact is frequently present, other diagnostic possibilities should be carefully excluded as benign lymphoid aggregates, inflammatory processes, lymphoma, and other small blue cell tumors may produce similar crush artifact and be confused with SCLC.

The only widely recognized SCLC variant is *combined small cell carcinoma*, in which small cell carcinoma is admixed with non–small cell elements (adenocarcinoma, squamous carcinoma, large cell carcinoma). No reproducible data are available to suggest any difference in prognosis or therapy compared to pure SCLC.

Large Cell Carcinoma

Large cell carcinoma (LCC) of the lung is essentially a default diagnosis. The tumor is a non–small cell lung cancer (NSCLC) that lacks the diagnostic features of small cell carcinoma, adenocarcinoma, or squamous cell carcinoma by light microscopy. In prior series, LCC comprised 9% of lung cancers; however, more recent reports utilizing immunohistochemical subtyping suggest that the proportion now approaches 3%. LCC is associated with smoking. The tumors often originate in the periphery of the lung but some may be centrally located (e.g., basaloid carcinoma). They are often large, tan masses with necrosis and hemorrhage; invasion of local structures such as pleura or chest wall is common.

Pathologic Diagnosis

The diagnosis of LCC requires a surgical resection specimen because small biopsies do not allow for the exclusion of other foci of differentiation within the tumor. As this category is largely a diagnosis of exclusion, by light microscopy these tumors are undifferentiated non–small cell carcinomas. Histology generally reveals sheets of large polygonal cells with ample cytoplasm, large vesicular nuclei, and prominent nucleoli (Fig. 3.6). By electron microscopy, this group consists of tumors with large epithelial cells, many of which show minimal evidence of glandular differentiation (adenocarcinoma), some with weak squamous differentiation and yet others that appear to be truly undifferentiated. There is considerable debate as to whether immunohistochemistry should be utilized to reclassify many of the resected tumors as poorly differentiated adenocarcinoma or poorly differentiated squamous carcinoma.

In the 2004 WHO classification, there are five variants of large cell carcinoma:

- Large cell neuroendocrine carcinoma (LCNEC)
- Basaloid carcinoma
- Lymphoepithelioma-like carcinoma
- Clear cell carcinoma
- Large cell carcinoma with rhabdoid phenotype.

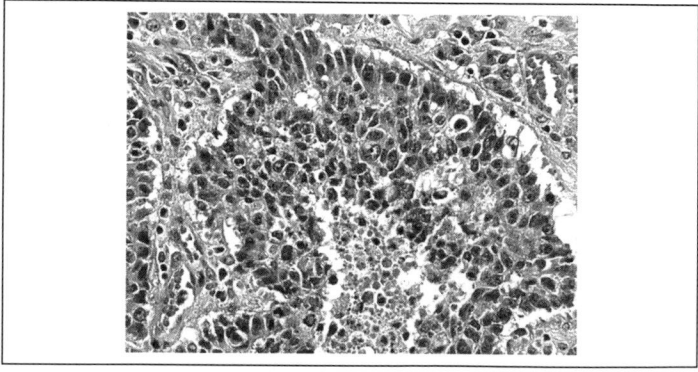

Figure 3.6 Large cell neuroendocrine carcinoma with peripheral palisading, highly atypical nuclei with nucleoli, and prominent zone of tumor necrosis (H&E stain, 400×). (Image courtesy of William W. West, MD.)

LCNEC comprises a group of high-grade lung tumors with a neuroendocrine growth pattern and unequivocal staining for at least one neuroendocrine marker (synaptophysin, chromogranin, CD56) by immunoperoxidase. The larger cell size, prominent nucleoli, vescicular chromatin pattern, and ample cytoplasm help to separate LCNEC from SCLC, although this can be problematic in small crushed specimens. Mitotic counts are high (average = 70 mitoses/2 mm^2), and there is usually extensive necrosis. LCNEC is an aggressive tumor with reported survival rates that are generally worse than other NSCLC subtypes and approach the poor prognosis of SCLC. The pathologic differential diagnosis of LCNEC includes SCLC and atypical carcinoid.

The Spectrum of Neuroendocrine Tumors of Lung

Neuroendocrine tumors of the lung include a spectrum of neoplasms that range from the low-grade carcinoid tumor (typical carcinoid, TC) to intermediate-grade atypical carcinoid (AC) tumor to two high-grade malignancies—large cell neuroendocrine carcinoma (LCNEC) and small cell carcinoma (SCLC).[5,22] This wide spectrum of pulmonary neuroendocrine neoplasia is also reflected in the range of clinicopathologic characteristics, biologic behavior, and therapeutic approaches to these tumors, making accurate classification important.

Carcinoid tumors are often found in younger individuals and are generally not related to smoking, while the high-grade neuroendocrine tumors occur in an older age group (mean age, 65 years) and are highly smoking related, especially SCLC. Genetic and molecular studies suggest that typical and atypical carcinoid tumors are likely related, but carcinoids are not closely related to LCNEC or SCLC.

Pulmonary neuroendocrine malignancies are uncommon tumors, with SCLC the most frequent:

- Small cell lung cancer (14% of all lung cancers)
- Large cell neuroendocrine carcinoma (3%)
- Typical carcinoid (2%)
- Atypical carcinoid (0.2%)

Accurate pathologic classification of pulmonary neuroendocrine tumors depends upon adequate sampling or resection of the tumor, properly preserved tissue, and adequate histologic processing and cutting. While pathologists are generally able to separate typical carcinoid from SCLC reliably in adequately sampled, well-preserved specimens, the separation of LCNEC from SCLC is more problematic, especially in limited samples with artifact.

While precursor lesions have not been identified for the high-grade neuroendocrine carcinomas, diffuse idiopathic pulmonary neuroendocrine cell hyperplasia (DIPNECH) is recognized as a preinvasive lesion for carcinoid tumors.

The separation of neuroendocrine lung tumors relies on differences in histologic growth patterns, cytopathologic features, mitotic activity, and evaluation for necrosis (Table 3.2).

- *Low-grade neuroendocrine tumors (typical carcinoid)*: characterized by prominent neuroendocrine histologic growth patterns, low-grade cytology, minimal mitotic activity, and lack of necrosis.

Table 3.2 Features of Neuroendocrine Lung Tumors

	Typical Carcinoid	Atypical Carcinoid	LCNEC	SCLC
NE features	Well differentiated	Well differentiated	Poorly differentiated	Poorly differentiated
Cell size	Intermediate	Intermediate	Large to intermediate	Small to intermediate
Mitotic rate	Low <2 Mitosis/2 mm^2	Intermediate 2–10 Mitosis/ 2 mm^2	High Median 70 Mitosis/ 2 mm^2	High Median 80 Mitosis/ 2 mm^2
NE markers by IHC	+++	++ to +++	+ to +++	+/-
Necrosis	–	+ (focal)	+++	+++
KI-67 Index	≤5%	5%–20%	50%–100%	80%–100%
5-Year survival	90%–95%	60%–70%	10%–40%	≤5%–10%

IHC, immunohistochemistry; LCNEC, large cell neuroendocrine carcinioma; NE, neuroendocrine; SCLC, small cell lung cancer.

- *Intermediate-grade neuroendocrine tumors (atypical carcinoid)*: also displays a prominent neuroendocrine growth pattern but includes increased mitotic figures (2–10 mitoses/2 mm^2) and/or focal necrosis.
- *High-grade neuroendocrine tumors (large cell neuroendocrine carcinoma and SCLC)*: aggressive carcinomas with high-grade cytology, extensive necrosis, and substantial mitotic activity (average = 60–80 mitoses/2 mm^2).

(For mitotic counts, 2 mm^2 is approximately 10 high-power fields [hpf] on a standard microscope with a 40× objective. Eyepiece field of view may vary significantly between models of microscopes; thus, each microscope should be calibrated to cover 2 mm^2.)

NSCLC with neuroendocrine features includes tumors that produce discordant results between the histologic and the immunohistochemical assessment for neuroendocrine differentiation. This category is controversial, suffers from confusing nomenclature, and lacks consensus regarding treatment and prognostic implications.

- *Non–small cell lung carcinoma with neuroendocrine morphology* (NSCLC-NEM) refers to NSCLC that has a growth pattern suggestive of neuroendocrine carcinoma but fails to stain with neuroendocrine markers by immunohistochemistry.
- *Non–small cell carcinoma with neuroendocrine differentiation* (NSCLC-NED) consists of NSCLC that morphologically appears as conventional NSCLC, lacks evidence of a neuroendocrine growth pattern by histology, but stains positively for neuroendocrine markers by immunohistochemistry.

At this time the significance of these categories is not known and the tumors should be classified as in Table 3.1 and the neuroendocrine features noted.

Carcinoid Tumors

Carcinoid tumors are subdivided into low-grade typical carcinoid tumors (Fig. 3.7) and intermediate-grade atypical carcinoid tumors (Fig. 3.8). These tumors display prominent neuroendocrine differentiation (well to intermediate differentiation) at the light microscopic, immunohistochemical, and electron microscopy levels. Organoid, trabecular, palisading, insular, and/or ribbon-like "neuroendocrine" growth patterns are evident on well-preserved and prepared H&E stained slides. Cells are relatively uniform, have a modest amount of granular cytoplasm, uniform to mildly pleomorphic nuclei with a finely granular chromatin pattern, and generally inconspicuous to absent nucleoli.

Tumors with this well-developed neuroendocrine histologic pattern that are ≥5 mm in greatest dimension are separated into typical carcinoid and

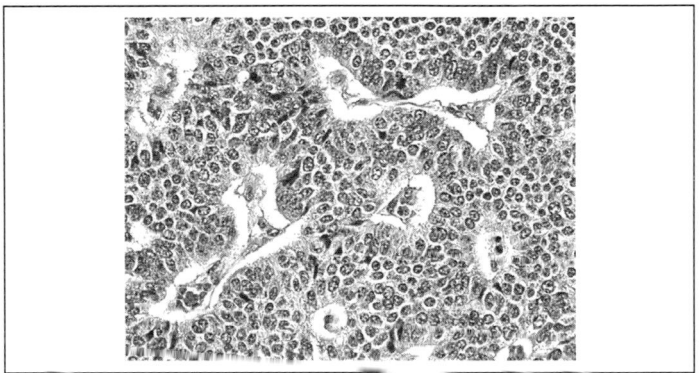

Figure 3.7 Typical carcinoid with relatively uniform cells, no necrosis and no mitotic activity (H&E stain, 400×). (Image courtesy of William W. West, MD.)

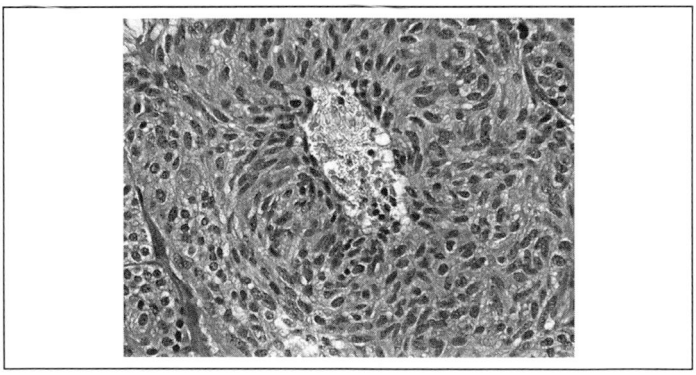

Figure 3.8 Atypical carcinoid with spindle cell pattern, demonstrating punctate zone of necrosis (H&E stain, 400×). (Image courtesy of William W. West, MD.)

atypical carcinoid on the basis of the number of mitoses and/or the presence or absence of necrosis. Low-grade neuroendocrine tumors <5 mm are designated as carcinoid tumorlets and are not included in this discussion of carcinoid tumors.

- *Typical carcinoid* has uncommon to rare mitotic figures (<2 mitoses/2 mm^2). Immunohistochemical staining for Ki-67 is generally low (<5%)
- *Atypical carcinoid* has 2–10 mitoses/2 mm^2 and/or focal necrosis (often in a punctate pattern). Ki-67 staining is usually intermediate (5%–20%) Ki-67 staining may be helpful in small biopsy specimens with considerable artifact, where the separation of low- to intermediate-grade neuroendocrine tumors from the high-grade neuroendocrine carcinomas (SCLC, large cell neuroendocrine carcinoma) may be problematic. High-grade neuroendocrine carcinomas often average 60%–80% by Ki-67 staining.

Immunohistochemistry demonstrates robust staining for one or more neuroendocrine markers (chromogranin, synaptophysin, CD56) in typical carcinoid and to a lesser extent in atypical carcinoid. Keratin stains are positive in 80%–90% of carcinoid tumors. The pathologic diagnosis of carcinoid tumor may be made on fine-needle aspiration or brushing cytology specimens as well as biopsy specimens; however, the separation of atypical carcinoid from typical carcinoid most often requires the pathologic assessment of the resection specimen, if mitotic activity or necrosis is not evident in the biopsy.

Typical Carcinoid

Typical carcinoids are often (60%–80%) centrally located, where they arise as tan-yellow luminal and/or mural tumors involving a major bronchus frequently with an endobronchial growth pattern. Tumors vary from 2–4 cm and are grossly circumscribed. Central bronchial involvement accounts for the clinical presentations of obstruction, hemoptysis, dyspnea, and/or persistent cough, although up to 50% of patients with carcinoid tumors are asymptomatic. Some carcinoid tumors are located in the periphery. These tumors are often asymptomatic, and this group has a higher incidence of spindle cell tumors. Typical carcinoid occurs over a wide age range, affects both sexes equally, and is not smoking related. These tumors are rarely associated with carcinoid syndrome, Cushing syndrome, or MEN1. Typical carcinoid has an excellent prognosis with surgical resection; 5- and 10-year survival rates approach 95% and 90%, respectively. Regional nodal metastases (5%–15% of patients) usually only minimally affect overall prognosis when resected. Subsequent metastases to liver and/or bone occur and negatively affect survival in 5%–10% of typical carcinoids. When dealing with metastatic well-differentiated neuroendocrine tumor, a lung primary is more likely if there are isolated skeletal metastases, while gastrointestinal primaries predominate if the metastases are in the liver.

Atypical Carcinoid

Atypical carcinoids share many of the gross findings and clinical features of carcinoid tumors, although they are often larger and more frequently peripherally located. Reports suggest a weak smoking association. The pathologic difference between typical and atypical carcinoid largely lies in the higher mitotic rate and/or presence of necrosis. Although there are often more atypical nuclei, occasional conspicuous nucleoli, and more evidence of invasive properties (vascular invasion, nodal involvement) in atypical carcinoid compared to typical carcinoid, the mitotic rate and presence or absence of necrosis define the distinction between the two. The prognosis in atypical carcinoid is more guarded, as these tumors have a higher rate of nodal metastases (40%–60%), a higher rate of distant metastases (20%–30%) and significantly lower overall survival. Five- and ten-year survival rates for atypical carcinoid approach 60% and 40%, respectively.

Immunohistochemistry in Lung Tumors

The use of special stains (immunohistochemistry, mucin) is frequently helpful in further classifying NSCLC, especially in cases of small specimens or poorly differentiated tumors (see Table 3.3)[3,12,23]:

- Squamous cell carcinoma (SCC) is often distinctly positive for p63 and CK5/6 but generally negative for TTF-1 and napsin A.
- Adenocarcinoma is generally positive for TTF-1 and napsin A but usually negative or only weakly positive for p63 and negative for CK5/6.[22, 24]
- Mucin histochemical stains (PAS, mucicarmine) can be performed to identify features of adenocarcinoma; however, these stains are generally

Table 3.3 Immunohistochemical Staining Patterns of Primary Lung Cancers

	Adenocarcinoma Nonmucinous	Adenocarcinoma Mucinous	Squamous Carcinoma	Small Cell Carcinoma
	(% positive cases)	(% positive cases)	(% positive cases)	(% positive cases)
CK7	>95	90	40	35
CK20	10	50	<5	<5
TTF-1	80	30	5	85
Napsin A	85	<5	20	<5
p63	25	N/A	>95	<5
CK 5/6	15	N/A	90	<5
34βE12	55	N/A	>95	<5
CDX-2	<5	45	<5	<5
Synaptophysin	15	N/A	5	55
Chromogranin A	<5	N/A	5	40
CD56	<5	N/A	10	95

Notes: Figures listed are estimates only. Staining must be interpreted in light of the specificity and sensitivity of the individual antibodies utilized in the immunohistochemical procedures as well as the profusion and intensity of the staining within the tumor. Immunoprofiles should always be interpreted in light of the H&E morphology and available cytopathologic material.

CD56, cluster of differentiation 56 (neural cell adhesion molecule, NCAM); CDX-2, homeobox protein CDX-2; CK, cytokeratin; N/A, not applicable; TTF-1, thyroid transcription factor-1; 34βE12, high molecular weight keratin.

less sensitive than the immunohistochemical studies for evidence of glandular differentiation.

Differential staining patterns allow reasonable separation of most poorly differentiated squamous cell carcinomas from poorly differentiated adenocarcinomas.[25,26] However, up to 5% of tumors will likely remain as NSCLC-not otherwise specified (NOS) even after evaluation with additional stains. Furthermore, several studies have demonstrated that a small proportion of tumors (<5%) with only limited biopsy samples will be misclassified even after special studies due to the technical vagaries of the special stain procedures, the heterogeneity of the tumor, and/or a severely limited sample.

To conserve tissue, one squamous marker and one adenocarcinoma marker are suggested (see Fig. 3.1), although the panel can be expanded in equivocal cases. The pathology report should state whether the final classification of the NSCLC is based upon the light microscopic H&E findings and/or the immunohistochemistry results. Sarcomatoid carcinoma and adenosquamous carcinoma are more difficult to identify on small biopsies even with immunostains.

A wide variety of malignant tumors may metastasize to the lung (breast, colon, upper gastrointestinal tract, kidney, melanoma, prostate, sarcomas, and others). Likewise, individuals with cancers in other organ systems may develop primary lung cancer. Separation of metastatic tumor to the lung from primary lung cancer can be problematic, especially in small biopsy/ cytology specimens, highlighting the essential requirement for adequate clinical, radiologic, and historical data. Failure to provide such information can lead to the mistaken diagnosis of primary lung cancer when in fact the patient suffers from metastatic disease. If there is sufficient well-preserved tumor for assessment, the pathologist may recognize histologic features to suggest metastatic disease.

Immunoprofiles can be invaluable in many of these cases and may provide suggestions for potential primary sites. The basic immunohistochemical panel utilized to separate lung squamous cell carcinoma from adenocarcinoma is not sufficient to reliably separate metastatic tumors from lung primaries, thus confirming the need to integrate the pathologic morphology on routine stains with the clinical and radiologic data in the assessment of a newly discovered lung tumor. If the patient has a history of carcinoma in another organ system, morphologic comparison of prior biopsy/resection material can be integral to the accurate classification of a lung tumor.

Pathologic Staging of Lung Tumors

The extent of tumor as delineated in the internationally accepted TNM system (seventh edition of American Joint Committee on Cancer Staging Manual) is the most powerful prognostic factor in lung cancer and frequently determines treatment strategies.[27] The staging system is used for NSCLC, SCLC, and carcinoid tumors.

For *localized* NSCLC and carcinoids, *pathologic* staging is usually assessed after surgical resection of the primary tumor or following examination of biopsy tissue if the lesion is more advanced. Most cases of SCLC (>90%) are metastatic or locally advanced at presentation; these are generally biopsied and *clinically* staged via imaging studies.

Pathologic examination of a resection specimen should include the following:

- Accurate measurement of tumor size (gross measurement confirmed by microscopic exam)
- Tumor location and any invasion of adjacent structures
- Margin status
- Nodal status (both peripheral nodes submitted with the specimen and mediastinal nodes usually submitted separately)

Central tumors require close attention to the bronchial margin(s), while parenchymal margins and evidence of pleural invasion are often more important in peripheral tumors.[11] Accurate assessment for visceral pleural invasion often requires a histochemical stain to delineate the visceral pleural elastica (see Fig. 3.9).[25,28]

Many resection specimens will produce N1 nodes within the specimen (stations 12–14) and the surgeon often separately submits and labels mediastinal nodes. Nodal status is determined by complete microscopic examination of submitted lymph nodes, including any samples from mediastinoscopy. Six nodes and/or nodal stations should be sampled in most cases in order to assign the pN0 category.

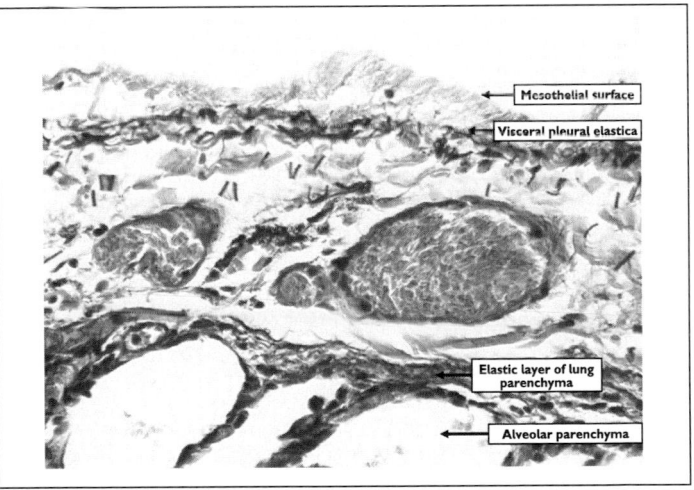

Figure 3.9 Visceral pleura. Stain for elastic tissue highlights the visceral pleural elastica as well as the underlying elastic layer associated with the lung parenchyma. Tumor should penetrate the visceral pleural elastica to qualify as visceral pleural invasion (PLI1). (400× original magnification) (Image courtesy of William W. West, MD.)

References

1. West H, Harpole D, Travis W. Histologic considerations for individualized systemic therapy approaches for the management of non-small cell lung cancer. *Chest* 2009;136:1112–8.

2. Travis WD, Brambilla E, Muller-Hermelink HK, Harris CC. *WHO: Pathology and Genetics of Tumours of the Lung, Pleura, Thymus and Heart.* Lyon: IARC Press; 2004.

3. Travis WD, Brambilla E, Noguchi M, et al. International Association for the Study of Lung Cancer/American Thoracic Society/European Respiratory Society International Multidisciplinary Classification of Lung Adenocarcinoma. *J Thorac Oncol* 2011;6:244–85.

4. Travis WD, Rekhtman N, Riley GJ, et al. Pathologic diagnosis of advanced lung cancer based on small biopsies and cytology: a paradigm shift. *J Thorac Oncol* 2010;5:411–4.

5. Franks TJ, Galvin JR. Lung tumors with neuroendocrine morphology: essential radiologic and pathologic features. *Arch Pathol Lab Med* 2008;132:1055–61.

6. Kerr KM. Pulmonary preinvasive neoplasia. *J Clin Pathol* 2001;54:257–71.

7. Lantuejoul S, Salameire D, Salon C, Brambilla E. Pulmonary preneoplasia—sequential molecular carcinogenetic events. *Histopathology* 2009;54:43–54.

8. Banerjee AK. Preinvasive lesions of the bronchus. *J Thorac Oncol* 2009;4:545–51.

9. Kennedy TC, McWilliams A, Edell E, et al. Bronchial intraepithelial neoplasia/early central airways lung cancer: ACCP evidence-based clinical practice guidelines (2nd edition). *Chest* 2007;132:221S–33S.

10. Alaa M, Shibuya K, Fujiwara T, et al. Risk of lung cancer in patients with preinvasive bronchial lesions followed by autofluorescence bronchoscopy and chest computed tomography. *Lung Cancer* 2011;72:303–8.

11. Butnor KJ, Beasley MB, Cagle PT, et al. Protocol for the examination of specimens from patients with primary non-small cell carcinoma, small cell carcinoma, or carcinoid tumor of the lung. *Cancer Protocol* 2009;133(10):1552–9.

12. Maeshima AM, Tochigi N, Yoshida A, Asamura H, Tsuta K, Tsuda H. Clinicopathologic analysis of multiple (five or more) atypical adenomatous hyperplasias (AAHs) of the lung: evidence for the AAH-adenocarcinoma sequence. *J Thorac Oncol* 2010;5:466–71.

13. Godoy MC, Naidich DP. Overview and strategic management of subsolid pulmonary nodules. *J Thorac Imaging* 2012;27:240–8.

14. Godoy MC, Sabloff B, Naidich DP. Subsolid pulmonary nodules: imaging evaluation and strategic management. *Curr Opin Pulm Med* 2009;18:304–12.

15. Noguchi M. Stepwise progression of pulmonary adenocarcinoma—clinical and molecular implications. *Cancer Metastasis Rev* 2010;29:15–21.

16. Nassar AA, Jaroszewski DE, Helmers RA, Colby TV, Patel BM, Mookadam F. Diffuse idiopathic pulmonary neuroendocrine cell hyperplasia: a systematic overview. *Am J Respir Crit Care Med* 2011;184:8–16.

17. Gorshtein A, Gross DJ, Barak D, et al. Diffuse idiopathic pulmonary neuroendocrine cell hyperplasia and the associated lung neuroendocrine tumors: clinical experience with a rare entity. *Cancer* 2012;118:612–9.

18. Davies SJ, Gosney JR, Hansell DM, et al. Diffuse idiopathic pulmonary neuroendocrine cell hyperplasia: an under-recognised spectrum of disease. *Thorax* 2007;62:248–52.

19. Kadota K, Suzuki K, Kachala SS, et al. A grading system combining architectural features and mitotic count predicts recurrence in stage I lung adenocarcinoma. *Mod Pathol* 2012;25:1117–27.

20. Yoshizawa A, Motoi N, Riely GJ, et al. Impact of proposed IASLC/ATS/ERS classification of lung adenocarcinoma: prognostic subgroups and implications for further revision of staging based on analysis of 514 stage I cases. *Mod Pathol* 2011;24:653–64.

21. Travis WD. Update on small cell carcinoma and its differentiation from squamous cell carcinoma and other non-small cell carcinomas. *Mod Pathol* 2012;25(Suppl 1):S18–30.

22. Moran CA, Suster S, Coppola D, Wick MR. Neuroendocrine carcinomas of the lung: a critical analysis. *Am J Clin Pathol* 2009;131:206–21.

23. Rossi G, Pelosi G, Graziano P, Barbareschi M, Papotti M. A reevaluation of the clinical significance of histological subtyping of non–small-cell lung carcinoma: diagnostic algorithms in the era of personalized treatments. *Int J Surg Pathol* 2009;17:206–18.

24. Rekhtman N, Ang DC, Sima CS, Travis WD, Moreira AL. Immunohistochemical algorithm for differentiation of lung adenocarcinoma and squamous cell carcinoma based on large series of whole-tissue sections with validation in small specimens. *Mod Pathol* 2011;24:1348–59.

25. Travis WD, Brambilla E, Rami-Porta R, et al. Visceral pleural invasion: pathologic criteria and use of elastic stains: proposal for the 7th edition of the TNM classification for lung cancer. *J Thorac Oncol* 2008;3:1384–90.

26. Pelosi G, Rossi G, Bianchi F, et al. Immunhistochemistry by means of widely agreed-upon markers (cytokeratins 5/6 and 7, p63, thyroid transcription factor-1, and vimentin) on small biopsies of non-small cell lung cancer effectively parallels the corresponding profiling and eventual diagnoses on surgical specimens. *J Thorac Oncol* 2011;6:1039–49.

27. Edge SB, Byrd DR, Comptom CC, Fritz AG, Greene FL, Trotti A. *AJCC Cancer Staging Manual.* 7th ed. New York: Springer; 2010.

28. Marchevsky AM. Problems in pathologic staging of lung cancer. *Arch Pathol Lab Med* 2006;130:292–302.

Chapter 4

Lung Cancer Screening

Apar Kishor Ganti and David E. Gerber

One of the major reasons for the poor outcomes from lung cancer is that most patients are diagnosed at a stage when their disease is no longer curable. In contrast, the 5-year survival for patients diagnosed at an early, resectable stage is almost 70%.[1–3] This would suggest early diagnosis could improve lung cancer outcomes to an extent and hence screening for early-stage disease could be potentially useful.

The gold standard for a screening tool is that it should improve the disease-related mortality. In addition, an ideal screening tool should fulfill the criteria proposed by Wilson and Jungner[4] in order to be widely utilized:

- The disease being screened for should be a major public health problem.
- There should be a clear understanding of the natural history and an obvious latent phase.
- There should be a suitable, safe, sensitive, acceptable, and cost-effective method to detect preclinical disease.
- There should be effective treatment available for the early disease detected.

The public health impact of lung cancer is obvious. Also, treatment of early-stage lung cancer is very effective. Until recently, the major debate over lung cancer screening has been the availability of a suitable diagnostic technique. However, with the recent publication of the results of the National Lung Screening Trial, these concerns also appear to have been addressed.

Historical Aspects

In the 1960s and 1970s, multiple large randomized trials of chest X-rays with or without sputum cytology were conducted in the United States and Europe (Table 4.1).[5–10] While there was an increased incidence of early-stage disease in the screening groups, there was no decrease in lung cancer–related mortality. These results led to the abandonment of chest radiographs and sputum cytology as potential screening options.

Rapid advances in computed tomography (CT) scan technology in the early 1990s rekindled an interest in screening for lung cancer.[11] Preliminary studies from Japan demonstrated that low-dose CT scans were highly effective in detecting early-stage lung cancer.[12,13] The Early Lung Cancer Action Project (ELCAP) suggested that low-dose CT scan improved the likelihood of detection

Table 4.1 Characteristics of Lung Cancer Detected by Screening with Chest X-Rays

Study	Intervention	Early Stage	Late Stage	5-year Survival	
				Test	Control
Johns Hopkins[5]	CXR annually ± sputum cytology every 4 months	139 (37%)	240 (63%)	20%	20%*
Czechoslovakia[6]	CXR + sputum cytology every 6 months vs. observation; initial CXR and sputum examination in both groups	20 (51%)	19 (49%)	No significant difference	
MSKCC[7]	CXR annually ± sputum cytology every 4 months	108 (46%)	127 (54%)	No significant difference	
Mayo Clinic[8]	CXR + sputum cytology every 4 months vs. observation; after an initial CXR in both groups	99 (48%)	107 (52%)	33%	15%
London[9]	CXR every 6 months vs. observation	44 (43%)	57 (57%)	15%	6%
PLCO[10]	CXR at baseline and annually for 3 years	68 (54%)†	58 (46%)	No difference. RR of death: 0.99 (95% CI 0.87–1.22)	

*8-year survival.

†Stages I and II.

CXR, chest X-ray; MSKCC, Memorial Sloan Kettering Cancer Center; PLCO, Prostate, Lung, Colorectal, and Ovarian Screening Trial.

of lung cancer at an earlier stage and the estimated 5-year survival in this group of patients was 60%–80%.[14] The results of these and other similar studies[15–17] have demonstrated that the vast majority of lung cancers detected by screening are stage I at diagnosis (Table 4.2).

National Lung Screening Trial

The National Lung Screening Trial (NLST) was a randomized multicenter study comparing low-dose CT scans with chest X-rays in the screening of 53,454 participants for early detection of lung cancer. The eligibility criteria for this study were as follows:

- Age 55–74 years
- ≥30 pack-year history of cigarette smoking
- Former smokers must have quit smoking within the previous 15 years.

Table 4.2 Characteristics of Lung Cancer Detected by Screening with Low-Dose Computed Tomography Scans in Nonrandomized Trials

Institution		% of Screened Patients With Cancer	Mean/Median Size (mm)	% Stage I
Matsumoto Research Center, Japan[12,13]	Prevalence	0.41	17/13.5	100
	Incidence	0.44	12/≈11	86
Cornell University[14,29]	Prevalence	2.7	≈14/≤10	85
	Incidence	0.7	12/8	71
Mayo Clinic[15]	Prevalence	1.9	14.7/14	67
	Incidence	2.1	14.6/8	60
National Cancer Center, Japan[17]	Prevalence	0.86	20/20	79
	Incidence	2.8	15/20	82
Milan[16]	Prevalence	1.06	21/NA	55
	Incidence	1.1	15/NA	100
Pittsburgh[30]	Prevalence	1.45	NA	60
	Incidence	0.78	NA	53

NA, not available.

Source: Adapted from Ganti and Mulshine.[11]

Participants were randomized to either low-dose CT or chest X-ray at baseline and two annual follow-up examinations. The primary endpoint was lung cancer mortality. Secondary endpoints included all-cause mortality, incidence of lung cancer, lung cancer case survival, and lung cancer stage distribution.

An interim analysis of this trial found a statistically significant survival benefit for CT scanning.[18] At a median follow-up of 6.5 years, there were 645 cases of lung cancer per 100,000 person years in the CT group compared to 572 cases in the chest X-ray group (incidence rate ratio: 1.13; 95% CI 1.03–1.23). There were 247 lung cancer deaths in the CT group compared to 309 in the X-ray group, that is, a relative reduction in lung cancer mortality of 20.0% (95% CI, 6.8% to 26.7%; $P = 0.004$). There was also a 6.7% (95% CI 1.2%–13.6%) reduction in all-cause mortality in the CT group.

Questions Raised by Computed Tomography Scan Screening

Lead-Time, Length-Time, and Overdiagnosis Bias

Although screening trials commonly report survival from the time of diagnosis, this parameter can be misleading due to lead-time, length-time, and overdiagnosis bias (see Figure 4.1).

- **Lead-time bias:** occurs when screening results in earlier detection of disease but does not change patient's lifespan (Figure 4.1a)
- **Length-time bias:** screening tests are more likely to detect indolent tumors than aggressive tumors that would result in clinical symptoms (Figure 4.1b)

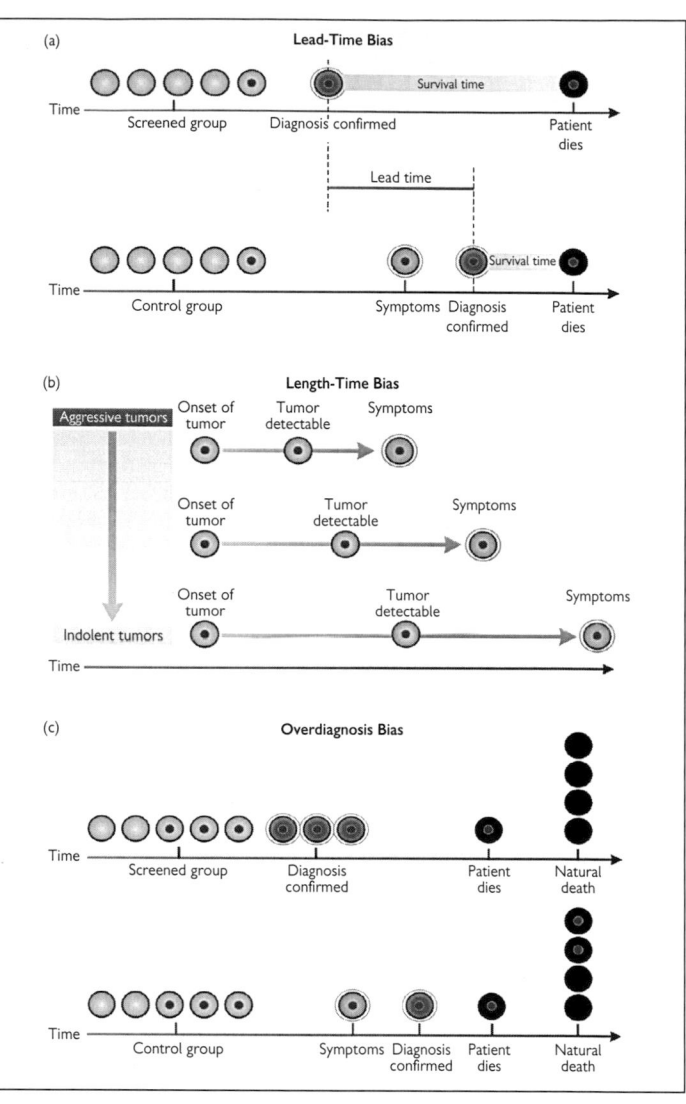

Figure 4.1 (a) *Lead-Time Bias.* Diagnosis of disease occurs earlier in the screened group, so these patients appear to live longer with disease than patients diagnosed clinically. However, the time of death is the same in the screened and control groups. (b) *Length-Time Bias.* Tumors identified by intermittent screening are more likely to be indolent, while aggressive tumors are more likely to present with symptoms. (c) *Overdiagnosis Bias.* Screening may detect tumors that would otherwise have remained clinically silent and not impacted patients' lifespans. Reprinted with permission from Patz EF et al. Screening for lung cancer. *N Engl J Med* 2000;343:1627–1633.

- **Overdiagnosis bias:** an extreme form of length-time bias, in which a screening test identifies a tumor that never would have affected the patient's life in the absence of screening (Figure 4.1c)

Examples of these biases are apparent from single-institution CT screening trials. Although over 80% of the screen-detected tumors in most of these studies represented stage I disease, there was no stage shift,[19] that is, no corresponding decrease in late-stage disease, raising the possibility of overdiagnosis. Nevertheless, the gene expression profile of screen-detected lung carcinomas appears to be similar to that of lung cancer diagnosed in symptomatic patients,[20] thereby inferring similar biologic behavior. By employing a primary endpoint of lung cancer-related *mortality,* rather than *survival,* the randomized NLST was less subject to these potential biases than earlier single-arm trials.

False-Positive Rates

In the Mayo Clinic study, ≈70% of subjects had noncalcified pulmonary nodules. The false-positive rates in this study ranged from 93% for nodules >4 mm in diameter, to 96% for all nodules.[19] In the NLST, 96% of the abnormalities in the low-dose CT group were false positive.[18] Although the perioperative mortality in the centers of excellence where the initial trials were conducted was low,[21] the concern is that if screening is made widely available, high complication rates may be an issue.

The approach to an abnormal screening chest CT is complex. Depending on the nature of the abnormality, subsequent steps may include interval CT, positron emission tomography (PET) scan, biopsy, or resection. The recommended algorithm in the NLST is depicted in Figure 4.2.

To minimize the number of invasive procedures required, Libby et al. have created an algorithm for nodules discovered incidentally on CT scan,[22] based upon the size, number, and density of the nodule(s), and patient characteristics, such as age, gender, smoking history, occupational history, and antecedent granulomatous disease.

Cost-Effectiveness

Mahadevia et al. used a model based on the Mayo clinic study and estimated the cost of screening to be $116,300 per quality-adjusted life-year (QALY) for current smokers.[23] However, Wisnivesky and associates estimated the same amount to be $2,500/year of life saved under favorable conditions based on the ELCAP data.[24] Another analysis modeled the potential cost-effectiveness of screening by CT scan for patient cohorts based on age and smoking history.[25] This projected that CT screening would decrease lung cancer mortality at 10 years by ≈20% at a cost ranging from $126,000 to $269,000 per QALY saved. Costs seemed to be related to the extent of smoking cessation associated with the screening program. Caution should be exercised while interpreting the results of such studies, due to the variable methodologies employed.[26]

Radiation Exposure

If half of the high-risk population in the United States were screened with low-dose CT scans annually for 20–25 years, there would be an estimated 36,000 new lung cancers due to radiation exposure.[27] This is a dynamic issue

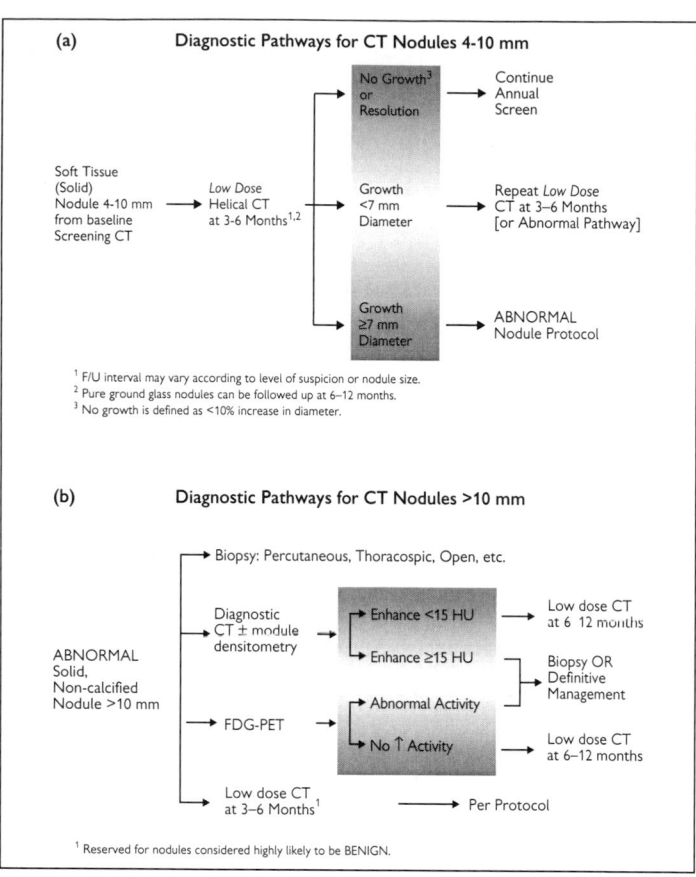

Figure 4.2 Algorithm for evaluation of abnormal screening chest CT scans: (a) nodules 4–10 mm; (b) nodules >10 mm. Nodules <4 mm are generally considered too small to characterize; follow-up low-dose CT is recommended in 12 months until nodule ≥4 mm, at which point the appropriate algorithm is followed. CT, computed tomography; FDG-PET, fluorodeoxyglucose-positron emission tomography; HU, Hounsfield units. Based on guidelines from the Fleschner Society and adapted from American College of Radiology Imaging Network ACRIN #6654 Contemporary Screening for the Detection of Lung Cancer. [http://www.acrin.org/Portals/0/Protocols/6654/Protocol-ACRIN%206654%20 Amendment%2010,%2011.1.04.pdf]

that must be considered when discussing the issue of lung cancer screening with the individual patient.

Recommendations

Updated guidelines from the National Comprehensive Cancer Network, American Society of Clinical Oncology, the American Cancer Society and the American College of Chest Physicians state that lung cancer screening should be discussed with individuals who are in good health and meet the NLST inclusion criteria. In addition, the NCCN guidelines[28] recommend consideration of screening in individuals ≥50 years and having ≥20 pack-year history of smoking and an additional risk factor, such as radon exposure, occupational exposure, cancer history, family history of lung cancer, and preexisting lung disease (i.e., chronic obstructive pulmonary disease or pulmonary fibrosis).

In addition, individuals who fit the aforementioned criteria and are motivated to seek out screening should be counseled regarding the risks and benefits of screening. They must be advised about the importance of repeat screening after a negative baseline study. Smoking cessation education should form an important part of this discussion in current smokers.

References

1. Shimizu J, Watanabe Y, Oda M, et al. Results of surgical treatment of stage I lung cancer. *Nippon Geka Gakkai Zasshi* 1993;94:505–10.

2. Williams DE, Pairolero PC, Davis CS, et al. Survival of patients surgically treated for stage I lung cancer. *J Thorac Cardiovasc Surg* 1981;82:70–6.

3. Shah R, Sabanathan S, Richardson J, Mearns AJ, Goulden C. Results of surgical treatment of stage I and II lung cancer. *J Cardiovasc Surg (Torino)* 1996;37:169–72.

4. Wilson JM, Jungner YG. [Principles and practice of mass screening for disease]. *Boletin de la Oficina Sanitaria Panamericana* 1968;65:281–393.

5. Tockman MS. Survival and mortality from lung cancer in a screened population. *Chest* 1986;89:324S–5S.

6. Kubik A, Polak J. Lung cancer detection. Results of a randomized prospective study in Czechoslovakia. *Cancer* 1986;57:2427–37.

7. Melamed MR, Flehinger BJ, Zaman MB, Heelan RT, Perchick WA, Martini N. Screening for early lung cancer. Results of the Memorial Sloan-Kettering study in New York. *Chest* 1984;86:44–53.

8. Fontana RS, Sanderson DR, Woolner LB, Taylor WF, Miller WE, Muhm JR. Lung cancer screening: the Mayo program. *J Occup Med* 1986;28:746–50.

9. Brett GZ. Earlier diagnosis and survival in lung cancer. *Br Med J* 1969;4:260–2.

10. Oken MM, Marcus PM, Hu P, et al. Baseline chest radiograph for lung cancer detection in the randomized Prostate, Lung, Colorectal and Ovarian Cancer Screening Trial. *J Natl Cancer Inst* 2005;97:1832–9.

11. Ganti AK, Mulshine JL. Lung cancer screening: panacea or pipe dream? *Ann Oncol* 2005;16 (Suppl 2):ii215–9.

12. Kaneko M, Eguchi K, Ohmatsu H, et al. Peripheral lung cancer: screening and detection with low-dose spiral CT versus radiography. *Radiology* 1996;201:798–802.

13. Sone S, Takashima S, Li F, et al. Mass screening for lung cancer with mobile spiral computed tomography scanner. *Lancet* 1998;351:1242–5.

14. Henschke CI. Early lung cancer action project: overall design and findings from baseline screening. *Cancer* 2000;89:2474–82.

15. Swensen SJ, Jett JR, Sloan JA, et al. Screening for lung cancer with low-dose spiral computed tomography. *Am J Respir Crit Care Med* 2002;165:508–13.

16. Pastorino U, Bellomi M, Landoni C, et al. Early lung-cancer detection with spiral CT and positron emission tomography in heavy smokers: 2-year results. *Lancet* 2003;362:593–7.

17. Sobue T, Moriyama N, Kaneko M, et al. Screening for lung cancer with low-dose helical computed tomography: anti-lung cancer association project. *J Clin Oncol* 2002;20:911–20.

18. National Lung Screening Trial Research Team. Reduced lung-cancer mortality with low-dose computed tomographic screening. *N Engl J Med* 2011;365:395–409.

19. Swensen SJ, Jett JR, Hartman TE, et al. CT screening for lung cancer: five-year prospective experience. *Radiology* 2005;235:259–65.

20. Bianchi F, Hu J, Pelosi G, et al. Lung cancers detected by screening with spiral computed tomography have a malignant phenotype when analyzed by cDNA microarray. *Clin Cancer Res* 2004;10:6023–8.

21. Crestanello JA, Allen MS, Jett JR, et al. Thoracic surgical operations in patients enrolled in a computed tomographic screening trial. *J Thorac Cardiovasc Surg* 2004;128:254–9.

22. Libby DM, Smith JP, Altorki NK, et al. Managing the small pulmonary nodule discovered by CT. *Chest* 2004;125:1522–9.

23. Mahadevia PJ, Fleisher LA, Frick KD, Eng J, Goodman SN, Powe NR. Lung cancer screening with helical computed tomography in older adult smokers: a decision and cost-effectiveness analysis. *JAMA* 2003;289:313–22.

24. Wisnivesky JP, Mushlin AI, Sicherman N, Henschke C. The cost-effectiveness of low-dose CT screening for lung cancer: preliminary results of baseline screening. *Chest* 2003;124:614–21.

25. McMahon PM, Kong CY, Bouzan C, et al. Cost-effectiveness of computed tomography screening for lung cancer in the United States. *J Thorac Oncol* 2011;6:1841–8.

26. Mulshine JL, Sullivan DC. Clinical practice. Lung cancer screening. *N Engl J Med* 2005;352:2714–20.

27. Brenner DJ. Radiation risks potentially associated with low-dose CT screening of adult smokers for lung cancer. *Radiology* 2004;231:440–5.

28. Wood DE, Eapen GA, Ettinger DS, et al. Lung cancer screening. *J Natl Compr Canc Netw* 2012;10:240–65.

29. Henschke CI, McCauley DI, Yankelevitz DF, et al. Early Lung Cancer Action Project: overall design and findings from baseline screening. *Lancet* 1999;354:99–105.

30. Wilson DO, Weissfeld JL, Fuhrman CR, et al. The Pittsburgh Lung Screening Study (PLuSS): outcomes within 3 years of a first computed tomography scan. *Am J Respir Crit Care Med* 2008;178:956–61.

Chapter 5

Clinical Manifestations of Lung Cancer

Apar Kishor Ganti

The majority of patients with lung cancer present with symptoms associated with the disease. Fewer than 5% of patients are completely asymptomatic at presentation.[1] In addition to constitutional symptoms such as weight loss and fatigue, patients can present with symptoms related either to the primary tumor, regional spread, or distant metastases. A small but significant number of patients, especially those with small cell lung cancer, may present with symptoms related to paraneoplastic syndromes.

Constitutional Symptoms

Constitutional symptoms are the most common symptoms reported by patients with lung cancer.[2] Weight loss is seen in 40%–70% of patients,[3–5] while fatigue is seen in almost 45%.[5] In a survey of 650 patients, the most common constitutional symptoms noted were tiredness and lack of appetite.[2]

Symptoms of Loco-Regional Disease

The most common symptoms seen with locoregional disease are cough, dyspnea, chest pain, and hemoptysis.

Cough

Cough is the most common symptom seen in patients with lung cancer.[5,6] Cough is more often seen in squamous cell carcinoma and small cell carcinoma, presumably due to the more frequent involvement of the central airways.

Dyspnea

The incidence of dyspnea varies from about 25% to 70% of lung cancer patients.[2,4–6] The causes of dyspnea include extrinsic compression of intraluminal obstruction of the airways, development of pleural (Fig. 5.1a-c) or pericardial effusion (Fig. 5.2a-d), phrenic nerve paralysis, and lymphangitic intraparenchymal spread of tumor.[7,8] In addition, anxiety, anemia, and cachexia associated with the tumor can also result in the development of dyspnea.[9]

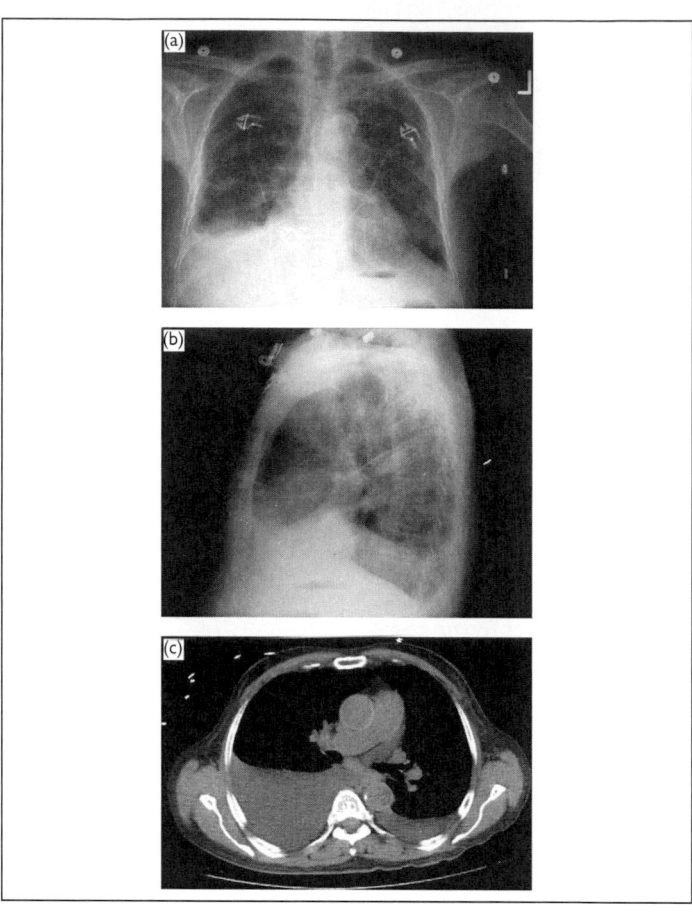

Figure 5.1 Pleural effusion. Chest X-ray with posterior-anterior (*a*) and lateral (*b*) views shows blunting of the right costo-phrenic angle; computed tomography scan (*c*) shows large right-sided and small left-sided pleural effusions. (Courtesy of Matthew J. DeVries, MD.)

Chest Pain

Lung cancer–associated chest pain is due to involvement of the pleura, chest wall, or mediastinum. The pain is usually dull, aching, and persistent, although involvement of the thoracic spine can give rise to a sharp neuropathic pain. The presence of chest pain, while suspicious for local spread, does not always preclude curative surgical resection. Occasionally patients can present with sharp pleuritic chest pain associated with lung infarction secondary to a pulmonary embolus. The incidence of chest pain in lung cancer varies from 20% to 70%.[2,5,8,10]

Hemoptysis

Hemoptysis is seen in 25%–50% of patients with lung cancer.[3,4,8] It is most often seen with small cell lung cancer, followed by squamous cell carcinoma and adenocarcinoma.[11]

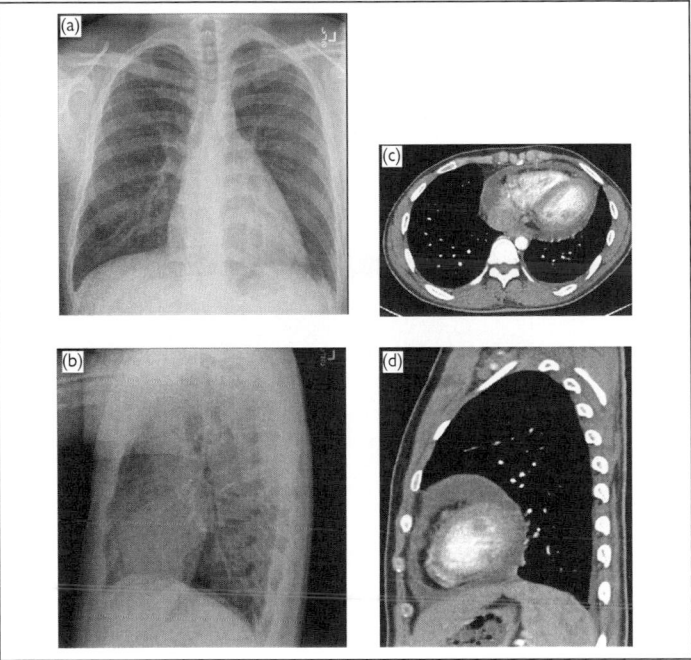

Figure 5.2 Pericardial effusion. Chest X-ray with posterior anterior (a) and lateral (b) views show cardiomegaly (cardio/thoracic ratio >50%). On the lateral view, there is a black-white-black stripe (sandwich/Oreo cookie sign) over the cardiac border—consistent with a pericardial effusion. The black stripes represent the epipericardial and epicardial fat, while the white stripe in the middle represents the pericardial effusion. Axial (c) and sagittal (d) views on the computed tomography scan show fluid in the pericardial space. Note that on sagittal image the sandwich/Oreo cookie sign is depicted by the epipericardial and epicardial fat pad with interposed pericardial fluid. (Courtesy of Matthew J. DeVries, MD.)

Hoarseness

This is usually seen with left-sided cancers that have either primary tumor or mediastinal lymph node involvement compressing the recurrent laryngeal nerve. Lung cancer is the most common malignant cause of vocal cord paralysis.[12]

Superior Vena Cava Syndrome

The superior vena cava syndrome comprises a constellation of symptoms arising as a result of compression of the superior vena cava (Fig. 5.3a-b). The most common cause of this syndrome is malignancy, and lung cancer accounts for almost 75% of all malignant causes of this syndrome.[13]

Patients present with swelling of the face, neck, and upper extremities and distended veins of the neck and upper extremities. Other symptoms include dyspnea, cough, plethora, hoarseness, dizziness, and headaches. These clinical features are due to decreased drainage of blood from the upper part of the body through the compressed superior vena cava.[13] While this represents a relative oncologic emergency, rarely is immediate intervention without a diagnosis indicated.

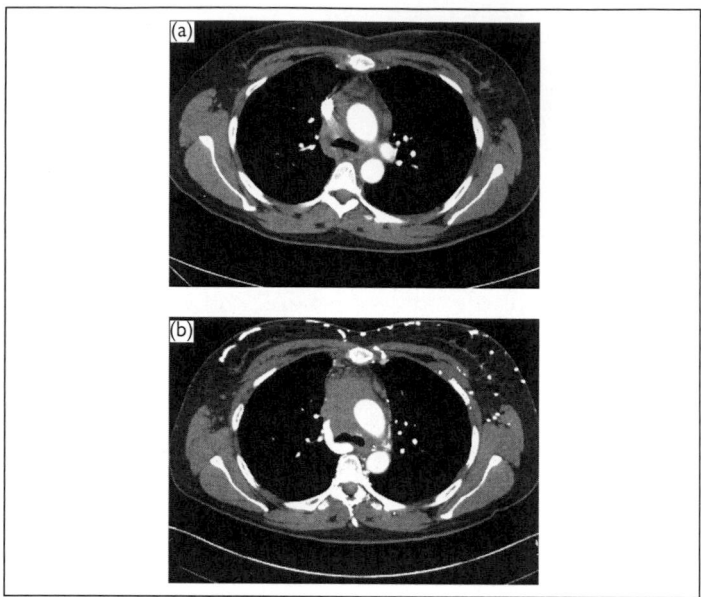

Figure 5.3 Superior vena cava syndrome. Initial computed tomography (*a*) shows mediastinal soft tissue prominence with patent superior vena cava; computed tomography from the same patient 8 months later (*b*) showing occlusion of the superior vena cava. Note the multiple body wall collateral vessels and contrast extending through the collateral azygos venous pathway. (Courtesy of Matthew J. DeVries, MD.)

Pleural Effusions

Pleural effusion in patients with lung cancer can either be malignant with cancer cells in the fluid or nonmalignant as a result of lymphatic obstruction, postobstructive pneumonitis, or atelectasis (Fig. 5.1). This distinction is important as it has significant therapeutic implications. Patients with a malignant effusion are considered to have stage IVA disease and are hence incurable, while a patient with a benign effusion may be curable depending on the other characteristics of the tumor. Hence, malignancy should be pathologically confirmed in every patient with a pleural effusion before deeming the patient incurable for this reason.

Pancoast Tumors

These are tumors involving the superior sulcus of the lung that often present with symptoms associated with invasion of surrounding structures, including the brachial plexus, subclavian vessels, and the spine (Fig. 5.4a-c).[14] Although non–small cell lung cancer (NSCLC) accounts for the majority of cases, a similar presentation may rarely be seen with small cell lung cancer, lymphoma, chest wall tumors, and tuberculosis.

Common symptoms in this setting include shoulder pain (although patients may occasionally present with pain in the forearm, scapula, and fingers), Horner's syndrome (ipsilateral ptosis, miosis, anhidrosis), bony destruction, and weakness and atrophy of intrinsic hand muscles.

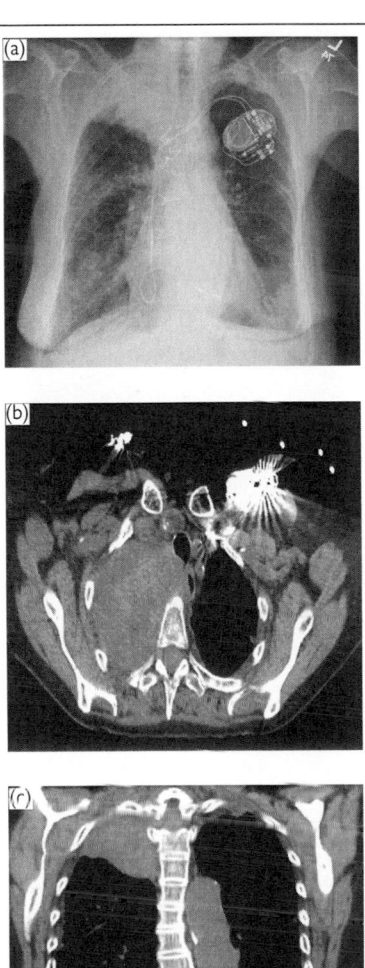

Figure 5.4 Pancoast tumor. Chest X-ray (*a*), computed tomography scan axial (*b*), and coronal (*c*) views show asymmetric right apical mass and/or pleural thickening consistent with a Pancoast/superior sulcus tumor. The patient also has an automated implantable cardioverter-defibrillator in place. (Courtesy of Matthew J. DeVries, MD.)

Symptoms of Distant Disease

Brain

Brain metastases are seen in 16%–20% of patients with lung cancer.[15,16] Small cell lung cancer and adenocarcinomas appear to have the greatest propensity to metastasize to the brain.[17,18] The risk of developing brain metastases in NSCLC appears to be related to the tumor size and lymph node metastases.[18] Symptoms of brain metastases in NSCLC include headaches, vomiting, seizures, and focal neurologic deficits, which may include sensory, motor, and cranial nerve involvement (Fig. 5.5a-b).

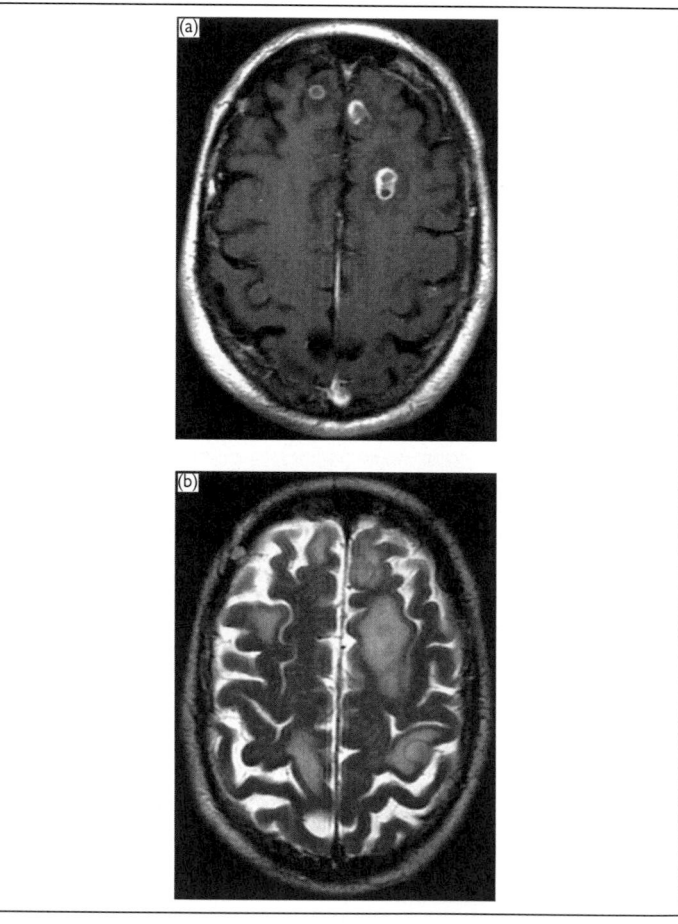

Figure 5.5 Brain metastases. Post-contrast T1-weighted (a) and corresponding T2-weighted (b) magnetic resonance imaging (MRI) are shown. Images show multiple areas of vasogenic edema on T2 images (which may also be seen with abscesses or hematomas) with corresponding multiple ring enhancing lesions on post-contrast T1-weighted images. Findings are most consistent with multiple metastases. (Courtesy of Matthew J. DeVries, MD.)

Adrenal

Although the adrenal glands are a common site for metastases from lung cancer, they are often asymptomatic. Usually they are detected during routine imaging for staging purposes as unilateral enlargement of an adrenal gland. Biopsy confirmation is preferred if the adrenal lesion is the only site of metastasis because only about 25% of isolated adrenal masses are malignant.[19]

Bone

Approximately 1 in 5 patients with NSCLC and 1 in 3 patients with SCLC develop bone metastases.[20,21] Most of these are symptomatic, presenting as localized pain. These are often osteolytic lesions, although osteoblastic lesions are not uncommon. The most common site of development of bone metastases appears to be the vertebral column. This can lead to complications such as cord compression with associated neurological deficits and fractures, leading to pain.

Liver

Asymptomatic liver metastases are often detected during the evaluation of abnormal liver chemistries or by imaging studies during the standard staging evaluation. Approximately 2% of patients with otherwise early-stage disease will have asymptomatic liver involvement, making them ineligible for curative resection.[22]

Paraneoplastic Syndromes

Paraneoplastic syndromes are a constellation of signs and symptoms that are not due to direct invasion or metastasis of the tumor. Instead, they are caused by the secretion of hormones, peptides, or cytokines by the tumor cells or from immune cross-reactivity between malignant and normal tissues.[23] Paraneoplastic syndromes can affect various organ systems. Lung cancer, especially small cell lung cancer, is the most common cancer associated with the development of paraneoplastic syndromes (Table 5.1). Treatment of paraneoplastic syndromes revolves mainly around the treatment of the underlying malignancy, but certain paraneoplastic syndromes may need specific treatments. The following section will discuss certain specific paraneoplastic presentations of lung cancer.

Endocrine

Hypercalcemia

Lung cancer cells secrete cytokines that promote bone resorption, for example, PTH-related peptide (PTHrP), IL-1, IL-2, prostaglandin E, transforming growth factors (TGF)-α and β, tumor necrosis factor (TNF)-β, and calcitriol. Approximately 6% of patients with lung cancer have hypercalcemia at the time of diagnosis and about 10%–25% of patients develop hypercalcemia during the course of their disease.[24] Among patients who present with hypercalcemia, squamous cell carcinoma is the most common subtype. The common symptoms of hypercalcemia include anorexia, nausea, vomiting, constipation, lethargy, polyuria, and polydipsia. The severity of the symptoms is associated not only with the degree but also with the rate of rise of the serum calcium level. Hypercalcemia at diagnosis confers a worse prognosis (median OS: 3.8 vs. 9.5 months; $P < 0.001$).[24]

Table 5.1 Common Paraneoplastic Syndromes Associated with Lung Cancer

Organ System	Syndrome	Specific Investigations	Specific Treatment
Systemic	Cachexia		
	Fever	Evaluate for infectious causes	
Endocrine	Syndrome of inappropriate antidiuretic hormone (SIADH)	Serum sodium level (low), urine sodium (increased/normal), urine osmolality (inappropriately normal or elevated)	Fluid restriction, demeclocycline, vasopressin antagonists, hypertonic saline
	Cushing's syndrome	High-dose dexamethasone suppression test (no response)	Drugs that inhibit steroid production—ketoconazole, mitotane, metyrapone, aminoglutethimide
	Hypercalcemia	Serum calcium (high), PTH (low), PTHrP (high)	Vigorous hydration, bisphosphonates
	Carcinoid syndrome		Octreotide
Neurologic	Lambert-Eaton myasthenic syndrome	Anti-VGCC	IV immunoglobulin, plasma exchange, steroids
	Peripheral neuropathy	Anti-Hu antibody	Steroids
	Cerebellar degeneration	Anti-Ri, anti-CV2, anti-Zic4 antibodies	
	Opsoclonus ataxia	Anti-Ri antibodies	Immunosuppression (steroids, cyclophosphamide), clonazepam, thiamine
	Limbic encephalitis	Anti-Hu, anti-Ma1, anti-Ma2(Ta), anti-GABA (B) antibodies	IV immunoglobulin, steroids
	Cancer-associated retinopathy; optic neuropathy	Anti-recoverin antibody	
	Encephalomyelitis	Anti-CV2 antibodies	
	Autonomic neuropathy	Anti-Hu, anti-nACh receptor antibodies	

Hematologic	Anemia	Erythropoietin level	Erythropoietic stimulating agents may be useful if erythropoietin level is <500 IU/mL
	Leukocytosis		
	Thrombocytosis		
	Hypercoagulable disorders		Anticoagulation; low molecular weight heparins have increased efficacy over warfarin
Cutaneous/ musculoskeletal	Clubbing		
	Hypertrophic osteoarthropathy	Imaging studies (can be avid on nuclear bone scan or PET scan*)	
	Acanthosis nigricans		
	Dermatomyositis/polymyositis		IV immunoglobulin, immunosuppression
	Pemphigus vulgaris		

*Uptake on nuclear bone scan or PET does not necessarily indicate metastatic disease.

GABA, gamma amino butyric acid; IV, intravenous; PET, positron emission tomography; PTH, parathyroid hormone; PTHrP, parathyroid hormone–related peptide; VGCC, voltage-gated calcium channel.

Syndrome of Inappropriate ADH Secretion

Syndrome of inappropriate ADH secretion (SIADH) is commonly seen in small cell lung cancer (15%), but it also occurs to a lesser extent in NSCLC (1%).[25] The development of clinical SIADH in SCLC patients does not appear to be dependent on the tumor burden or site of metastasis.[26] The symptoms of SIADH are related to the serum sodium level and the rapidity of the decline in these levels. Symptoms may include nonspecific anorexia, nausea, and vomiting. Cerebral edema can occur with a rapid drop in levels and presents with irritability, restlessness, personality changes, confusion, coma, and seizures. Treatment of the underlying SCLC can lead to a rapid normalization of the sodium levels. The hyponatremia associated with SIADH may rarely be mistaken for cisplatin-induced salt wasting.

Cushing's Syndrome

Neuroendocrine lung tumors (small cell lung cancer and bronchial carcinoids) account for almost half of these cases.[23] Secretion of adrenocorticotropic hormone or corticotropin-releasing factor by the tumor[23] leads to the release of cortisol from the adrenal glands. Patients present with hypertension, hypokalemia, muscle weakness, weight gain, psychiatric disorders, bruising, infections, and generalized edema.[27]

Neurologic

Neurologic paraneoplastic syndromes can affect either a single type of neuronal cell or diffusely involve the nervous system. These symptoms can develop in the presence of known cancer or may precede a cancer diagnosis by months to years. The diagnosis of neurologic paraneoplastic syndromes is often made by the presence of specific antibodies, but these are neither sensitive nor specific. The common syndromes seen are discussed in Table 5.1.

Neurologic paraneoplastic syndromes are difficult to treat, and stabilization of the deficit upon treatment of the underlying tumor is often the best outcome achieved. The most likely reason for this poor response is that irreversible neuronal damage has often occurred before the onset of treatment.

Hematologic

Anemia

Anemia is seen in almost 40% of patients with untreated lung cancer, and the incidence can be as high as 80% in patients undergoing chemotherapy.[28] As there are multiple causes of anemia in cancer patients, potentially reversible etiologies such as bleeding, bone marrow replacement by the tumor, and treatment-related causes should be excluded before making a diagnosis of paraneoplastic anemia.

Leukocytosis

Tumor-associated leukocytosis has been attributed to overproduction of G-CSF and IL-6[29] and confers a worse prognosis in patients with lung cancer.

Thrombocytosis

Almost 14% percent of patients with lung cancer will have elevated platelet counts at presentation.[30] Thrombocytosis at presentation also appears to be an independent predictor of decreased survival.[31]

Hypercoagulable Disorders

A variety of hypercoagulable disorders have been associated with lung cancer, including migratory superficial thrombophlebitis (Trousseau's syndrome), deep venous thrombosis, disseminated intravascular coagulopathy, and thrombotic microangiopathy. Low molecular weight heparins appear to be more effective than warfarin in the treatment of venous thromboembolism in cancer patients.[32]

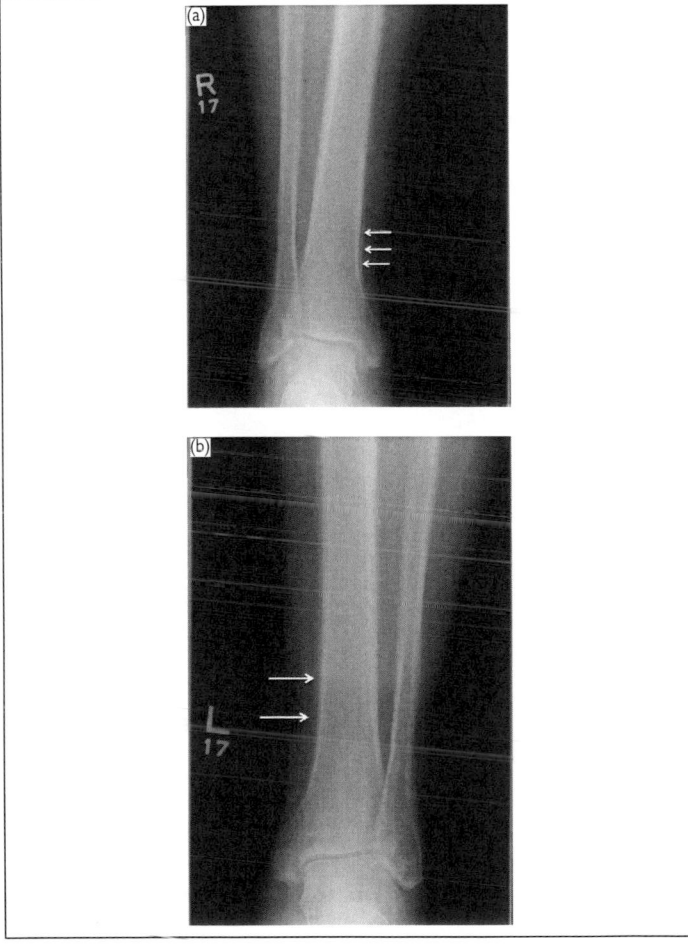

Figure 5.6 Hypertrophic osteoarthropathy. Bilateral [right (a) and left (b)] plain films show diffuse bilateral periosteal reaction of the distal tibia/fibula. Among other multiple etiologies (cystic fibrosis, right-to-left cardiac shunts), findings are consistent with hypertrophic pulmonary osteoarthropathy. (Courtesy of Matthew J. DeVries, MD.)

Rheumatologic

Hypertrophic Pulmonary Osteoarthropathy

Hypertrophic pulmonary osteoarthropathy (HPOA) is caused by periosteal proliferation of long bones. HPOA presents with a painful arthropathy involving the major joints of the appendicular skeleton. Involvement of the small bones of the hands and feet can present as clubbing. X-rays show periosteal new bone formation (Fig. 5.6 a-b), while bone scan and positron emission tomography scan may show diffuse uptake. The symptoms may resolve with resection, but nonsteroidal anti-inflammatory drugs and bisphosphonates may be useful in patients who are not surgical candidates.[33]

References

1. Kuo CW, Chen YM, Chao JY, Tsai CM, Perng RP. Non-small cell lung cancer in very young and very old patients. *Chest* 2000;117:354–7.

2. Hopwood P, Stephens RJ. Symptoms at presentation for treatment in patients with lung cancer: implications for the evaluation of palliative treatment. The Medical Research Council (MRC) Lung Cancer Working Party. *Br J Cancer* 1995;71:633–6.

3. Hyde L, Hyde CI. Clinical manifestations of lung cancer. *Chest* 1974;65:299–306.

4. Chute CG, Greenberg ER, Baron J, Korson R, Baker J, Yates J. Presenting conditions of 1539 population-based lung cancer patients by cell type and stage in New Hampshire and Vermont. *Cancer* 1985;56:2107–11.

5. Cohen S, Hossain SA. Primary carcinoma of the lung. A review of 417 histologically proved cases. *Dis Chest* 1966;49:67–74.

6. Martins SJ, Pereira JR. Clinical factors and prognosis in non-small cell lung cancer. *Am J Clin Oncol* 1999;22:453–7.

7. Piehler JM, Pairolero PC, Gracey DR, Bernatz PE. Unexplained diaphragmatic paralysis: a harbinger of malignant disease? *J Thorac Cardiovasc Surg* 1982;84:861–4.

8. Dudgeon DJ, Rosenthal S. Management of dyspnea and cough in patients with cancer. *Hematol/Oncol Clin North Am* 1996;10:157–71.

9. Jantarakupt P, Porock D. Dyspnea management in lung cancer: applying the evidence from chronic obstructive pulmonary disease. *Oncol Nurs Forum* 2005;32:785–97.

10. Inoperable non-small-cell lung cancer (NSCLC): a Medical Research Council randomised trial of palliative radiotherapy with two fractions or ten fractions. Report to the Medical Research Council by its Lung Cancer Working Party. *Br J Cancer* 1991;63:265–70.

11. Hirshberg B, Biran I, Glazer M, Kramer MR. Hemoptysis: etiology, evaluation, and outcome in a tertiary referral hospital. *Chest* 1997;112:440–4.

12. Chen HC, Jen YM, Wang CH, Lee JC, Lin YS. Etiology of vocal cord paralysis. *ORL J Otorhinolaryngol Relat Spec* 2007;69:167–71.

13. Wilson LD, Detterbeck FC, Yahalom J. Clinical practice. Superior vena cava syndrome with malignant causes. *N Engl J Med* 2007;356:1862–9.

14. Rusch VW. Management of Pancoast tumours. *Lancet Oncol* 2006;7:997–1005.

15. Schouten LJ, Rutten J, Huveneers HA, Twijnstra A. Incidence of brain metastases in a cohort of patients with carcinoma of the breast, colon, kidney, and lung and melanoma. *Cancer* 2002;94:2698–705.

16. Barnholtz-Sloan JS, Sloan AE, Davis FG, Vigneau FD, Lai P, Sawaya RE. Incidence proportions of brain metastases in patients diagnosed (1973 to 2001) in the Metropolitan Detroit Cancer Surveillance System. *J Clin Oncol* 2004;22:2865–72.

17. Doyle TJ. Brain metastasis in the natural history of small-cell lung cancer: 1972–1979. *Cancer* 1982;50:752–4.

18. Mujoomdar A, Austin JH, Malhorta R, et al. Clinical predictors of metastatic disease to the brain from non-small cell lung carcinoma: primary tumor size, cell type, and lymph node metastases. *Radiology* 2007;242:882–8.

19. Oliver TW, Jr., Bernardino ME, Miller JI, Mansour K, Greene D, Davis WA. Isolated adrenal masses in nonsmall-cell bronchogenic carcinoma. *Radiology* 1984;153:217–8.

20. Toloza EM, Harpole L, McCrory DC. Noninvasive staging of non-small cell lung cancer: a review of the current evidence. *Chest* 2003;123:137S–46S.

21. Schumacher T, Brink I, Mix M, et al. FDG-PET imaging for the staging and follow-up of small cell lung cancer. *Eur J Nucl Med* 2001;28:483–8.

22. Hillers TK, Sauve MD, Guyatt GH. Analysis of published studies on the detection of extrathoracic metastases in patients presumed to have operable non-small cell lung cancer. *Thorax* 1994;49:14–9.

23. Pelosof LC, Gerber DE. Paraneoplastic syndromes: an approach to diagnosis and treatment. *Mayo Clin Proc* 2010;85:838–54.

24. Hiraki A, Ueoka H, Takata I, et al. Hypercalcemia-leukocytosis syndrome associated with lung cancer. *Lung Cancer* 2004;43:301–7.

25. Sorensen JB, Andersen MK, Hansen HH. Syndrome of inappropriate secretion of antidiuretic hormone (SIADH) in malignant disease. *J Intern Med* 1995;238:97–110.

26. List AF, Hainsworth JD, Davis BW, Hande KR, Greco FA, Johnson DH. The syndrome of inappropriate secretion of antidiuretic hormone (SIADH) in small-cell lung cancer. *J Clin Oncol* 1986;4:1191–8.

27. Ilias I, Torpy DJ, Pacak K, Mullen N, Wesley RA, Nieman LK. Cushing's syndrome due to ectopic corticotropin secretion: twenty years' experience at the National Institutes of Health. *J Clin Endocrinol Metab* 2005;90:4955–62.

28. Kosmidis P, Krzakowski M. Anemia profiles in patients with lung cancer: what have we learned from the European Cancer Anaemia Survey (ECAS)? *Lung Cancer* 2005;50:401–12.

29. Kasuga I, Makino S, Kiyokawa H, Katoh H, Ebihara Y, Ohyashiki K. Tumor-related leukocytosis is linked with poor prognosis in patients with lung carcinoma. *Cancer* 2001;92:2399–405.

30. Hamilton W, Peters TJ, Round A, Sharp D. What are the clinical features of lung cancer before the diagnosis is made? A population based case-control study. *Thorax* 2005;60:1059–65.

31. Aoe K, Hiraki A, Ueoka H, et al. Thrombocytosis as a useful prognostic indicator in patients with lung cancer. *Respiration* 2004;71:170–3.

32. Akl EA, Labedi N, Barba M, et al. Anticoagulation for the long term treatment of venous thromboembolism in patients with cancer. *Cochrane Database Syst Rev* 2008;6:CD006650.

33. Amital H, Applbaum YH, Vasiliev L, Rubinow A. Hypertrophic pulmonary osteoarthropathy: control of pain and symptoms with pamidronate. *Clin Rheumatol* 2004;23:330–2.

Chapter 6

Diagnostic Evaluation and Staging of Lung Cancer

Apar Kishor Ganti, David E. Gerber, Matthew DeVries, and Rudy P. Lackner

The first step in the management of a patient diagnosed with lung cancer is to determine the extent of the disease, as this dictates the treatment approach. The diagnostic evaluation includes a thorough physical examination, laboratory testing, imaging studies, and occasionally invasive techniques to accurately identify the stage of the patient. Table 6.1 shows the tumor-node-metastasis (TNM) descriptors for lung cancer staging, while Table 6.2 shows the stage grouping for lung cancer based on the American Joint Committee on Cancer, seventh edition.[1]

Physical Examination

The main symptoms and signs commonly associated with lung cancer are reviewed in Chapter 5 (Clinical Presentation). Although most symptoms and signs are nonspecific, certain features may help identify clinically relevant disease; for example, hoarseness due to recurrent laryngeal nerve involvement, dyspnea and decreased breath sounds secondary to a pleural effusion, and worsening headaches or seizures as a result of brain metastases. In addition, a physical examination will help identify relevant comorbidities that could potentially affect management decisions.

Laboratory Investigations

Every patient diagnosed with lung cancer should have a complete blood count and a comprehensive metabolic panel, including liver and kidney function tests. Any abnormalities seen in these investigations could either be a marker of underlying comorbidities or may provide an estimate of the extent of disease spread. These results may provide guidance for further testing, such as a nuclear bone scan for elevated alkaline phosphatase or calcium, or a contrasted computerized tomography (CT) scan of the liver for abnormal liver chemistries. Figure 6.1 describes a possible approach to staging a patient with lung cancer.

Table 6.1 Tumor-Node-Metastasis Classification of Lung Cancer

Primary tumor (T)	
T0	No evidence of primary tumor
Tx	Positive cytology
Tis	Carcinoma *in situ*
T1	≤3 cm, no invasion of visceral pleura, no invasion more proximal than lobar bronchus
T1a	≤2 cm
T1b	>2 cm but ≤3 cm
T2	Involvement of a main-stem bronchus, with proximal extent ≥2 cm from the carina; invasion of visceral pleura; atelectasis or obstructive pneumonitis that does not involve the entire lung
T2a	>3 cm but ≤5 cm
T2b	>5 but ≤7 cm
T3	>7 cm; invasion of the chest wall, diaphragm, mediastinal pleura, or parietal pericardium; involvement of main-stem bronchus <2 cm of the carina, but without invasion of the carina; atelectasis/obstructive pneumonitis of entire lung; satellite tumor nodule(s) within the same lobe of lung as the primary tumor
T4	Invasion of the mediastinum, heart, great vessels, trachea, esophagus, vertebral body, or carina; satellite tumor nodule(s) within a different lobe of the ipsilateral lung as the primary tumor
Lymph nodes (N)	
N0	No regional lymph node involvement
N1	Involvement of ipsilateral peribronchial, intrapulmonary, and/or ipsilateral hilar lymph nodes
N2	Involvement of ipsilateral mediastinal and/or subcarinal lymph nodes
N3	Metastasis to contralateral mediastinal or contralateral hilar nodes, or involvement of scalene or supraclavicular lymph nodes
Metastasis (M)	
M1	Distant metastases
M1a	Malignant pleural or pericardial effusions; pleural nodules; nodules in contralateral lung
M1b	Distant metastases

Source: Adapted from Goldstraw P, et al. The IASLC Lung Cancer Staging Project: proposals for the revision of the TNM stage groupings in the forthcoming (seventh) edition of the TNM Classification of malignant tumours. *J Thoracic Oncol*. 2007;2:706–14.

Chest X-Ray

Chest radiography (CXR) is routinely available and inexpensive. It plays a key role in identifying the nature of a lung nodule by comparison with previous films. A new/enlarging lesion is more likely to represent malignancy than a

Table 6.2 Stage Grouping of Lung Cancer

Occult carcinoma	TxN0M0
Stage 0	TisN0M0
Stage IA	T1aN0M0; T1bN0M0
Stage IB	T2aN0M0
Stage IIA	T2bN0M0; T1aN1M0; T1bN1M0; T2aN1M0
Stage IIB	T2bN1M0; T3N0M0
Stage IIIA	T1aN2M0; T1bN2M0; T2aN2M0; T2bN2M0; T3N1M0; T3N2M0; T4N0M0; T4N1M0
Stage IIIB	T4N2M0; any T, N3M0
Stage IVA	Any T, any N, M1a
Stage IVB	Any T, any N, M1b

Source: Adapted from: Goldstraw P, et al. The IASLC Lung Cancer Staging Project: proposals for the revision of the TNM stage groupings in the forthcoming (seventh) edition of the TNM Classification of malignant tumours. *J Thoracic Oncol.* 2007;2:706–14.

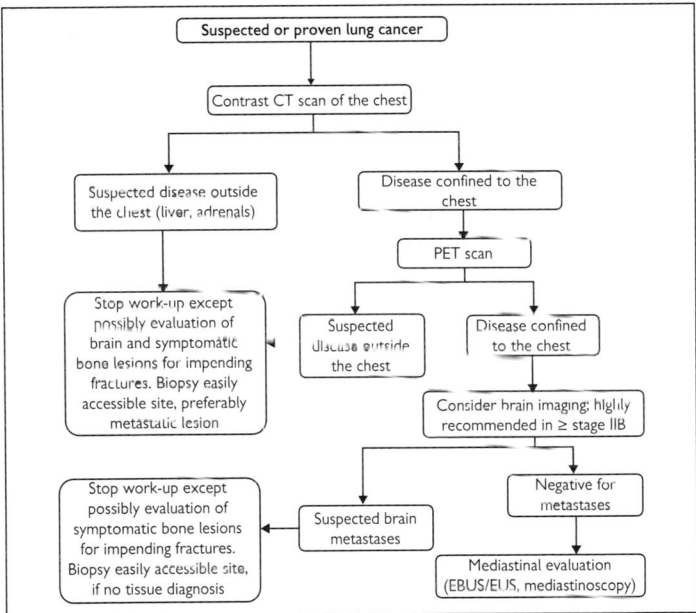

Figure 6.1 Suggested evaluation for a patient with suspected lung cancer. CT, computed tomography; EBUS, endobronchial ultrasound; EUS, endoscopic ultrasound; PET, positron emission tomography.

lesion that has been stable for years (Fig. 6.2). However, CXR cannot accurately detect lymph node, chest wall, or mediastinal involvement.

Chest Computed Tomography

A contrasted CT scan of the chest is mandatory in all patients diagnosed with or suspected of having lung cancer. A routine CT scan of the chest often includes

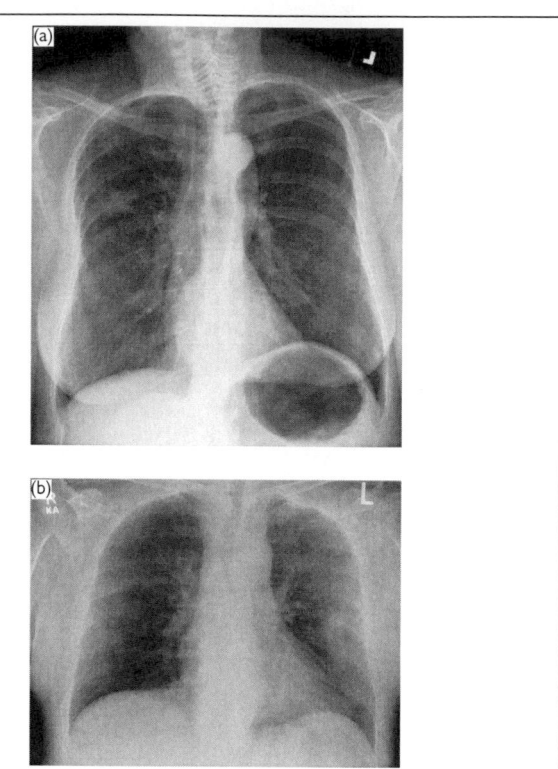

Figure 6.2 Chest radiograph. Chest X-rays showing a right upper lobe spiculated nodular opacity (a) and a left midlung mass (b). Both lesions are concerning for malignancy. (Courtesy of Matthew J. DeVries, MD.)

all the thoracic structures from the base of the neck, including the chest wall, the liver, and adrenal glands.

Positron Emission Tomography

The positron emission tomography (PET) scan provides metabolic information regarding the tumor. It is based on the principle that malignant cells are metabolically more active than normal cells and hence take up more glucose. Cells with increased metabolic activity appear brighter than the surrounding tissues because they take up more 18-fluoro 2-deoxyglucose (^{18}FDG), the tracer used in these scans. PET scan is approved for the evaluation of a solitary pulmonary nodule in addition to the staging of non–small cell lung cancer.

Integrated Computed Tomography-Positron Emission Tomography

CT-PET integrates both CT and PET, thereby providing both anatomic (CT) and metabolic (PET) characterization of the malignancy.

Magnetic Resonance Imaging

Magnetic resonance imaging (MRI) is not routinely used in the chest, but it is useful in the evaluation of the brain and adrenal glands for metastatic disease.

Nuclear Bone Scan

Bone scans help identify osseous metastases using technetium 99m methylene-diphosphonate (^{99m}Tc-MDP). Evaluation for bone metastases is indicated in patients with elevated alkaline phosphatase, especially in the setting of normal bilirubin and other liver enzymes and patients with bone pain or difficulty in bearing weight. In general, osteoblastic bone metastases are better visualized on nuclear bone scan, while osteolytic bone metastases are better visualized on PET-CT.

A more detailed utility of these different modalities in lung cancer staging is described in the next section.

Utility of the Various Modalities in Staging

Primary Tumor

- CT scan is often sufficient for characterization of the primary tumor (Fig. 6.3).
  - CT provides an estimate of the size, presence or absence of other nodules, presence of postobstructive pneumonia (although a PET scan may help demarcate the tumor from the atelectatic lung), and invasion of surrounding structures.
  - Use of intravenous contrast helps distinguish vasculature from non-vascular mediastinal structures such as lymph nodes.
  - CT facilitates assessment of potential involvement by the tumor of the superior vena cava, pulmonary vessels, and cardiac structures.
- PET scan does not help categorize the accurate T stage of the tumor, but it helps distinguish malignancy from other nonmalignant abnormalities seen within the chest.
- The main utility of the MRI of the chest in lung cancer staging is in determining mediastinal invasion of the primary tumor and involvement of the vertebral bodies or brachial plexus.

Mediastinal Lymph Nodes

Thoracic lymph nodes are described according to station (see Fig. 6.4). Stations 1–9 (mediastinal) are N2 (ipsilateral) or N3 (contralateral) nodes. Ipsilateral stations 10–14 (hilar) are N1 nodes.

An understanding of expected lymphatic drainage patterns is relevant to planning mediastinal lymph node evaluation. Nodal pathways are largely dependent on the lobar origin of the tumor and do not differ according to histologic subtype. In general, primary lung cancers drain initially to interlobar and hilar nodes. Subsequent lymphatic drainage is commonly as follows[2]:

- Right Upper Lobe: Right paratracheal, anterior mediastinal
- Right Middle Lobe, Right Lower Lobe: subcarinal → Right paratracheal, anterior mediastinal

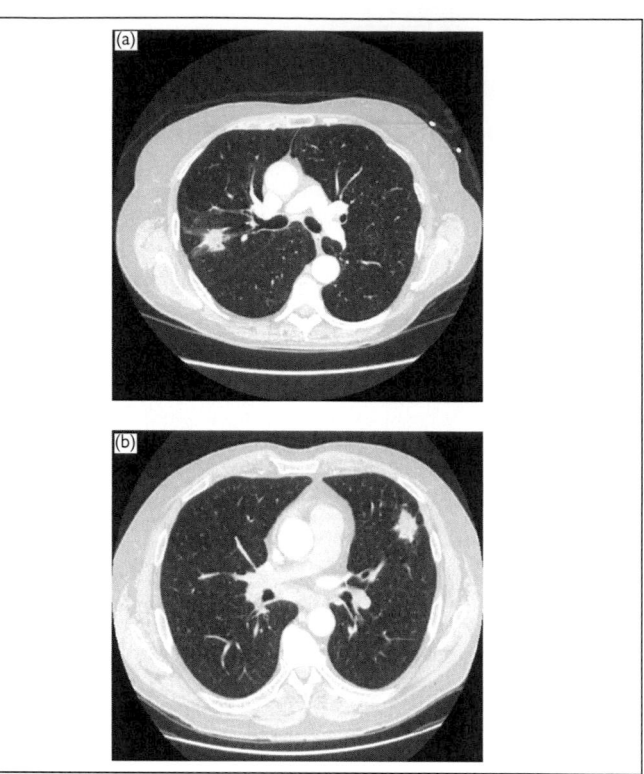

Figure 6.3 Computed tomography (CT) scan characteristics of malignancy. CT images showing right-sided (*a*) and left-sided (*b*) lesions with multiple features suggestive of malignancy: spiculated margins, tethering of the adjacent fissures and pleura, and ectasia of the small airways (bronchiolectasis) (arrow). (Courtesy of Matthew J. DeVries, MD.)

- Left Upper Lobe: subaortic, para-aortic
- Left Lower Lobe: subcarinal, subaortic

In up to 25% of cases, most commonly upper lobe tumors, direct mediastinal nodal involvement may occur without hilar nodal involvement. In rare instances, direct spread to contralateral mediastinal nodal basins has been documented, primarily with lower lobe basal segment tumors. In general, at a minimum, it is recommended that stations 4 and 7 be sampled for right-sided tumors and that stations 5/6 and 7 be sampled for left-sided tumors.

Based on expected lymphatic drainage patterns and radiographic findings, cytologic and/or pathologic evaluation of mediastinal lymph nodes may be performed via a number of techniques:

Noninvasive Staging

CT scans are often the first step in evaluation of the mediastinum (Fig. 6.5). Increased size of mediastinal lymph nodes raises the suspicion of involvement by tumor.

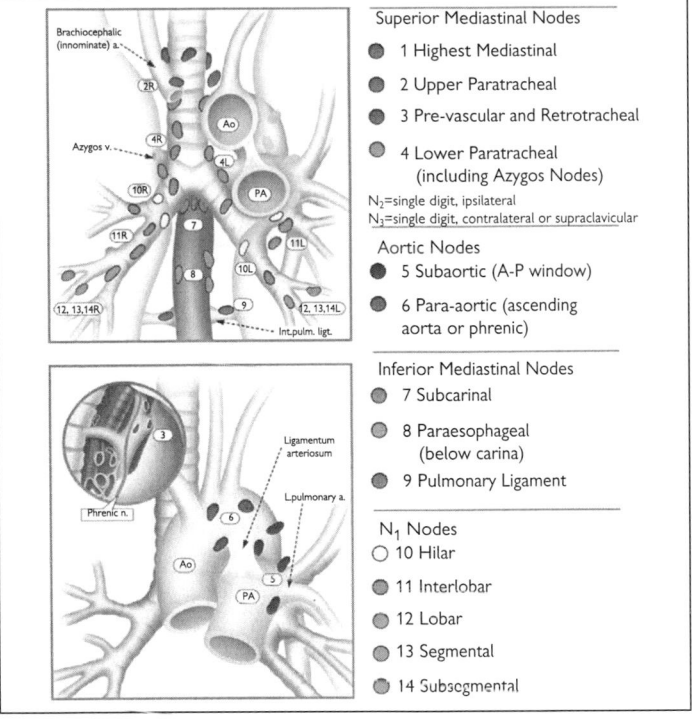

Superior Mediastinal Nodes

● 1 Highest Mediastinal

● 2 Upper Paratracheal

● 3 Pre-vascular and Retrotracheal

○ 4 Lower Paratracheal
(including Azygos Nodes)

N_2=single digit, ipsilateral
N_3=single digit, contralateral or supraclavicular

Aortic Nodes

● 5 Subaortic (A-P window)

● 6 Para-aortic (ascending
aorta or phrenic)

Inferior Mediastinal Nodes

● 7 Subcarinal

● 8 Paraesophageal
(below carina)

● 9 Pulmonary Ligament

N_1 Nodes

○ 10 Hilar

● 11 Interlobar

● 12 Lobar

● 13 Segmental

● 14 Subsegmental

Figure 6.4 Thoracic lymph node stations. Reproduced with permission from the American College of Chest Physicians.[3]

- In a large meta-analysis, CT scans were neither sensitive (51%; 95% confidence interval [CI], 47% to 54%) nor highly specific (85%; 95% CI, 84% to 88%) for identifying mediastinal lymph node involvement.[4]
- PET scans were 74% (95% CI, 69% to 79%) sensitive and 85% (95% CI, 82% to 88%) specific. Thus, PET scans are more accurate in mediastinal evaluation.

Many infectious or inflammatory conditions may lead to false-positive findings. Conversely, radiographically normal nodes may harbor malignancy, even with small, peripheral primary tumors. Approximately 7% of patients with T1 primary tumors and negative CT and PET of the mediastinum harbor occult N2 disease.[5] Accordingly, radiographic assessment alone with CT and PET-CT is often insufficient to confirm mediastinal lymph node status, and cytologic/pathologic evaluation is recommended.

Invasive Mediastinal Staging

Based on expected lymphatic drainage patterns and radiographic findings, cytologic and/or pathologic evaluation of mediastinal lymph nodes may be performed via a number of techniques:

- *Cervical mediastinal exploration (CME)/cervical mediastinoscopy.* This procedure requires general anesthesia and a 1.5-inch anterior incision at the

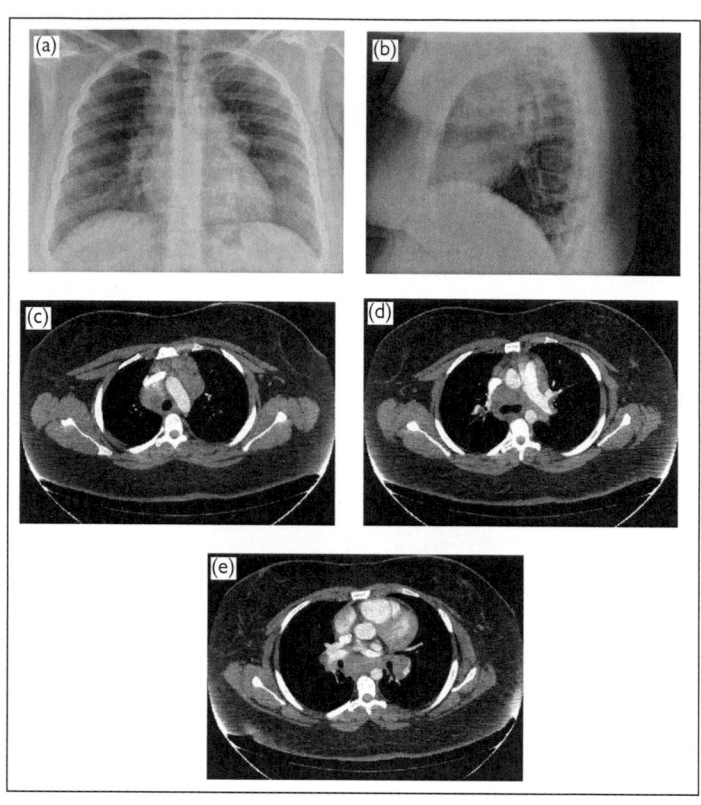

Figure 6.5 Imaging of the mediastinum. Postero-anterior (*a*) and lateral (*b*) chest X-ray shows prominent right paratracheal and bilateral hilar soft tissue consistent with mediastinal and hilar adenopathy. Computed tomography images (*c, d,* and *e*) show adenopathy throughout the mediastinum. (Courtesy of Matthew J. DeVries, MD.)

base of the neck; mediastinoscopy permits direct visualization and biopsy of paratracheal lymph node stations (2R, 2L, 3, 4R, 4L) and usually the anterior subcarinal lymph node (station 7); access to aortopulmonary (AP) window, posterior and inferior mediastinal lymph nodes may be limited; the principal complication is bleeding.

- *Endobronchial ultrasound (EBUS).* With this technique, an ultrasound probe is placed via bronchoscopy and permits US-guided imaging and transbronchial biopsy of lymph node stations 2, 3, 4, 7, 10, and 11; these are performed under conscious sedation or general anesthesia. False-negative findings have been reported, especially at stations 4R and 7.

- *Endoscopic ultrasound (EUS).* This technique is similar to EBUS, but the probe is placed via the esophagus and the procedure is usually performed by a gastroenterologist. It is most useful for assessment of postero-inferior mediastinal lymph node stations (4L, 5, 7, 8, 9).

- *Video-assisted thoracoscopic surgery (VATS)/thoracoscopy.* This is a minimally invasive surgical technique that requires general anesthesia and has higher complication rates than CME. These approaches are most commonly used in settings where (1) lymph node sampling is not feasible by other methods and/or (2) proceeding to surgical resection (wedge resection or lobectomy) is planned during the same operation;

- *Anterior mediastinotomy (Chamberlain procedure).* This procedure requires general anesthesia and a 2-inch incision at the junction of the left 2nd rib and sternum; it provides access to lymph nodes in aortopulmonary window (stations 5 and 6). The main complications include bleeding and pneumothorax.

In a study of 117 patients with potentially operable non–small cell lung cancer, the sensitivity, specificity, and accuracy of PET-CT were 70%, 60%, and 62% versus 90%, 100%, and 97%, respectively, for endobronchial ultrasound (EBUS)–guided transbronchial biopsy.[6] A combination of endosonography (EBUS/EUS) plus mediastinoscopy is more sensitive for detecting mediastinal involvement compared to mediastinoscopy alone (94% vs. 79%).[7] More patients who underwent mediastinoscopy alone had unnecessary thoracotomy as compared to those who underwent endosonography and mediastinoscopy (18% vs. 7%).

In some centers, patients with suspected early-stage, resectable lung cancer may be taken directly to surgery. If mediastinal lymph node sampling is not routinely performed in all patients prior to surgery, generally accepted criteria for mediastinal sampling include the following:

- Clinical stage II disease (i.e., enlarged N1 hilar lymph nodes)
- Enlarged (>1 cm in short axis) mediastinal nodes on CT
- FDG-avid nodes on PET

If mediastinal lymph node sampling is not performed prior to surgery, it may be performed at the time of surgery, prior to resection, as a staged procedure. If not performed prior to surgery, an adequate mediastinal lymph node dissection must be performed with the resection itself.

Distant Metastases

Intrathoracic Lesions

- CT scans can identify pleural nodules, pleural and pericardial effusions, and contralateral lung nodules, all of which may signify M1a disease.

- Pleural effusions seen on a CT scan need to be confirmed cytologically, especially if there is no evidence of disease outside the ipsilateral hemithorax.

- Multiple cytologic examinations of the pleural fluid should be performed before determining the nonmalignant nature of the pleural effusion.

Extrathoracic Soft Tissue Metastases

- A PET scan is more accurate than a CT scan in identifying distant metastases (Fig. 6.6). An integrated PET-CT has higher sensitivity, positive predictive value, and negative predictive value for detecting malignant extrathoracic lesions (92%, 89%, and 98%, respectively) compared to a CT scan (18%, 71%, and 89%, respectively).[7]

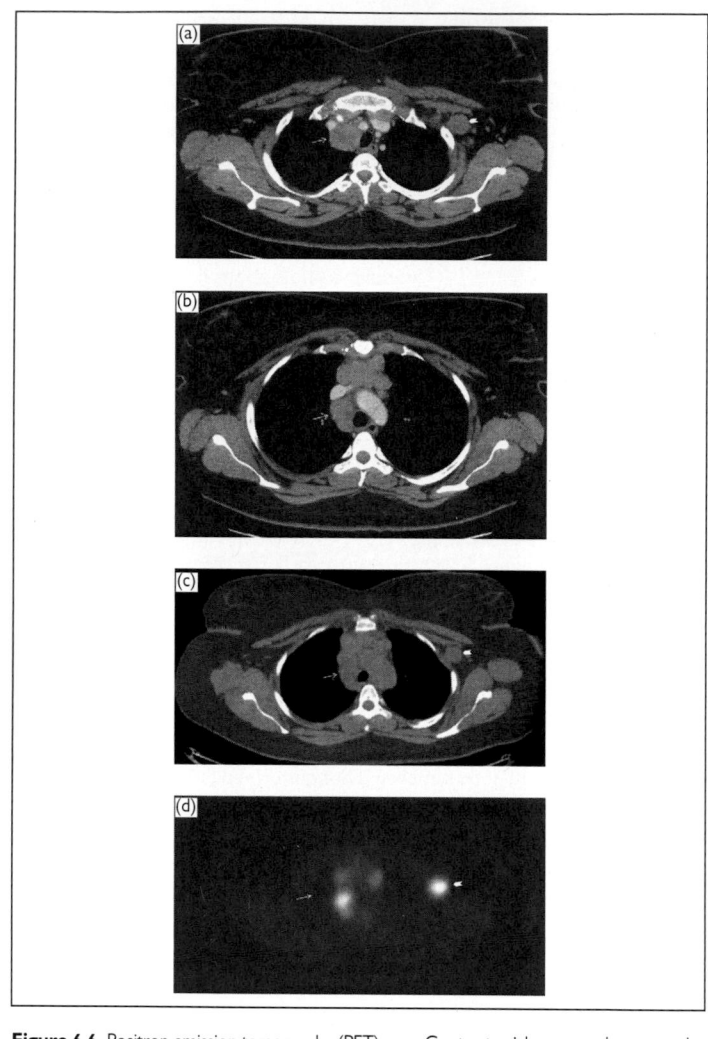

Figure 6.6 Positron emission tomography (PET) scan. Contrast axial computed tomography (CT) images (*a* and *b*) show adenopathy involving the mediastinum (arrow) and left axilla (arrowhead). Non-contrast CT from a PET/CT exam (*c*) shows adenopathy involving the mediastinum (arrow) and left axilla (arrowhead). Attenuation corrected PET images from a PET/CT exam (*d*) show increased glucose avidity correlating with adenopathy involving the mediastinum (arrow) and left axilla (arrowhead). (Courtesy of Matthew J. DeVries, MD.)

- In patients with solitary adrenal lesions, MRI may also be helpful in distinguishing adrenal adenomas from adrenal metastases. However, with the advent of the PET scan the use of MRI in this setting is diminishing.

Brain Metastases

Brain imaging is recommended in all patients with neurological signs and symptoms. In addition, patients who have a large primary lesion or suspected nodal involvement and are candidates for resection, should be offered brain imaging to identify asymptomatic metastatic lesions.

- MRI of the brain (Fig. 6.7) is more sensitive than a contrasted CT scan in identifying brain lesions and is preferred.[4] Approximately 19% of patients who have a solitary metastasis on CT scan will have multiple lesions on an MRI.[9]

- In patients who cannot tolerate an MRI, a CT scan with contrast may be obtained.

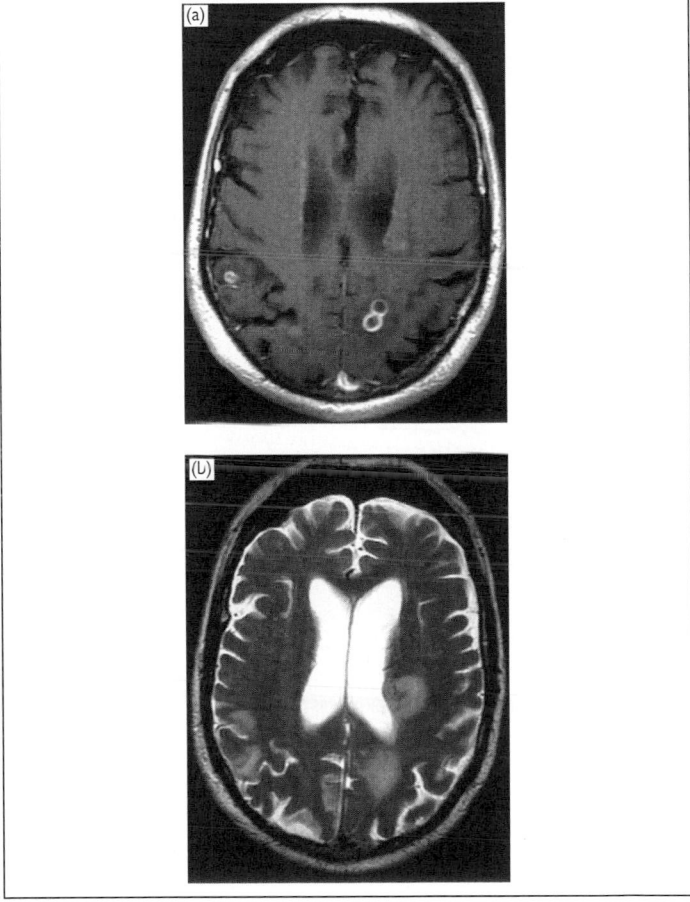

Figure 6.7 Brain magnetic resonance imaging. Post-contrast T1-weighted (*a*) and corresponding T2-weighted (*b*) images are shown. Images show multiple ring enhancing lesions on T1-post-contrast-weighted images with corresponding areas of vasogenic edema on T2-weighted images. (Courtesy of Matthew J. DeVries, MD.)

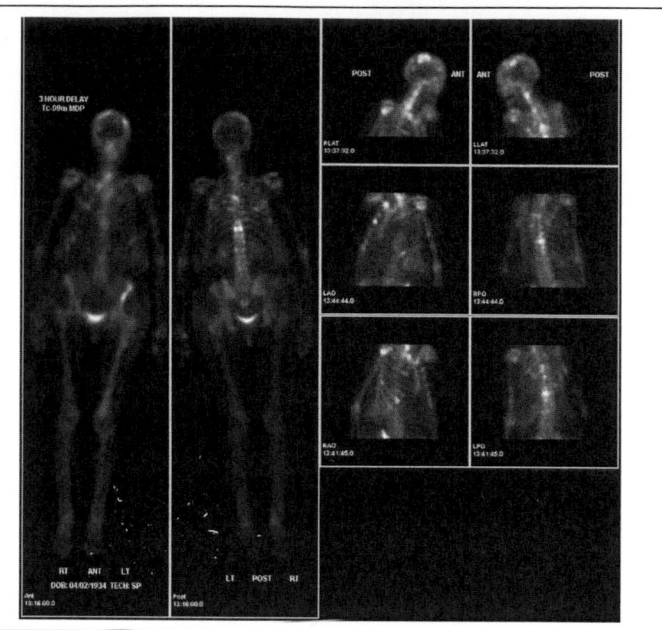

Figure 6.8 Bone scan. Whole-body frontal, posterior, and spot planar image projections from a 3-hour delayed bone scan show multiple foci of increased radiotracer accumulation within the skull, ribs, vertebral bodies, pelvis, left humerus, and left femur consistent with metastases. (Courtesy of Matthew J. DeVries, MD.)

Bone Metastases

Bone imaging is recommended in any patient who has an elevated alkaline phosphatase (in the setting of a normal γ-glutamyl transpeptidase) or symptoms (e.g., focal bone pain) and signs (e.g., inability to bear weight).

- Bone metastases can be identified with a technetium 99m MDP nuclear medicine scan (Fig. 6.8). They are less time consuming and less likely to have false-negative results from osteoblastic lesions.
- PET scans have a similar sensitivity and better specificity at identifying bone metastases compared to bone scans.[10] Moreover, PET scans have the advantage of being able to identify soft tissue metastases as well.

Assessment of Medical Fitness in Patients with Resectable Non–Small Cell Lung Cancer

Patients with suspected early-stage disease should be evaluated for their ability to tolerate surgery (Fig. 6.9). The preoperative evaluation of patients should provide an adequate assessment of the individual's cardiopulmonary capacity, allowing an accurate assessment of the perioperative risk associated with these procedures.

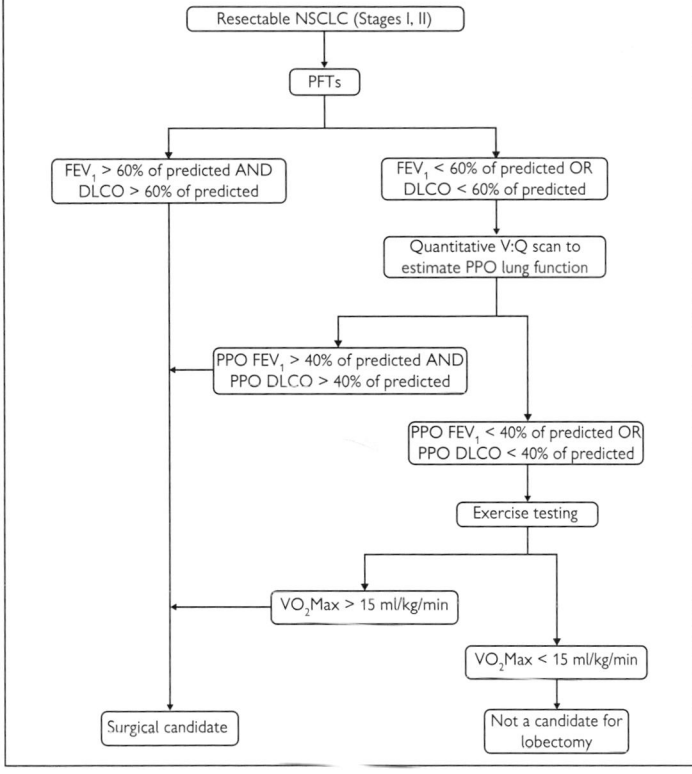

Figure 6.9 Suggested preoperative evaluation for a patient with suspected early-stage (stage I or stage II) disease. DLCO, diffusion capacity for carbon monoxide, FEV₁, forced expiratory volume in 1 second; NSCLC, non–small cell lung cancer; PFTs, pulmonary function tests; PPO, predicted postoperative; VO₂Max, maximum oxygen consumption; V:Q, ventilation perfusion.

Ideally, the operative mortality for patients undergoing a lobectomy should be <5%, and for those undergoing a pneumonectomy, <9%. Therefore, it is recommended that all patients undergoing potentially curative resection be evaluated by a multidisciplinary team that includes a dedicated thoracic surgeon specializing in lung cancer, a medical oncologist, radiation oncologist, and a pulmonologist.

Pulmonary Function Tests

Patients undergoing major thoracic surgical procedures should have baseline pulmonary function tests (PFTs) performed. The information obtained from these tests should include an FEV_1, DLCO, and an arterial blood gas.

FEV_1

- Spirometry, including an FEV_1, is the most commonly utilized test to determine suitability for lung cancer surgery and should be performed when the patient is clinically stable.

- Bronchodilator therapy should be maximized when indicated.
- Operative mortalities <5% have been observed when the preoperative FEV_1 is >1.5 L in patients planned for a lobectomy and >2.0 L in pneumo-nectomy patients.
- Using absolute values may introduce some bias against older patients, those of smaller stature, and women, so patients with an FEV_1 >80% of predicted can tolerate a pneumonectomy when indicated.[11]

In patients whose FEV_1 is <80% of predicted, the predicted postoperative (PPO) lung function can be calculated using a number of methods.

- The easiest method is an anatomic estimation of the number of anatomic lung segments to be resected.[12]
- Ventilation-perfusion scans[13]: In the ventilation phase of the test, a gas-eous radionuclide (technetium diethylene triamine pentaacetic acid [DTPA]) aerosol is inhaled. The perfusion phase of the test involves the intravenous injection of radioactive technetium macroaggregated albumin (Tc99m-MAA). A gamma camera acquires the images for both phases of the study.
- Quantitative perfusion scans: This method is strongly recommended in patients planned for a pneumonectomy as the anatomic method may underestimate the postoperative FEV_1.[12,14]
- Quantitative CT scans: This technique involves spirometry and a conven-tional CT scan. A computer program is then used to quantify the ventila-tion to different parts of the lung.[15]

The lower limit of predicted postoperative FEV_1 is suggested to be ≥0.8 L. Again, use of an absolute number might preclude offering a potentially curative resection to those who are older, of smaller stature, and women, so use of %PPO FEV_1 can be considered in selected patients.[16]

Diffusion Capacity for Carbon Monoxide

- An increased mortality in patients undergoing lung resection was observed in patients having a diffusion capacity for carbon monoxide (DLCO) <60% of predicted.
- Patients with a PPO DLCO <40% have a higher mortality and require further testing prior to undergoing surgical resection.[11,17]

Arterial Blood Gas

- Preoperative hypoxemia, or an arterial oxygen saturation (SaO_2) <90%, has been associated with an increased risk of perioperative respiratory complications.[18]
- Patients with hypercapnea, or a $PaCO_2$ >45mm Hg, are deemed to be at an increased risk of perioperative complications, but recent stud-ies have suggested that hypercapnea is not an independent predictor of complications.[19]

Cardiopulmonary Exercise Stress Testing

In those patients deemed to be marginal, or high-risk candidates based on the above data (PPO FEV_1 and/or PPO DLCO <40%), cardiopulmonary stress test-ing should be performed. This examination measures a number of parameters, including electrocardiogram, heart rate response to exercise, minute ventilation, and oxygen uptake per minute. The test also allows the determination of the maximum oxygen consumption (VO_2 max).

- Patients found to have a VO_2 max between 15 and 20 mL/kg per minute can undergo anatomic lung resection with an acceptably low mortality.[20]
- Patients with a VO_2 max between 10 and 15 mL/kg per minute have an increased perioperative mortality.[21]
- A VO_2 max <10 mL/kg per minute is associated with a very high operative mortality.[22] While surgery can be performed successfully in this group of patients, a thorough discussion of the operative risks and alternative treatment options should be provided to the patient.

Preoperative Cardiac Evaluation

Little data exist regarding the cardiac risk in patients undergoing thoracic surgical procedures.

- Most thoracic procedures fall into the intermediate cardiac risk category, meaning an expected cardiac complication rate of <5%, although some procedures, especially pneumonectomy, convey higher risk.
- The most widely used system for predicting cardiac risk is the Revised Cardiac Risk Index (RCRI). The risk predictors in this index include ischemic heart disease, heart failure, cerebrovascular disease, chronic renal insufficiency (serum creatinine >2), insulin-dependent diabetes mellitus, and high-risk surgery.[23] Patients with three or more risk factors are considered to be at high risk, those with 0–1 risk factors would be at low risk, and the remainder in the intermediate risk group. Postoperative cardiac complications would be expected in 10%, 5%, and 1%, in the high-, intermediate-, and low-risk groups, respectively.
- Formal cardiac stress testing should be obtained in those patients felt to be at higher risk for perioperative cardiac complications.[24]

References

1. Goldstraw P, Crowley J, Chansky K, et al. The IASLC Lung Cancer Staging Project: proposals for the revision of the TNM stage groupings in the forthcoming (seventh) edition of the TNM Classification of malignant tumours. *J Thorac Oncol* 2007;2:706–14.

2. Sharma A, Fidias P, Hayman LA, Loomis SL, Taber KH, Aquino SL. Patterns of lymphadenopathy in thoracic malignancies. *Radiographics* 2004;24:419–34.

3. Mountain CF, Dresler CM. Regional lymph node classification for lung cancer staging. *Chest* 1997;111:1718–23.

4. Silvestri GA, Gould MK, Margolis ML, et al. Noninvasive staging of non-small cell lung cancer: ACCP evidenced-based clinical practice guidelines (2nd edition). *Chest* 2007;132:178S–201S.

5. Lee PC, Port JL, Korst RJ, et al. Risk factors for occult mediastinal metastases in clinical stage I non-small cell lung cancer. *Ann Thorac Surg* 2007;84:177–81.

6. Hwangbo B, Kim SK, Lee HS, et al. Application of endobronchial ultrasound-guided transbronchial needle aspiration following integrated PET/CT in mediastinal staging of potentially operable non-small cell lung cancer. *Chest* 2009;135:1280–7.

7. Annema JT, van Meerbeeck JP, Rintoul RC, et al. Mediastinoscopy vs endo-sonography for mediastinal nodal staging of lung cancer: a randomized trial. *JAMA* 2010;304:2245–52.

8. De Wever W, Vankan Y, Stroobants S, Verschakelen J. Detection of extrapul-monary lesions with integrated PET/CT in the staging of lung cancer. *Eur Respir J* 2007;29:995–1002.

9. Schellinger PD, Meinck HM, Thron A. Diagnostic accuracy of MRI compared to CCT in patients with brain metastases. *J Neurooncol* 1999;44:275–81.

10. Bury T, Barreto A, Daenen F, Barthelemy N, Ghaye B, Rigo P. Fluorine-18 deox-yglucose positron emission tomography for the detection of bone metastases in patients with non-small cell lung cancer. *Eur J Nuclear Med* 1998;25:1244–7.

11. Wyser C, Stulz P, Solèr M, et al. Prospective evaluation of an algorithm for the functional assessment of lung resection candidates. *Am J Respir Crit Care Med* 1999;159:1450–6.

12. Zeiher BG, Gross TJ, Kern JA, Lanza LA, Peterson MW. Predicting postop-erative pulmonary function in patients undergoing lung resection. *Chest* 1995;108:68–72.

13. Wernly JA, DeMeester TR, Kirchner PT, Myerowitz PD, Oxford DE, Golomb HM. Clinical value of quantitative ventilation-perfusion lung scans in the sur-gical management of bronchogenic carcinoma. *J Thorac Cardiovasc Surg* 1980;80:535–43.

14. Smulders SA, Smeenk FW, Janssen-Heijnen ML, Postmus PE. Actual and pre-dicted postoperative changes in lung function after pneumonectomy: a retro-spective analysis. *Chest* 2004;125:1735–41.

15. Wu MT, Chang JM, Chiang AA, et al. Use of quantitative CT to predict postop-erative lung function in patients with lung cancer. *Radiology* 1994;191:257–62.

16. Bolliger CT, Wyser C, Roser H, Solèr M, Perruchoud AP. Lung scanning and exercise testing for the prediction of postoperative performance in lung resec-tion candidates at increased risk for complications. *Chest* 1995;108:341–8.

17. Ferguson MK, Little L, Rizzo L, et al. Diffusing capacity predicts morbidity and mortality after pulmonary resection. *J Thorac Cardiovasc Surg* 1988;96:894–900.

18. Turner SE, Eastwood PR, Cecins NM, Hillman DR, Jenkins SC. Physiologic responses to incremental and self-paced exercise in COPD: a comparison of three tests. *Chest* 2004;126:766–73.

19. Harpole DH, Liptay MJ, DeCamp MM Jr., et al. Prospective analysis of pneumo-nectomy: risk factors for major morbidity and cardiac dysrhythmias. *Ann Thorac Surg* 1996;61:977–82.

20. Win T, Jackson A, Sharples L, et al. Cardiopulmonary exercise tests and lung cancer surgical outcome. *Chest* 2005;127:1159–65.

21. Wang J, Olak J, Ultmann RE, Ferguson MK. Assessment of pulmonary complica-tions after lung resection. *Ann Thorac Surg* 1999;67:1444–7.

22. Bechard D, Wetstein L. Assessment of exercise oxygen consumption as preop-erative criterion for lung resection. *Ann Thorac Surg* 1987;44:344–9.

23. Lee TH, Marcantonio ER, Mangione CM, et al. Derivation and prospective vali-dation of a simple index for prediction of cardiac risk of major noncardiac sur-gery. *Circulation* 1999;100:1043–9.

24. Cohn SL. Preoperative cardiac evaluation of lung resection candidates. *Thorac Surg Clin* 2008;18:45–59.

Chapter 7

Early Stage Non–Small Cell Lung Cancer

Rudy P. Lackner, Raghav Murthy, Kemp H. Kernstine, Puneeth Iyengar, and Apar Kishor Ganti

Approximately 40% of all patients with non–small cell lung cancer (NSCLC) present at an early stage, where cure is the goal of treatment. Surgery is the mainstay of the treatment of these patients. Patients with resected stages II and IIIA NSCLC benefit from adjuvant chemotherapy following resection. Radiation therapy is recommended for patients who are either not candidates for or decline surgical options.

Preoperative Evaluation

The detailed preoperative evaluation of patients undergoing surgical resection has been discussed in Chapter 6. In summary, patients who are considered for resection must have adequate pulmonary reserve demonstrated by pulmonary function tests (PFTs), arterial blood gas (ABG), and—in some cases— cardiopulmonary exercise stress testing. Typical requirements for resection include the following criteria:

- Predicted postoperative 1-second forced expiratory volume (FEV_1) >0.8 L
- FEV_1 and carbon monoxide diffusing capacity (DLCO) >60% of predicted
- Maximal oxygen uptake (VO_{2max}) >15 mL/kg per minute

These criteria roughly correspond to the ability to walk up more than one flight of stairs without stopping.

Thoracic Surgeon and Facility

Whenever possible, lung resections should be performed by a thoracic surgeon with a dedicated interest in lung cancer, as these cases have the lowest operative mortality and are associated with better long-term survival.[1] Also the procedure should be performed at a facility that is sufficiently staffed, equipped, and has appropriate experience to provide optimal care.[2,3]

Diagnostic Thoracoscopy

In an attempt to minimize the number of futile thoracotomies, a diagnostic video-assisted thoracoscopy (VATS) should be considered an integral component of any planned open resection.

- This procedure will permit a thorough examination of the pleural space and will allow for biopsies of any unexpected intraoperative findings.
- In cases where computed tomography (CT) findings of invasion are raised, a diagnostic thoracoscopy can facilitate inspection of these areas, which may change the planned surgical approach.[4,5]

Surgical Management

Multiple options exist for the surgical management of patients diagnosed with lung cancer. The surgical procedures span the spectrum to include those considered limited resections, as well as more complex extended operations, which may require a multispecialty team. The extent of surgical resection represents a balance between obtaining appropriate surgical margins and maintaining adequate residual pulmonary reserve.

Lobectomy

- A lobectomy, or bilobectomy, should be considered the indicated operation for those patients diagnosed with lung cancer.[6] The operative mortality for a lobectomy should be <2%. Bilobectomy involves the resection of the right upper and middle lobes (for a tumor that crosses the minor fissure or abuts an incomplete fissure) or the right middle and lower lobes (for a centrally located lower lobe tumor in close proximity to the middle lobe bronchus).
- These procedures may be accomplished via a muscle-sparing thoracotomy, but a standard posterolateral thoracotomy is an acceptable approach. Other approaches include an anterolateral thoracotomy, axillary thoracotomy, median sternotomy, VATS, and robotic approaches.
- When the surgical expertise is available, a VATS lung resection is the preferred choice for a lobectomy, as it is associated with lower morbidity.[7]

Sublobar Resections

- Patients undergoing limited surgical resection have a higher local recurrence rate compared to a lobectomy: 3 times higher for a wedge resection and 2.4 times higher for a segmentectomy.[8]
- Sublobar resections can be considered in those patients with marginal lung function. An anatomic segmentectomy via VATS is the preferred option to further minimize the risks of local recurrence. Surgical margins should be at least equal to the size of the tumor resected.[9]

Pneumonectomy and Sleeve Lobectomy

- Patients with larger, more centrally located tumors may require a pneumonectomy in order to accomplish a complete resection. However, the operative mortality for a pneumonectomy is 5%–6% for left-sided and 10%–15% in patients undergoing a right-sided pneumonectomy.[10]
- Hence, whenever possible, consideration should be given to lung-conserving procedures, including sleeve lobectomy. In this setting, if the primary tumor originates from or invades the airway, rather than perform a pneumonectomy, the involved airway is resected and then a primary reconstruction is performed. Mortality from sleeve lobectomy is about 4%.[11]

Extended Resections

These resections are not commonly performed and should only be performed by a team thoroughly familiar with these complex operations. Included in this group are patients with the following:

- Large tumors needing lung resection plus chest wall resection and reconstruction
- Pancoast tumors
- Tumors involving the trachea or carina
- Superior vena cava involvement requiring resection and reconstruction of the superior vena cava
- Large T4 tumors that will need resection of the atrium, main pulmonary artery, aorta, esophagus, or vertebral bodies.[12,13]

Mediastinal Nodal Evaluation

- A thorough evaluation of the mediastinal lymph nodes is required in all patients undergoing anatomic lung resections to stage the patient accurately and to allow for more informed recommendations regarding adjuvant therapy.
- A formal mediastinal lymph node dissection is recommended, but at the very least, a systematic sampling of the mediastinal nodes should be performed.
- On the right-side levels, 2R, 4R, 7, 8, and 9 should be included, while on the left-side levels 4L, 5, 6, 7, 8, and 9 are targeted.[14]

Surgical Complications

With the median age of patients diagnosed with lung cancer approximately 70 years, multiple comorbidities can be expected. As one would anticipate in this patient population, the range of complications is wide.

- *Pulmonary*: Atelectasis, pneumonia, respiratory distress syndrome/failure, noncardiogenic pulmonary edema, prolonged air leaks, subcutaneous emphysema, and broncho-pleural fistulas.

- *Pleural space*: Effusions, hemothorax, chylothorax, and empyema.
- *Cardiovascular*: Myocardial infarction and atrial fibrillation are the most common; the latter being encountered more commonly in patients over the age of 70 years.
- *Neurological*: Phrenic and recurrent laryngeal nerve injury. Transient ischemic attacks and strokes are relatively uncommon following lobectomy.
- *Drug induced*: The use of narcotic analgesics is associated with mental status changes and severe constipation, especially in older patients.
- *Other*: Deep venous thrombosis (DVT)/pulmonary embolism (PE) and urinary tract infections are seen infrequently with the careful use of DVT prophylaxis and early removal of indwelling bladder catheters.

Radiation Therapy for Patients with Inoperable Lung Cancer

Conventional Fractionated Radiation Therapy

As previously stated, for patients with early-stage NSCLC who are operable candidates, lobectomy is the preferred treatment modality. For patients who are not operable for medical reasons, external beam radiation should then be considered. Five-year lung cancer disease-specific survival for stage I, medically inoperable NSCLC group is 10%–25%, suggesting that despite other medical comorbidities, these individuals will succumb to malignancy more often than not.[15,16]

For medically inoperable patients treated with fractionated radiation for local therapy for early-stage NSCLC, outcomes are better than no treatment but worse than lobectomy. Median overall survival (OS) for these patients is 1.5 years, with 20% 5-year survival. Data from the Surveillance Epidemiology and End Results (SEER) database have demonstrated that radiation offers a survival benefit of 5–7 months over no treatment.[16] The attempted fractionated doses delivered to these lung tumors ranged from 45 Gray (Gy) to 66 Gy. For further details on general approaches to conventional thoracic radiation, see Chapter 8 (Locally Advanced Non–Small Cell Lung Cancer).

The take-home message from these evaluations was that while standard fractionation radiation offered a clear benefit to this patient population versus no treatment, it was still inferior to optimal surgical resection. Studies with radiation alone did not achieve a maximum tolerated dose (MTD) in a majority of these studies, making it difficult to determine an optimal total dose and schedule.[17]

Stereotactic Body Radiation Therapy

Stereotactic body radiation therapy (SBRT) is a type of external beam radiation that employs higher doses per fraction in a more limited number of treatments as a means of "ablating" disease. SBRT is considered biologically more effective in promoting tumor kill due to the higher doses delivered per treatment. This form of "hypofractionated" radiotherapy is gaining momentum as a means of controlling local disease for a variety of malignancies, including NSCLC. Typical doses used in SBRT range from 12 to 20 Gy per fraction and are approximately

8–10 times that of conventional radiation fractions. These higher doses are permissible without an increase in normal tissue toxicity through the following advances:

- High-definition imaging for better target delineation
- Ability to image tumors immediately prior to treatment for assessing accuracy of radiation delivery
- Techniques to account for tumor motion during treatment and more effective patient immobilization to limit tumor motion during treatment.[18]

Multiple studies have provided impetus for the mainstream use of SBRT for NSCLC in medically inoperable candidates. Table 7.1 provides comparative primary tumor control rates for stage I NSCLC treated with various SBRT regimens.[19–28]

A Phase II study at Indiana University included 70 medically inoperable, clinical T1N0 NSCLC patients treated with SBRT to a dose of 60 Gy in three fractions and T2N0 (less than 7 cm) patients treated to 66 Gy in three fractions.[19] Two-year local control was 95%, median OS was 2.7 years, and 2-year OS was 55%. At 50 months, 3-year local control was 88% and OS was 42%. The study also showed, however, that patients with centrally located lesions (within 2 cm of the proximal bronchial tree) had 46% severe (grade 3–5) toxicities (including six treatment-related deaths) versus 17% for patients with peripheral tumors.[29] Four of the six deaths were attributed to pneumonia, potentially as a result of reduced pulmonary toilet capabilities from radiation.

The Radiation Therapy Oncology Group (RTOG) undertook a Phase II, multicenter trial to assess the efficacy of stereotactic treatments for peripheral early-stage NSCLC.[20] Fifty-five patients with medically inoperable T1-T2 N0 NSCLC disease were included with lesions <5 cm. Mediastinal staging was based on imaging studies only. All patients were treated with 54 Gy in three fractions.

Table 7.1 Primary Tumor Control Results Following Stereotactic Body Radiation Therapy of Stage I Lung Tumors

Author	Primary Tumor Control	Treatment Dose
Zimmermann[21]	87% (3 years)	12.5 Gy × 3
Nyman[23]	80% (crude)	15 Gy × 3
Fritz[26]	80% (3 years)	30 Gy × 1
Baumann[28]	92% (3 years)	15 Gy × 3
Timmerman[29]	95% (2 years)	20–22 Gy × 3
Nagata[25]	94% (3 years)	12 Gy × 4
Hara[24]	80% (3 years)	30–34 Gy × 1
Xia[22]	95% (3 years)	5 Gy × 10
Lagerwaard[27]	93% (crude)	20 Gy × 3, 12 Gy × 5, or 7.5 Gy × 8
Timmerman[20]	98% (3 years)	18 Gy × 3
Gy, gray.		

The 3-year tumor control rate was 98% with a median follow-up of 2.9 years. At three years, local (tumor plus lobe) control was 91%, loco-regional control was 87%, distant metastasis rate was 22%, and median OS was 48 months. No deaths were attributed to treatment. Three-year disease-free survival was 48%; 3-yr OS was 56%.[20]

Future Directions

Currently, several studies are attempting to identify optimal total dose and dose per fraction for SBRT treatment of NSCLC. Efforts are also being made to determine the largest lesions that can safely and effectively be treated and the ultimate limitations that tumor location places on total dose and dose per fraction for NSCLC. Studies are also underway evaluating the role of SBRT in medically operable patients with early-stage NSCLC.

Recommendations

- For peripheral T1 or T2 lesions up to 5 cm, SBRT to a dose of 54 Gy over three fractions is a standard approach.
- For lesions closer to the chest wall, 12 Gy given five times to a total dose of 60 Gy is reasonable as the higher dose per fraction may increase the risk of musculoskeletal pain and rib fractures.
- For lesions larger than 5 cm and for central lesions, SBRT is not recommended. Instead, fractionated radiation to 60–70 Gy at 2 Gy per fraction is considered appropriate.

Adjuvant Chemotherapy Following Resection of Early-Stage Non–Small Cell Lung Cancer

Despite complete resection, a substantial proportion of early-stage NSCLC will recur.[30,31] Hence, the 5-year survival of such cases is only between 45% and 70%.[32–37] To improve outcomes, both chemotherapy and radiation therapy have been given after surgery.

Role of Chemotherapy

In 1995, a meta-analysis showed that the use of cisplatin-based chemotherapy following surgical resection of NSCLC resulted in a 13% decreased risk of death (5% overall survival [OS] benefit) at 5 years.[38] This led to the conduct of multiple phase III trials comparing platinum-based doublets to observation following resection (Table 7.2).[39–42]

The Lung Adjuvant Cisplatin Evaluation (LACE) was a meta-analysis of these newer trials.[43] This analysis, which included five trials and 4584 patients, found a benefit for chemotherapy for both OS (HR, 0.89; 95% CI, 0.82–0.96; $P = 0.005$) and DFS (HR, 0.84; 95% CI, 0.78-0.91; $P = 0.001$). This translated to an 11% reduction in the risk of death and absolute benefit of 5.4% at 5 years. Another meta-analysis of surgery plus chemotherapy versus surgery alone, based on 34 trials and 8447 patients, showed a benefit from chemotherapy after surgery (HR, 0.86, 95% CI 0.81–0.92, $P < 0.0001$), with a 4% absolute increase in survival at 5 years (64% vs. 60%).[44]

Table 7.2 Contemporary Trials of Adjuvant Chemotherapy

Study	n	Drug	Stage	Outcomes
IALT[39,51]	1867	Cisplatin + etoposide, vinblastine, vinorelbine, or vindesine × 3–4 cycles	I-IIIA	Benefit for adjuvant therapy on OS ($P = 0.10$) and DFS ($P = 0.02$). Significant difference between the results of OS before and after 5 years ($P = 0.01$ vs. $P = 0.04$); P-value for interaction = 0.006.
JBR 10[40]	482	Cisplatin 50 mg/m^2 days 1 and 8 every 4 weeks × 4 cycles; Vinorelbine 25 mg/m^2 weekly × 16 weeks	IB, II (excl. T3N0)	Benefit for chemotherapy at 9 years ($P = 0.04$). Benefit restricted to node positive patients. 73% grade 3/4 neutropenia.
CALGB 9633[41]	344	Paclitaxel 200 mg/m^2; Carboplatin AUC 6 every 3 weeks × 4 cycles	IB	No difference in OS. Significant benefit for subset of patients with tumors ≥4 cm ($P = 0.04$).
ANITA[42]	840	Vinorelbine 30 mg/m^2 weekly × 16 weeks; Cisplatin 100 mg/m^2 every 4 weeks × 4 cycles	IB-IIIA	5 yr OS: 51% with chemotherapy vs. 43% ($P = 0.017$). After 76 months of follow-up, median survival 66 vs. 44 months. 85% grade 3/4 neutropenia.

ANITA, Adjuvant Navelbine International Trialist Association; AUC, area under the curve; CALGB, Cancer and Leukemia Group B; DFS, disease-free survival; IALT, International Adjuvant Lung Cancer Trial; OS, overall survival.

Effect of Individual Agents

While many chemotherapy regimens have been assessed in the adjuvant setting, there have not been any head-to-head comparisons between different regimens. The LACE meta-analysis, which included only modern cisplatin-based regimens, possibly provides more relevant support for the selection of adjuvant treatment.[43]

A planned subgroup analysis of the LACE analysis showed that cisplatin-vinorelbine was marginally better than other combinations ($P = 0.11$ for OS; $P = 0.07$ for DFS). Higher planned doses of cisplatin (cumulative dose >300 mg/m^2) showed a favorable trend toward benefit. This may also have accounted for the beneficial effects seen with the cisplatin-vinorelbine combination, as the median planned dose of cisplatin when combined with vinorelbine was higher compared to cisplatin doses in other combinations. It is unlikely that the dose of vinorelbine has a major impact on the efficacy of adjuvant chemotherapy, as studies using different doses found similar benefit.

All but one of these trials used cisplatin, leading to a preference for cisplatin in the adjuvant setting. The only trial to use carboplatin (Cancer and Leukemia Group B [CALGB] 9633, which was limited to resected stage IB) did not show an OS benefit for carboplatin-based therapy. It may be argued, however, that cisplatin-based therapy has not demonstrated a benefit for stage IB patients either.

Although the majority of evidence is in favor of cisplatin-vinorelbine, a combination of cisplatin and any third-generation agent (paclitaxel, docetaxel, gemcitabine, pemetrexed, vinorelbine) is probably reasonable, given the equivalence in advanced-stage trials.[45] A recent phase II study showed that cisplatin-pemetrexed was better tolerated compared to cisplatin-vinorelbine.[46] The trial, however, is still ongoing, and outcome data are awaited.

Benefit of Chemotherapy by Stage

The benefits of adjuvant chemotherapy seem to be more pronounced in the more advanced stages. The benefit seen in the JBR.10 trial seemed to be confined to node-positive patients,[40] with a suggestion for a benefit in patients with node-negative tumors >4 cm. Similarly, the maximum benefit in the International Adjuvant Lung Cancer Trial (IALT)[39] and Adjuvant Navelbine International Trialist Association (ANITA)[42] trials was in patients with resected stage IIIA disease. While the overall results of CALGB 9633 did not show any advantage to adjuvant chemotherapy, an unplanned subset analysis showed that patients with tumors ≥4 cm in diameter who received adjuvant chemotherapy had a significant survival advantage.[11]

In the LACE meta-analysis[43] patients with stage IA appeared to do worse after adjuvant chemotherapy (HR, 1.40; 95% CI, 0.95–2.06), while patients with stages II and III seemed to benefit (HR for stage II, 0.83; 95% CI, 0.73–0.95; HR for stage III, 0.83; 95% CI, 0.72–0.94). Patients with stage IB did not seem to benefit from chemotherapy (HR, 0.93; 95% CI, 0.78–1.10). The results of the larger meta-analysis appear to be similar.[44] In that analysis, there seemed to be absolute improvements in 5-year survival of 3% for stage IA and 5% for stages IB–IIIA. However, the number of patients with stage IA in these trials is too small to make any definite conclusions.

Benefit of Chemotherapy by Performance Status

There appeared to be a detrimental effect of adjuvant chemotherapy for patients with a poor performance status (PS) in the trials that included this population. These findings have been further confirmed in the meta-analyses. Thus, although the number of PS 2 patients studied is low, the consistent harm seen suggests that these patients should not be offered adjuvant chemotherapy.

Benefit of Chemotherapy by Age

Although older patients seem to have more treatment delays, age did not seem to affect either chemotherapy tolerance or outcomes following adjuvant chemotherapy.[47] Hence, age should not be a limiting factor while making a decision regarding adjuvant chemotherapy.

Role of Targeted Therapy

The role of targeted agents in treatment of surgically resected lung cancer is still evolving. Currently there are no data suggesting a survival benefit with adjuvant molecularly targeted therapy, but results of the RADIANT trial (adjuvant erlotinib) (NCT00373425) are awaited. This trial included patients who have EGFR-positive tumors (by either immunohistochemistry and/or fluorescence *in situ* hybridization). Studies targeting molecularly defined populations (*EGFR* mutation and *ALK* rearrangement) are currently in development.

Commonly Used Adjuvant Chemotherapy Regimens

- Cisplatin + vinorelbine:
  - Cisplatin 75 mg/m^2 IV day 1; Vinorelbine 30 mg/m^2 IV days 1 and 8. Repeat every 3 weeks for four cycles.
  - Cisplatin 100 mg/m^2 IV day 1. Repeat every 4 weeks for four cycles; Vinorelbine 25 mg/m^2 IV weekly for 16 weeks.
- Cisplatin + gemcitabine: Cisplatin 75 mg/m^2 IV day 1; Gemcitabine 1200 mg/m^2 IV days 1 and 8. Repeat every 3 weeks for four cycles.
- Cisplatin + pemetrexed (nonsquamous histology): Cisplatin 75 mg/m^2 IV day 1; Pemetrexed 500 mg/m^2 IV day 1. Repeat every 3 weeks for four cycles. Start vitamin supplementation 1 week before initial dose of pemetrexed until 21 days after last dose of pemetrexed: folic acid 350–1000 mcg PO daily plus vitamin B12 1000 mcg IM every 9 weeks. Dexamethasone 4 mg bid the day before, the day of, and the day after pemetrexed.
- Cisplatin + docetaxel: Cisplatin 75 mg/m^2 IV day 1; Docetaxel 75 mg/m^2 IV day 1. Repeat every 3 weeks for four cycles. Dexamethasone 8 mg bid the day before, the day of, and the day after docetaxel.

Postoperative Radiation Therapy

For clinical stage I and II disease found to be pathologic stage III disease at the time of resection, postoperative external beam radiation may be recommended for improvement in local control. Specifically, the presence of mediastinal lymph node involvement in the resection specimen, positive margins (microscopic or gross), and/or lymphovascular space involvement (LVSI) could be reasons for offering radiation postoperatively. Postoperative radiotherapy (PORT) should be considered on a case-by-case basis for patients with these adverse pathologic features as it may be detrimental to patients without these pathologic features.

A meta-analysis including information on 2128 patients from 15 randomized trials assessed the effect of PORT.[48] The results of this analysis showed a significant adverse effect of postoperative radiotherapy on survival (HR, 1.21; 95% CI 1.08–1.34). This seemed to be more pronounced in earlier stage disease, with stage IIIA patients demonstrating no obvious adverse outcomes following postoperative radiation therapy. The results of the PORT meta-analysis have been questioned based on inappropriate patient selection (more than half of patients had N2 disease) and inadequate staging. Additionally, most of the included studies involved the use of obsolete radiotherapy devices (i.e., cobalt-60 units) and techniques, as well as high total (60 Gy) and daily radiotherapy (2.6–3.0 Gy) doses.

A SEER database analysis of T1-3N1-2 patients confirmed these observations.[49] Patients with N0 (HR, 1.18; 95% CI, 1.01–1.38; $P = 0.04$) and N1 (HR, 1.10; 95% CI, 1.02–1.19; $P = 0.02$) nodal disease had a significant decrease in survival with PORT. However, patients with N2 nodal disease seemed to have a significant benefit (HR, 0.86; 95% CI, 0.76–0.96; $P = 0.008$). The use of chemotherapy was not specified in the SEER analysis and therefore the role of PORT in the setting of systemic therapy was not addressed. The results of the ANITA study help address this question. The intent to use PORT was declared for each patient prospectively prior to study entry. Although only 28% of patients received PORT, patients with pN2 disease had improved overall survival if they received PORT following systemic therapy, while those with N1 disease did not.[42]

The Lung Cancer Study Group (LCSG) assessed the impact of adjuvant therapy in patients with incompletely resected lung cancer (positive surgical margins or metastasis in the highest paratracheal node sampled).[50] Patients were randomized to PORT given as two courses of 4 Gy/d x 5 days separated by 3 weeks or PORT with cyclophosphamide, doxorubicin, and cisplatin given on day 1 weekly during PORT. Patients who received concurrent chemotherapy and radiation had a significantly longer recurrence-free survival ($P = 0.004$) and a 14% improvement in survival compared to those who received radiation alone (68% vs. 54%). Although neither the chemotherapy nor the radiotherapy regimen is routinely used today, the data suggest a possible benefit to concurrent therapy for patients with incompletely resected disease.

The role of postoperative radiation is being evaluated in the European Lung Adjuvant Radiotherapy Trial (LungART) study, which is randomizing patients with completely resected NSCLC and N2 disease to radiation (54 Gy in 27–30 fractions) and chemotherapy or to chemotherapy alone.

References

1. Silvestri GA, Handy J, Lackland D, Corley E, Reed CE. Specialists achieve better outcomes than generalists for lung cancer surgery. *Chest* 1998;114:675–80.

2. Bach PB, Cramer LD, Schrag D, Downey RJ, Gelfand SE, Begg CB. The influence of hospital volume on survival after resection for lung cancer. *N Engl J Med* 2001;345:181–8.

3. Birkmeyer JD, Stukel TA, Siewers AE, Goodney PP, Wennberg DE, Lucas FL. Surgeon volume and operative mortality in the United States. *N Engl J Med* 2003;349:2117–27.

4. Massone PP, Lequaglie C, Magnani B, Ferro F, Cataldo I. The real impact and usefulness of video-assisted thoracoscopic surgery in the diagnosis and therapy of clinical lymphadenopathies of the mediastinum. *Ann Surg Oncol* 2003;10:1197–202.

5. Sebastian-Quetglas F, Molins L, Baldo X, Buitrago J, Vidal G. Clinical value of video-assisted thoracoscopy for preoperative staging of non-small cell lung cancer. A prospective study of 105 patients. *Lung Cancer* 2003;42:297–301.

6. Manser R, Wright G, Hart D, Byrnes G, Campbell DA. Surgery for early stage non-small cell lung cancer. *Cochrane Database Syst Rev* 2005;CD004699.

7. Villamizar NR, Darrabie MD, Burfiend WR, et al. Thoracoscopic lobectomy is associated with lower morbidity compared with thoracotomy. *J Thorac Cardiovasc Surg* 2009;138:419–25.

8. Ginsberg RJ, Rubinstein LV. Randomized trial of lobectomy versus limited resection for T1 N0 non-small cell lung cancer. Lung Cancer Study Group. *Ann Thorac Surg* 1995;60:615–22.

9. El-Sherif A, Gooding WE, Santos R, et al. Outcomes of sublobar resection versus lobectomy for stage I non-small cell lung cancer: a 13-year analysis. *Ann Thorac Surg* 2006;82:408–16.

10. Watanabe S, Asamura H, Suzuki K, Tsuchiya R. Recent results of postoperative mortality for surgical resections in lung cancer. *Ann Thorac Surg* 2004;78:999–1002.

11. Yildizeli B, Fadel E, Mussot S, Fabre D, Chataigner O, Dartevelle PG. Morbidity, mortality, and long-term survival after sleeve lobectomy for non-small cell lung cancer. *Eur J Cardiothorac Surg* 2007;31:95–102.

12. Osaki T, Sugio K, Hanagiri T, et al. Survival and prognostic factors of surgically resected T4 non-small cell lung cancer. *Ann Thorac Surg* 2003;75:1745–51.

13. Shargall Y, de Perrot M, Keshavjee S, et al. 15 years single center experience with surgical resection of the superior vena cava for non-small cell lung cancer. *Lung Cancer* 2004;45:357–63.

14. Allen MS, Darling GE, Decker PA, et al. Number of lymph nodes harvested from a mediastinal lymphadenectomy: results of the randomized, prospective ACOSOG Z0030 trial. ASCO Meeting Abstracts 2007;25: abstr 7555.

15. Kaskowitz L, Graham MV, Emami B, Halverson KJ, Rush C. Radiation therapy alone for stage I non-small cell lung cancer. *Int J Radiat Oncol Biol Phys* 1993;27:517–23.

16. Wisnivesky JP, Bonomi M, Henschke C, Iannuzzi M, McGinn T. Radiation therapy for the treatment of unresected stage I-II non-small cell lung cancer. *Chest* 2005;128:1461–7.

17 Sura S, Yorke E, Jackson A, Rosenzweig KE. High-dose radiotherapy for the treatment of inoperable non-small cell lung cancer. *Cancer J* 2007;13:238 42.

18. Potters L, Steinberg M, Rose C, et al. American Society for Therapeutic Radiology and Oncology and American College of Radiology practice guideline for the performance of stereotactic body radiation therapy. *Int J Radiat Oncol Biol Phys* 2004;60:1026–32.

19. McGarry RC, Papiez L, Williams M, Whitford T, Timmerman RD. Stereotactic body radiation therapy of early stage non-small-cell lung carcinoma: phase I study. *Int J Radiat Oncol Biol Phys* 2005;63:1010–15.

20. Timmerman R, Paulus R, Galvin J, et al. Stereotactic body radiation therapy for inoperable early stage lung cancer. *JAMA* 2010;303:1070–6.

21. Zimmermann FB, Geinitz H, Schill S, et al. Stereotactic hypofractionated radiation therapy for stage I non-small cell lung cancer. *Lung Cancer* 2005;48:107–14.

22. Xia T, Li H, Sun Q, et al. Promising clinical outcome of stereotactic body radiation therapy for patients with inoperable Stage I/II non-small-cell lung cancer. *Int J Radiat Oncol Biol Phys* 2006;66(1):117–25.

23. Nyman J, Johansson KA, Hulten U. Stereotactic hypofractionated radiotherapy for stage I non-small cell lung cancer—mature results for medically inoperable patients. *Lung Cancer* 2006;51:97–103.

24. Hara R, Itami J, Kondo T, et al. Clinical outcomes of single-fraction stereotactic radiation therapy of lung tumors. *Cancer* 2006;106:1347–52.

25. Nagata Y, Takayama K, Matsuo Y, et al. Clinical outcomes of a phase I/II study of 48 Gy of stereotactic body radiotherapy in 4 fractions for primary lung cancer using a stereotactic body frame. *Int J Radiat Oncol Biol Phys* 2005;63:1427–31.

26. Fritz P, Kraus HJ, Mühlnickel W, et al. Stereotactic, single-dose irradiation of stage I non-small cell lung cancer and lung metastases. *Radiat Oncol* 2006;1:30.

27. Lagerwaard FJ, Haasbeek CJ, Smit EF, Slotman BJ, Senan S. Outcomes of risk-adapted fractionated stereotactic radiotherapy for stage I non-small-cell lung cancer. *Int J Radiat Oncol Biol Phys* 2008;70:685–92.

28. Baumann P, Nyman J, Hoyer M, et al. Outcome in a prospective phase II trial of medically inoperable stage I non-small-cell lung cancer patients treated with stereotactic body radiotherapy. *J Clin Oncol* 2009;27:3290–6.

29. Timmerman R, McGarry R, Yiannoutsos C, et al. Excessive toxicity when treating central tumors in a phase II study of stereotactic body radiation therapy for medically inoperable early-stage lung cancer. *J Clin Oncol* 2006;24:4833–9.

30. Feld R, Rubinstein LV, Weisenberger TH. Sites of recurrence in resected stage I non-small-cell lung cancer: a guide for future studies. *J Clin Oncol* 1984;2:1352–8.

31. Immerman SC, Vanecko RM, Fry WA, Head LR, Shields TW. Site of recurrence in patients with stages I and II carcinoma of the lung resected for cure. *Ann Thorac Surg* 1981;32:23–7.

32. Mountain CF. A new international staging system for lung cancer. *Chest* 1986;89:225S–33S.

33. Holmes EC. Treatment of stage II lung cancer (T1N1 and T2N1). *Surg Clin North Am* 1987;67:945–9.

34. Naruke T, Goya T, Tsuchiya R, Suemasu K. Prognosis and survival in resected lung carcinoma based on the new international staging system. *J Thorac Cardiovasc Surg* 1988;96:440–7.

35. Williams DE, Pairolero PC, Davis CS, et al. Survival of patients surgically treated for stage I lung cancer. *J Thorac Cardiovasc Surg* 1981;82:70–6.

36. Shimizu J, Watanabe Y, Oda M, et al. [Results of surgical treatment of stage I lung cancer]. *Nippon Geka Gakkai Zasshi* 1993;94:505–10.

37. Shah R, Sabanathan S, Richardson J, Mearns AJ, Goulden C. Results of surgical treatment of stage I and II lung cancer. *J Cardiovasc Surg (Torino)* 1996;37:169–72.

38. Non-small Cell Lung Cancer Collaborative Group. Chemotherapy in non-small cell lung cancer: a meta-analysis using updated data on individual patients from 52 randomised clinical trials. Non-small Cell Lung Cancer Collaborative Group. *BMJ* 1995;311:899–909.

39. Arriagada R, Bergman B, Dunant A, et al. Cisplatin-based adjuvant chemotherapy in patients with completely resected non-small-cell lung cancer. *N Engl J Med* 2004;350:351–60.

40. Butts CA, Ding K, Seymour L, et al. Randomized phase III trial of vinorelbine plus cisplatin compared with observation in completely resected stage IB and II non-small-cell lung cancer: updated survival analysis of JBR-10. *J Clin Oncol* 2010;28:29–34.

41. Strauss GM, Herndon JE II, Maddaus MA, et al. Adjuvant paclitaxel plus carboplatin compared with observation in stage IB non-small-cell lung cancer: CALGB 9633 with the Cancer and Leukemia Group B, Radiation Therapy Oncology Group, and North Central Cancer Treatment Group Study Groups. *J Clin Oncol* 2008;26:5043–51.

42. Douillard JY, Rosell R, De Lena M, et al. Adjuvant vinorelbine plus cisplatin versus observation in patients with completely resected stage IB-IIIA non-small-cell

lung cancer (Adjuvant Navelbine International Trialist Association [ANITA]): a randomised controlled trial. *Lancet Oncol* 2006;7:719–27.

43. Pignon JP, Tribodet H, Scagliotti GV, et al. Lung adjuvant cisplatin evaluation: a pooled analysis by the LACE Collaborative Group. *J Clin Oncol* 2008;26:3552–9.

44. Arriagada R, Auperin A, Burdett S, et al. Adjuvant chemotherapy, with or without postoperative radiotherapy, in operable non-small-cell lung cancer: two meta-analyses of individual patient data. *Lancet* 2010;375:1267–7.

45. Kalemkerian GP. Adjuvant therapy for non-small-cell lung cancer. *Lancet* 2010;375:1230–1.

46. Kreuter M, Vansteenkiste J, Fischer JR, et al. Randomized phase II trial on refinement of early-stage NSCLC adjuvant chemotherapy with cisplatin and pemetrexed (CPx) versus cisplatin and vinorelbine (CVb): TREAT. *J Clin Oncol* 2011;29 (suppl; abstr 7002).

47. Arriagada R, Auperin A, Burdett S, et al. Adjuvant chemotherapy, with or without postoperative radiotherapy, in operable non-small-cell lung cancer: two meta-analyses of individual patient data. *Lancet* 2010;375:1267–77.

48. PORT Meta-analysis Trialists Group. Postoperative radiotherapy in non-small-cell lung cancer: systematic review and meta-analysis of individual patient data from nine randomised controlled trials. PORT Meta-analysis Trialists Group. *Lancet* 1998;352:257–63.

49. Lally BE, Zelterman D, Colasanto JM, Haffty BG, Detterbeck FC, Wilson LD. Postoperative radiotherapy for stage II or III non-small-cell lung cancer using the surveillance, epidemiology, and end results database. *J Clin Oncol* 2006;24:2998–3006.

50. The benefit of adjuvant treatment for resected locally advanced non-small-cell lung cancer. The Lung Cancer Study Group. *J Clin Oncol* 1988;6:9–17.

51. Le Chevalier T, Dunant, A, Arriagada, R, et al. Long-term results of the International Adjuvant Lung Cancer Trial (IALT) evaluating adjuvant cisplatin-based chemotherapy in resected non-small cell lung cancer (NSCLC). *J Clin Oncol* 2008;26 (suppl; abstr 7507).

Chapter 8

Locally Advanced Non–Small Cell Lung Cancer

David E. Gerber and Puneeth Iyengar

Locally advanced (stage III) non–small cell lung cancer (NSCLC) includes a diverse range of clinical scenarios, including the following:

- T4 primary tumors that invade the mediastinum, great vessels, vertebral column, or feature multiple nodules in separate ipsilateral lobes
- Any primary tumor with mediastinal or supraclavicular (N2 or N3) nodal involvement

The evaluation and treatment of locally advanced NSCLC is arguably the most controversial area in thoracic oncology. Debated points include the following:

- The role of invasive mediastinal staging techniques, including mediastinoscopy, endobronchial ultrasound (EBUS), and thoracoscopy
- The determination of what constitutes "operable" stage IIIA disease, with many experts questioning the role of surgery altogether for stage III disease
- The role and type of preoperative therapy
- The role of assessing pathologic response after preoperative therapy
- The optimal chemotherapy regimen
- The dose and technique of radiation therapy

Pretreatment Evaluation

Recommended radiographic studies include chest computed tomography (CT) (including adrenals), positron emission tomography (PET)-CT, and brain magnetic resonance imaging (MRI). Brain imaging is required even in the absence of symptoms, as approximately 20% of patients otherwise appearing to have stage III disease will have asymptomatic brain metastases.[1] In patients with superior sulcus tumors, an MRI of the thoracic inlet is useful to assess vertebral body and/or brachial plexus involvement.

Mediastinal Lymph Node Assessment

In patients with no evidence of extrathoracic disease radiographically (by CT, PET-CT, brain MRI), assessment of mediastinal nodal status is a key component of disease staging for suspected locally advance disease. In almost all instances, radiographic assessment alone with CT and PET-CT is insufficient to rule in or

out mediastinal lymph node involvement, and cytologic or pathologic evaluation is recommended. Mediastinal lymph node anatomy, drainage patterns, and
evaluation techniques are reviewed in Chapter 6.

Medical Fitness Assessment

As the case for early-stage NSCLC, patients with locally advanced disease who
are considered for resection must have adequate pulmonary reserve demonstrated by pulmonary function tests (PFTs) and arterial blood gas (ABG).
Typical requirements for resection are described in Chapter 6.

For definitive radiation therapy in patients with locally advanced disease, a
1-second forced expiratory volume (FEV_1) greater than 1–1.5 L is a commonly
used criterion. For both surgery and radiation therapy, ongoing smoking is associated with substantial increased risk of complications.

Treatment Selection

Given the complexity and heterogeneity of locally advanced NSCLC, multidisciplinary evaluation is critical. While there is no widely accepted standard treatment
for these patients, it is generally agreed that no single treatment modality—surgery, radiation, or chemotherapy—is itself sufficient therapy. Pivotal clinical trials
evaluating stage III NSCLC treatment are listed in Table 8.1. All studies listed
are phase III clinical trials, with the exception of the LAMP (Locally Advanced
Multimodality Protocol) trial (randomized phase II).

The initial management decision is resectability. In locally advanced NSCLC,
surgical resection is generally limited to patients with adequate medical fitness
and "non-bulky" stage IIIA disease.

"Bulky" disease is variably defined. A reasonable definition includes the
following:

- Lymph nodes greater than 2–3 cm in short-axis diameter, measured
  by CT
- Involvement of contralateral N3 lymph nodes
- Groupings of multiple smaller lymph nodes
- Involvement of more than two lymph node stations

"Non-Bulky" Stage IIIA Disease

Possible approaches to "non-bulky" stage IIIA NSCLC include the following:

- Neoadjuvant chemotherapy followed by surgery[11–13]
- Surgery followed by adjuvant chemotherapy (with or without sequential
  postoperative radiation therapy [PORT] to the mediastinum)[6]
- Radiation therapy plus chemotherapy (either concurrent [preferable] or
  sequential)[4,5]
- A trimodality approach[9]

Surgery

The incorporation of surgery into multimodality approaches has been shown
to prolong disease control rates but not overall survival. Surgical resection may

Table 8.1 Pivotal Clinical Trials for Locally Advanced Non–Small Cell Lung Cancer

Trial (year)	Treatment Radiation Therapy	Chemotherapy	Median PFS	HR P	Median OS	HR P	Conclusions
CALGB 8433[2] (1990)	60 Gy (2.0 Gy x 30 fx) (starting 2–3 weeks after completion of chemotherapy)	Cisplatin 100 mg/m² days 1, 29 plus Vinblastine 5 mg/m² days 1, 8, 15, 22, 29	8.2 months	P = 0.03	13.7 months (19% 5-yr OS)	P = 0.012	Sequential chemotherapy followed by radiation is superior to radiation alone
	60 Gy (2.0 Gy x 30 fx)	None	5.5 months		9.6 months (7% 5-yr OS)		
West Japan Lung Cancer Group[3] (1999)	56 Gy (2.0 Gy x 14 fx then 10 day rest then 2.0 Gy x 14 fx) (split-course) (concurrent with chemotherapy)	Cisplatin 80 mg/m² days 1, 29 plus Vindesine 3 mg/m² days 1, 8, 29, 36 plus Mitomycin 8 mg/m² days 1, 29	8.3 months	P = 0.15	16.5 months (15.8% 5-yr OS)	P = 0.039	Concurrent chemoradiotherapy is superior to sequential chemoradiotherapy
	56 Gy (2.0 Gy x 28 fx) (after completion of chemotherapy)	Sequential Cisplatin-Vindesine-Mitomycin C	8.0 months		13.3 months (8.9% 5-yr OS)		
RTOG 9410[4] (2003)	63 Gy (1.8 Gy x 25 fx then 2.0 Gy x 9 fx) (after completion of chemotherapy) [Arm 1]	Cisplatin 100 mg/m² days 1, 29 plus Vinblastine 5 mg/m² days 1, 8, 15, 22, 29	NR	No significant difference	14.6 months (10% 5-yr OS)	HR 0.81, P = 0.046 (Arm 2 vs. Arm 1)	Concurrent chemoradiotherapy is superior to sequential chemoradiotherapy
	63 Gy (1.8 Gy x 25 fx then 2.0 Gy x 9 fx) (concurrent with chemotherapy) [Arm 2]	Cisplatin 100 mg/m² days 1, 29 plus Vinblastine 5 mg/m² days 1, 8, 15, 22, 29			17.0 months (16% 5-yr OS)	HR 0.93, P = 0.46 (Arm 2 vs. Arm 3)	
	69.6 Gy (1.2 Gy twice daily x 58 fx) (concurrent with chemotherapy) [Arm 3]	Cisplatin 50 mg/m2 days 1, 8, 29, 36 plus Etoposide 50 mg PO bid days 1–5 8–12, 25–33, 36–40			15.6 months (13% 5-yr OS)		

(continued)

Table 8.1 (Continued)

Trial (year)	Treatment		Median PFS	HR P	Median OS	HR P	Conclusions
	Radiation Therapy	Chemotherapy					
LAMP: ACR 427[5] (2005)	63.0 Gy (1.8 Gy x 25 fx then 2.0 Gy x 9 fx) (after completion of chemotherapy) [Arm 1: sequential]	Carboplatin AUC 6 day 1 plus paclitaxel 200 mg/m² day 1 x 2 cycles	9.0 months	NR (noncomparative study)	13.0 months (17% 3-yr OS)	NR (noncomparative study)	Concurrent chemoradiotherapy followed by consolidation chemotherapy seems to be associated with best outcomes
	63.0 Gy (1.8 Gy x 25 fx then 2.0 Gy x 9 fx) (concurrent with weekly chemotherapy) [Arm 2: induction/ concurrent]	Carboplatin AUC 6 day 1 plus paclitaxel 200 mg/m² day 1 x 2 cycles followed by weekly Carboplatin AUC 2 plus Paclitaxel 45 mg/m²	6.7 months		12.7 months (15% 3-yr OS)		
	63.0 Gy (1.8 Gy x 25 fx then 2.0 Gy x 9 fx) (concurrent with weekly chemotherapy) [Arm 3: concurrent/consolidation]	Weekly Carboplatin AUC 2 plus Paclitaxel 45 mg/m² followed by Carboplatin AUC 6 day 1 plus Paclitaxel 200 mg/m² day 1 x 2 cycles	8.7 months		16.3 months (17% 3-yr OS)		
ANITA[6] (2006) (stage IB-IIIA)	45–60 Gy (2.0 Gy fractions) administered to 22% of patients after chemotherapy (at discretion of treating physician—not randomized)	Cisplatin 100 mg/m² day 1 plus Vinorelbine 30 mg/m² days 1, 8, 15, 22 x 4 cycles	36.3 months	HR 0.76, P = 0.002	65.7 months (For stage IIIA, 42% 5-yr OS) (For N2 disease, 5-yr OS 47% with RT, 34% without RT)	HR 0.80, P = 0.017 (For stage IIIA, HR 0.69)	Adjuvant chemotherapy improves overall survival for resected stage IB-IIIA. The role of postoperative RT needs to be clearly defined.
	45–60 Gy (2.0 Gy fractions) administered to 33% of patients after surgery (at discretion of treating physician—not randomized)	None	20.7 months		43.7 months (For stage IIIA, 26% 5-yr OS) (For N2 disease, 5-yr OS 21% with RT, 17% without RT)		

HOG LUN 01–24/USO-023[7] (2008)	59.4 Gy (1.8 Gy × 33 fx)	Cisplatin 50 mg/m² days 1, 8, 29, 36 plus Etoposide 50 mg/m² days 1–5, 29–33 during radiotherapy followed by Docetaxel 75 mg/m² every 3 weeks x 3 cycles	NR	P = 0.960	21.2 months (26.1% 3-yr OS)	P = 0.88	Consolidation chemotherapy with docetaxel after concurrent chemoradiotherapy does not improve survival.
	59.4 Gy (1.8 Gy × 33 fx)	Cisplatin 50 mg/m² days 1, 8, 29, 36 plus Etoposide 50 mg/m² days 1–5, 29–33 during radiotherapy			23.2 months (27.1% 3-yr OS)		
SWOG 0023[8] (2008)	61.0 Gy (1.8- to 2.0-Gy fractions)	Cisplatin 50 mg/m² days 1, 8, 29, 36 plus Etoposide 50 mg/m² days 1–5, 29–33 during radiotherapy followed by Docetaxel 75 mg/m² every 3 weeks x 3 cycles followed by Gefitinib 250 mg PO daily until progression	8.3 months	HR 0.80, P = 0.17	23.0 months	HR 0.63, P = 0.013	Gefitinib results in inferior survival compared with placebo when delivered as maintenance therapy after concurrent chemoradiotherapy.
	61.0 Gy (1.8- to 2.0-Gy fractions)	Cisplatin 50 mg/m² days 1, 8, 29, 36 plus Etoposide 50 mg/m² days 1–5, 29–33 during radiotherapy followed by Docetaxel 75 mg/m² every 3 weeks x 3 cycles followed by placebo PO daily until progression	11.7 months		35.0 months		

(continued)

Table 8.1 (Continued)

Trial (year)	Treatment		Median PFS	HR P	Median OS	HR P	Conclusions
	Radiation Therapy	Chemotherapy					
INT 0139[9] (2009)	45 Gy (1.8 Gy x 25 fx) concurrent with chemotherapy before surgery (wedge resection 2%, lobectomy 63%, pneumonectomy 35%)	Cisplatin 50 mg/m² days 1, 8, 29, 36 plus Etoposide 50 mg/m² days 1–5, 29–33 during radiotherapy then repeated after surgery	12.8 months (22% 5-yr OS)	HR 0.77, P = 0.017	Overall: 23.6 months (27% 5-yr OS) Lobectomy: 33.6 months (36% 5-yr OS) Pneumonectomy: 18.9 months (22% 5-yr OS)	HR 0.87, P = 0.24 (Lobectomy vs. chemoradio-therapy: P = 0.02)	PFS improved with trimodality therapy (concurrent chemoradiotherapy followed by surgery) compared to chemoradiotherapy alone, but no difference in OS. In exploratory analysis, OS improved for patients who underwent lobectomy, but not pneumonectomy, versus chemoradiotherapy.
	61 Gy (1.8 Gy x 34 fx) concurrent with chemotherapy	Cisplatin 50 mg/m² days 1, 8, 29, 36 plus Etoposide 50 mg/m² days 1–5, 29–33 during radiotherapy then repeated after radiotherapy	10.5 months (11% 5-yr OS)		22.2 months (20% 5-yr OS)		

RTOG 0617 (2011) (10)	60 Gy concurrent with weekly chemotherapy	Weekly Carboplatin AUC 2 plus Paclitaxel 45 mg/m² followed by Carboplatin AUC 6 day 1 plus paclitaxel 200 mg/m² every 21 days x 2 cycles ± Cetuximab 400 mg/m² loading dose then 250 mg/m² weekly throughout treatment	NR	NR	NR	NR	At interim analysis, 74 Gy arms closed because higher dose of radiotherapy did not improve survival. 60 Gy arms remain open. Effect of cetuximab not yet known.
	74 Gy concurrent with weekly chemotherapy	Weekly Carboplatin AUC 2 plus Paclitaxel 45 mg/m² followed by Carboplatin AUC 6 day 1 plus paclitaxel 200 mg/m² every 21 days x 2 cycles ± Cetuximab 400 mg/m² loading dose then 250 mg/m² weekly throughout treatment	NR		NR		

ACR, American College of Radiology; ANITA, Adjuvant Navelbine International Trialist Association; CALGB, Cancer and Leukemia Group B; Gy, Gray; HOG LUN, Hoosier Oncology Group Lung; HR, hazard ratio; INT, intergroup; LAMP, Locally Advanced Multimodality Protocol; NR, not reported; OS, overall survival; PFS, progression-free survival; RT, radiation therapy; RTOG, Radiation Therapy Oncology Group; SWOG, Southwestern Oncology Group; USO, US Oncology.

be associated with considerable morbidity and mortality. In patients treated with this approach, the benefit of surgery appears greatest for patients who "clear" the mediastinum (i.e., have negative pathologic evaluation of sampled lymph nodes) after induction therapy; the toxicity of therapy appears greatest for patients who require a pneumonectomy.

The following are commonly recognized indications for pneumonectomy for the treatment of malignant disease[14]:

- Tumor located in a mainstem bronchus or proximal bronchus intermedius
- Tumor located adjacent to right upper lobe orifice
- Tumor extending across a major fissure

The phase III Intergroup 0139 trial provides several insights into the role of surgery in trimodality therapy.[9] In this study, 202 patients (median age 59 years) with stage IIIA (T1-T3pN2M0) NSCLC were randomized to concurrent chemoradiation with or without subsequent surgical resection. Specifically, all patients received thoracic radiation therapy to 45 Gy with two cycles of cisplatin-etoposide chemotherapy administered concurrently. Following this induction therapy, a repeat CT scan was performed. If there was no evidence of disease progression, patients in Group 1 underwent surgical resection, while patients in Group 2 received additional thoracic radiation therapy to a total dose of 61 Gy. Patients in both groups received two cycles of consolidation cisplatin-etoposide chemotherapy. The following results were observed:

- Progression-free survival was superior in the surgery arm: median 12.8 months versus 10.5 months ($P = 0.017$).
- There was not a significant difference in overall survival: median 25.6 months with surgery versus 22.2 months without surgery ($P = 0.24$); 5-year OS 27% with surgery versus 20% without surgery ($P = 0.10$).
- Treatment-related deaths were more common in the surgery arm: 8% versus 2%.
- Patients in the surgery arm who underwent lobectomy had numerically improved overall survival compared to matched patients in the no-surgery arm: median 33.6 months versus 21.7 months; 5-year overall survival 36% versus 18%.
- Patients in the surgery arm who underwent pneumonectomy had numerically inferior overall survival compared to matched patients in the no-surgery arm: median 18.9 months versus 29.4 months; 5-year overall survival 22% versus 24%.
- Among patients assigned to surgery, survival was greatest in the subset that had pathologically negative lymph nodes at the time of resection:
  - TxN0: median OS 34 months; 5-year OS 41%
  - TxN1-3 or unknown: median OS 26.4 months; 5-year OS 24%
  - No surgery: median OS 7.9 months; 5-year OS 8%

Radiation Therapy

Thoracic radiation therapy for locally advanced lung cancer is employed as a component of trimodality therapy, with chemotherapy for unresectable patients, or as monotherapy in certain patients with poor functional status. If radiation therapy is not administered before surgery, commonly used indications for postoperative radiation therapy (PORT) include positive surgical margins, N2 mediastinal disease, and lymphovascular space invasion. The benefit of PORT in resected N2 cases stands in contrast to resected N0 and N1 cases. In a SEER database analysis, patients with N0 (HR: 1.176; 95% CI, 1.005–1.376; P = 0.04) and N1 (HR: 1.097; 95% CI, 1.02–1.19; P = 0.0196) nodal disease had a significant *decrease* in survival with PORT. However, patients with N2 nodal disease seemed to have a significant survival *benefit* (HR: 0.855; 95% CI, 0.76–0.96; P = 0.0077).[15] In the ANITA trial, the use of PORT was not randomized but was specified prospectively by treating physicians. A survival advantage was seen among patients with N2 disease, but not among patients with N1 disease.[6]

Traditionally, radiation is offered in fractions or treatments. The dose for each of these fractions usually ranges from 1.8 Gray (Gy) to 2 Gy. The following are general recommendations for radiation therapy administration for patients with locally advanced lung cancer:

- In patients planned for surgery, a radiation therapy dose of 45 Gy in 25 fractions at 1.8 Gy per fraction is administered preoperatively. The radiation field encompasses gross disease seen on imaging and/ or bronchoscopic examination plus adequate margins for microscopic disease (typically 8 mm) and setup error (determined by the radiation oncologist).

- In unresectable patients, a radiation therapy dose of 60–63 Gy in 30–35 fractions (1.8–2.0 Gy per fraction) is administered with chemotherapy (concurrently or sequentially) or alone. The radiation field encompasses the same volumes as treatment in the preoperative setting. Higher radiation doses (e.g., 74 Gy) do not yield improved outcomes.[10]

- In patients with unresectable stage III disease for whom up-front radiation therapy is not feasible due to the extensive volume of disease and associated risk of pneumonitis or other significant toxicity, induction chemotherapy may be administered, followed by concurrent chemoradiation. The postinduction disease volume is used for radiation treatment planning.

- For patients with stage III disease identified at surgery, radiation therapy is administered postoperatively if there is pathologic N2 disease at the time of resection, a positive surgical margin, or—in some centers—nodal extracapsular extension. Radiation is typically given after adjuvant chemotherapy. The radiation field targets the ipsilateral hilum, the bronchial stump for a positive margin, and involved nodal stations (with perhaps one additional nodal station superiorly and inferiorly). A standard dose is 50.4 Gy in 1.8 Gy fractions or 50 Gy in 2 Gy fractions. The dose may be increased to 56 Gy for nodal extracapsular extension, to 60 Gy for a microscopic positive margin, and to 60–66 Gy for a grossly positive margin.

Basic radiation therapy parameters and definitions are described as follows:

- *Definitive treatment*: Total dose is commonly 63 Gy/35 fractions at 1.8 Gy per fraction (based on RTOG 9410[4]) or 60 Gy/30 fractions at 2 Gy per fraction (based on RTOG 0617 standard arm[10]). Many studies have used doses between 60 and 66 Gy in 30–33 fractions with equivalent benefit.

For superior sulcus lesions (Pancoast tumor), 1.8 Gy fractions to 63 Gy is recommended.[16]

- *Gross tumor volume (GTV)*: Volume representing disease evident radiographically and/or by physical examination, bronchoscopy, or other clinical tool.

- *Clinical target volume (CTV)*: Volume representing the best determination of the extent beyond GTV that microscopic disease may be present but is not visualized by imaging or physical examination. Commonly set at an 8 mm expansion from GTV out of bone, vessel, and adjacent normal structures of involvement such as heart, esophagus, and lung if dealing with mediastinal disease.

- *Planning target volume (PTV)*: Volume representing an expansion beyond the CTV which accounts for daily setup error in patient positioning and machine calibration. Generally set at 5 mm if daily imaging performed; otherwise set at up to 10 mm.

- The ultimate final treatment dose is prescribed and directed to the PTV. To adjudicate the quality of the radiation treatment plan created, standard goals include the following: (1) delivering 100% of the total dose to at least 95% of the total PTV, (2) not allowing any part of the PTV to receive more than 110% of the prescribed dose, and (3) not allowing any part of the PTV to receive less than 90% of the prescribed dose. For instance, if the PTV is to receive 60 Gy, at least 95% of the PTV should receive that dose. No portion of the PTV should receive higher than 66 Gy or lower than 54 Gy.

- For lung cancer treatment, 6 MV photon energies are preferred. Higher energy beams such as 18 MV photons may increase the risk of neutron contamination, which could lead to an increased rate of secondary malignancies and cause overshooting of dose due to lung interfaces with tumor.

- Recommended standard organ tolerances are as follows:
  - Total lung V20 (volume [excluding GTV] receiving 20 Gy) <35% with concurrent therapy, <40% with radiation alone
  - Mean lung dose <20 Gy
  - Spinal cord <45 Gy
  - Heart V40 (volume receiving 40 Gy) <50%
  - Esophagus mean dose <34 Gy

- *Proton therapy*, a form of particle therapy (versus standard X-ray or photon therapy), offers the theoretical advantage of equivalently conformal tumor targeting, but less toxicity due to the absence of radiation deposited distally to the tumor. Photons or X-rays will deposit some dose after entering the patient's body proximal to the tumor and some dose distal to the tumor when exiting the patient. Protons possess a unique Bragg peak, an intrinsic property that allows all of the proton's ionizing effects to be deposited where targeted, in this case at the site of the lung tumor. Distally, there is no subsequent deposition, potentially limiting normal tissue toxicity. However, proton therapy has not been directly compared to conventional photon therapy in a prospective trial. Retrospective studies suggest decreases in pneumonitis, esophagitis, and bone marrow suppression compared to photon-based therapy.[17]

- *Intensity modulated radiation therapy (IMRT)* can be utilized in lesions with limited motion to permit dose escalation while avoiding normal tissue toxicity to the spinal cord, esophagus, and other critical structures.[18] IMRT employs inverse planning, in which a radiation planning system generates a plan according to target and normal structure dose parameters set by the radiation oncologist.

- *Three-dimensional conformal radiation therapy (3D-CRT)* approaches can be utilized if there are concerns of excessive tumor motion or inadequate tumor coverage with IMRT.

- Most 3D-CRT and IMRT treatments employ *multileaf collimation (MLC)*. Multileaf collimators are devices attached to the radiation treatment machine head. They are made up of many high atomic number (e.g., tungsten) "leaves" that shift in and out of the radiation beam aperture. This process results in highly conformal radiation delivery that limits normal tissue exposure.

- *Four-dimensional (4D) planning* accounts for target movement (due to respiratory motion in the case of lung cancer). Respiratory motion and associated tumor movement can be measured by fluoroscopy or patient imaging systems tied in with CT imaging. These parameters are then incorporated into modified GTVs.

- *Hypofractionation* refers to administration of larger doses of radiation per fraction over fewer overall treatments to achieve similarly biologic effective doses to disease as standard fractionation. For the treatment of stage III NSCLC, fraction doses up to 3–4 Gy to total doses of 45–60 Gy are under investigation in clinical trials.

An example of a typical radiation treatment plan for stage III NSCLC is shown in Figures 8.1–8.3.

Chemotherapy

For stage III disease, chemotherapy may be administered before or after surgery, with radiation therapy (concurrently or sequentially), or—in instances of limited functional status and/or pulmonary reserve—as monotherapy.

Adjuvant Chemotherapy

Adjuvant chemotherapy has been shown to improve overall survival in stage IB-III NSCLC. Patients with locally advanced disease appear to derive the greatest incremental survival benefit (Table 8.2).

A number of adjuvant chemotherapy regimens are employed. Although the principal adjuvant chemotherapy trials employed cisplatin combined with either vinorelbine, vindesine, vinblastine, or etoposide, or carboplatin-paclitaxel, data for other agents (e.g., docetaxel, gemcitabine, pemetrexed) from the advanced disease setting has been extrapolated to the adjuvant setting. Commonly used chemotherapy regimens, including drugs, doses, and schedules, are listed in Chapter 7.

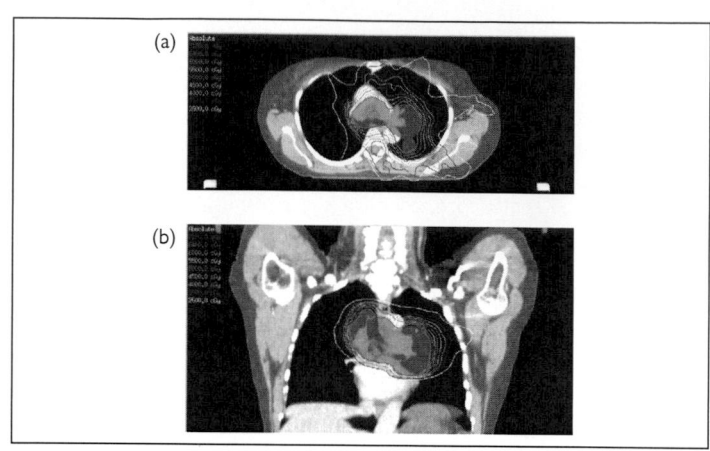

Figure 8.1 Axial (a) and coronal (b) images of a radiation treatment plan for a patient with stage IIIB non–small cell lung cancer (left lung parenchymal disease and bilateral mediastinal nodal metastases) treated with concurrent chemoradiation. Isodose curves display radiation doses delivered to specific volumes. (Images courtesy of Puneeth Iyengar, MD PhD.)

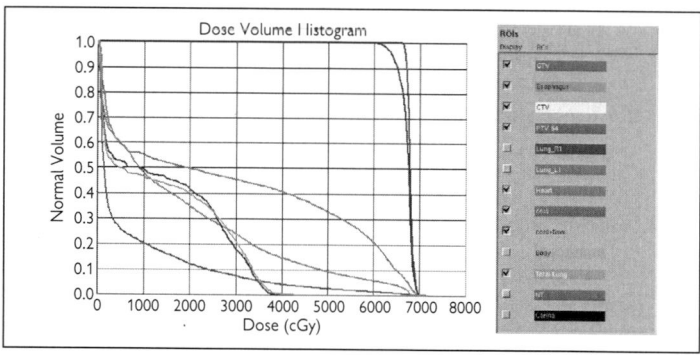

Figure 8.2 Dose–volume histogram (DVH) of the case in Figure 7.1. DVHs provide the radiation per volume received by individual structures/organs as a means of predicting toxicity and of evaluating coverage of disease by treatment. (Images courtesy of Puneeth Iyengar, MD, PhD.)

Neoadjuvant Chemotherapy

Compared to adjuvant chemotherapy, neoadjuvant chemotherapy offers the potential advantages of reducing tumor volume before surgery (which might simplify resection), demonstrating *in vivo* chemosensitivity, addressing micro-metastatic disease earlier, and possibly being better tolerated. While not widely used for early-stage disease, preoperative chemotherapy is a common approach to locally advanced tumors. Chemotherapy regimens are similar to those administered in the adjuvant setting.

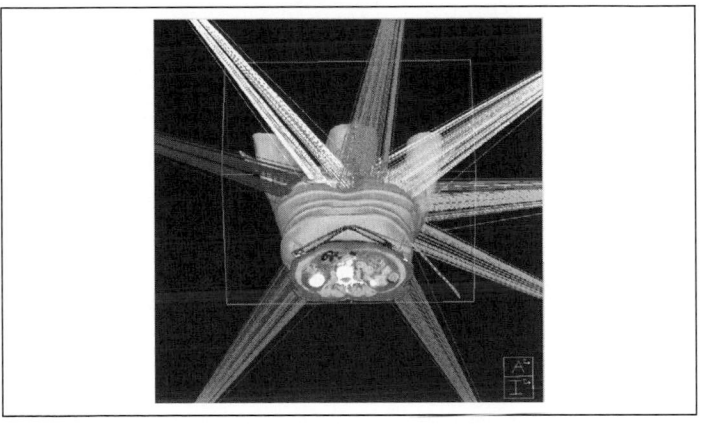

Figure 8.3 Skin rendering demonstrating angles at which radiation beams are entering patient to treat tumor. (Image courtesy of Puneeth Iyengar, MD, PhD.)

Table 8.2 Effect of Adjuvant Chemotherapy According to N Stage*

Nodal Status	5-Year Survival		HR (95% CI)
	No Chemotherapy	Chemotherapy	
N0	61%	58%	1.44 (0.83–1.57)
N1	36%	52%	0.67 (0.47–0.94)
N2	19%	40%	0.60 (0.44–0.82)

*Based on outcomes in the ANITA study (see ref. 6).

Chemoradiation

There is a 2- to 3-month survival advantage with concurrent chemoradiation over a sequential approach, albeit it with increased toxicities.[3,4] Accordingly, in patients with adequate functional status, concurrent therapy is preferred. The two most commonly employed regimens are cisplatin-etoposide and carboplatin-paclitaxel.

Cisplatin-Etoposide

Cisplatin 50 mg/m^2 IV days 1, 8, 29, 36
Etoposide 50 mg/m^2 IV days 1–5, 29–33 during radiation therapy

Carboplatin-Paclitaxel

Carboplatin AUC 2 IV weekly
Paclitaxel 45 mg/m^2 IV weekly during radiation therapy
followed by two cycles of consolidation therapy:

Carboplatin AUC 6 IV day 1
Paclitaxel 200 mg/m^2 IV day 1 every 21 days

These two regimens have not been compared directly in clinical trials. Because weekly carboplatin-paclitaxel is administered in "radiosensitizing" doses, full "systemic" doses are used for consolidation therapy to address possible microscopic disease outside the chest.

Randomized clinical trials have demonstrated that consolidation chemotherapy with docetaxel after concurrent cisplatin-etoposide chemoradiation does not prolong survival and is associated with increased rates of pneumonitis.[7] For reasons that remain unclear, the administration of the epidermal growth factor receptor inhibitor gefitinib as maintenance therapy after concurrent chemoradiation is associated with a statistically and clinically significant *decrease* in overall survival in a molecularly unselected population.[8] The role of molecular targeted therapies in the treatment of stage III NSCLC harboring driver kinase mutations (e.g., *EGFR* mutations, *EML4-ALK* fusions) has not been established. Currently, there is no role for antiangiogenic therapy (e.g., bevacizumab) in locally advanced NSCLC. In phase 2 studies, this treatment has been associated with increased rates of toxicities such as tracheoesophageal fistula.[19]

"Bulky" Stage III

These cases are treated with concurrent or sequential chemoradiation (as described earlier), without surgery.

Separate Tumor Nodules

Separate tumor nodules are classified as the following:

- Same lobe = T3
- Different ipsilateral lobe = T4
- Contralateral lung = M1a

Patients with separate tumor nodules within the same lobe (T3N0 [stage II] or T3N1, [stage III]) are considered candidates for upfront surgery. Patients with separate nodules in another ipsilateral lobe (T4N0 or T4N1) may also be considered for resection. While the presence of solitary pulmonary nodules in each lung is classified as stage IV disease, in selected cases with negative mediastinal evaluation, treatment as two separate primary tumors is reasonable. Adjuvant chemotherapy is generally recommended for all of these scenarios.

T3N1 Disease

In the current staging system, T3 tumors invade chest wall, involve proximal airways, or are greater than 7 cm in size. T3N1 tumors are classified as stage IIIA but have a more favorable prognosis than does N2 stage IIIA disease. If feasible, these patients should undergo surgical resection, followed by adjuvant chemotherapy.

For superior sulcus (Pancoast) tumors with hilar LN involvement (T3-4N1), induction chemoradiation followed by surgery is recommended. A commonly employed regimen is thoracic radiation therapy to 45 Gy in 25 fractions with concurrent cisplatin-etoposide chemotherapy, followed by resection if the patient remains a candidate at the time of reassessment. If the patient is not a candidate for surgery, radiation is continued to 63 Gy total. However, care must be taken to avoid a long interruption (ideally <2–3 days) in radiation while the assessment of resectability is made. If the patient is deemed unresectable up front, concurrent thoracic RT to 63 Gy plus concurrent cisplatin-etoposide chemotherapy is planned.

T4N0–1 Disease

Historically, T4 lesions were considered by definition, unresectable. However, in carefully selected patients, modern surgical techniques now permit resection of certain T4 primary tumors within a multimodality approach. Given the favorable outcomes (5-year survival rates up to 50%) with this approach, these tumors are classified as stage IIIA. However, most T4 lesions are not completely resectable and are best treated with chemoradiation.

Posttreatment Surveillance

A widely used posttreatment surveillance schedule is as follows:

- Diagnostic CT of the chest (including adrenals) every 3 months after treatment for 2 years, then every 6 months for 3 more years
- PET/CT may be performed for further characterization of radiographic abnormalities if there is a suspicion or concern for recurrence/residual disease; PET/CT is best performed at least 6 months after radiation therapy because posttreatment changes are frequently FDG avid. Routine PET/CT for surveillance is *not* recommended.
- Brain MRI if signs or symptoms concerning for brain metastases

Mediastinal Recurrence after Definitive Treatment of Early-Stage Disease

Loco-regional failures are three times as common (18% versus 6%) after wedge resection versus lobectomy for early stage disease.[20] If there is a mediastinal recurrence after definitive treatment for early-stage lung cancer, treatment options include chemotherapy alone, chemoradiation to areas of involved disease to a dose of 60 Gy in 30 fractions, or radiation therapy alone if chemotherapy cannot be offered (70 Gy in 35 fractions).

Treatment-Related Toxicities

Radiation- and chemotherapy-related toxicities are covered in detail in Chapter 14. Surgical complications are reviewed in Chapter 7.

References

1. Hochstenbag MM, Twijnstra A, Hofman P, Wouters EF, ten Velde GP. MR-imaging of the brain of neurologic asymptomatic patients with large cell or adenocarcinoma of the lung. Does it influence prognosis and treatment? *Lung Cancer* 2003;42:189–93.

2. Dillman RO, Herndon J, Seagren SL, Eaton WL, Jr., Green MR. Improved survival in stage III non-small-cell lung cancer: seven-year follow-up of cancer and leukemia group B (CALGB) 8433 trial. *J Natl Cancer Inst* 1996;88:1210–5.

3. Furuse K, Fukuoka M, Kawahara M, et al. Phase III study of concurrent versus sequential thoracic radiotherapy in combination with mitomycin, vindesine, and cisplatin in unresectable stage III non-small-cell lung cancer. *J Clin Oncol* 1999;17:2692–9.

4. Curran WJ, Jr., Paulus R, Langer CJ, et al. Sequential vs concurrent chemoradiation for stage III non-small cell lung cancer: randomized phase III trial RTOG 9410. *J Natl Cancer Inst* 2011;103:1452–60.

5. Belani CP, Choy H, Bonomi P, et al. Combined chemoradiotherapy regimens of paclitaxel and carboplatin for locally advanced non-small-cell lung cancer: a randomized phase II locally advanced multi-modality protocol. *J Clin Oncol* 2005;23:5883–91.

6. Douillard JY, Rosell R, De Lena M, et al. Adjuvant vinorelbine plus cisplatin versus observation in patients with completely resected stage IB-IIIA non-small-cell lung cancer (Adjuvant Navelbine International Trialist Association [ANITA]): a randomised controlled trial. *Lancet Oncol* 2006;7:719–27.

7. Hanna N, Neubauer M, Yiannoutsos C, et al. Phase III study of cisplatin, etoposide, and concurrent chest radiation with or without consolidation docetaxel in patients with inoperable stage III non-small-cell lung cancer: the Hoosier Oncology Group and U.S. Oncology. *J Clin Oncol* 2008;26:5755–60.

8. Kelly K, Chansky K, Gaspar LE, et al. Phase III trial of maintenance gefitinib or placebo after concurrent chemoradiotherapy and docetaxel consolidation in inoperable stage III non-small-cell lung cancer: SWOG S0023. *J Clin Oncol* 2008;26:2450–6.

9. Albain KS, Swann RS, Rusch VW, et al. Radiotherapy plus chemotherapy with or without surgical resection for stage III non-small-cell lung cancer: a phase III randomised controlled trial. *Lancet* 2009;374:379–86.

10. Bradley J, Paulus R, Komaki R. A randomized phase III comparison of standard dose (60 Gy) v high dose (74 Gy) conformal chemoradiotherapy +/- cetuximab in stage IIIA/B NSCLC: preliminary findings on radiation dose in RTOG 0617. *Proc Am Soc Therapeut Radiation Oncol* 2011.

11. Depierre A, Milleron B, Moro-Sibilot D, et al. Preoperative chemotherapy followed by surgery compared with primary surgery in resectable stage I (except T1N0), II, and IIIa non-small-cell lung cancer. *J Clin Oncol* 2002;20:247–53.

12. Roth JA, Fossella F, Komaki R, et al. A randomized trial comparing perioperative chemotherapy and surgery with surgery alone in resectable stage IIIA non-small-cell lung cancer. *J Natl Cancer Inst* 1994;86:673–80.

13. Rosell R, Gomez-Codina J, Camps C, et al. A randomized trial comparing preoperative chemotherapy plus surgery with surgery alone in patients with non-small-cell lung cancer. *N Engl J Med* 1994;330:153–8.

14. James TW, Faber LP. Indications for pneumonectomy. Pneumonectomy for malignant disease. *Chest Surg Clin N Am* 1999;9:291–309, ix.

15. Lally BE, Zelterman D, Colasanto JM, Haffty BG, Detterbeck FC, Wilson LD. Postoperative radiotherapy for stage II or III non-small-cell lung cancer using the surveillance, epidemiology, and end results database. *J Clin Oncol* 2006;24:2998–3006.

16. Rusch VW, Giroux DJ, Kraut MJ, et al. Induction chemoradiation and surgical resection for superior sulcus non-small-cell lung carcinomas: long-term results of Southwest Oncology Group Trial 9416 (Intergroup Trial 0160). *J Clin Oncol* 2007;25:313–8.

17. Sejpal S, Komaki R, Tsao A, et al. Early findings on toxicity of proton beam therapy with concurrent chemotherapy for nonsmall cell lung cancer. *Cancer* 2011;117:3004–13.

18. Zhang X, Li Y, Pan X, et al. Intensity-modulated proton therapy reduces the dose to normal tissue compared with intensity-modulated radiation therapy or passive scattering proton therapy and enables individualized radical radiotherapy for extensive stage IIIB non-small-cell lung cancer: a virtual clinical study. *Int J Radiat Oncol Biol Phys* 2010;77:357–66.

19. Spigel DR, Hainsworth JD, Yardley DA, et al. Tracheoesophageal fistula formation in patients with lung cancer treated with chemoradiation and bevacizumab. *J Clin Oncol* 2010;28:43–8.

20. Ginsberg RJ, Rubinstein LV. Randomized trial of lobectomy versus limited resection for T1 N0 non-small cell lung cancer. Lung Cancer Study Group. *Ann Thorac Surg* 1995;60:615–22.

Metastatic Non–Small Cell Lung Cancer

Apar Kishor Ganti

Almost 40% of patients with non–small cell lung cancer (NSCLC) present with stage IV disease.[1] Median survival of these patients in population-based databases is approximately 6–8 months, while the median survival of patients enrolled in clinical trials is ≈12 months. Systemic chemotherapy is the mainstay of treatment in these patients. The role of chemotherapy is mainly palliative in this setting. Advances in our understanding of the biology of NSCLC have led to the identification of certain populations with a relatively good prognosis despite presenting with advanced disease, such as individuals with tumors harboring activating epidermal growth factor receptor (EGFR) mutations.

First-Line Therapy for Metastatic Non–Small Cell Lung Cancer

The role of systemic chemotherapy in patients with advanced NSCLC is palliative; it not only improves survival compared to best supportive care[2] but also maintains quality of life.[3] A meta-analysis of 16 randomized trials involving 2714 patients found a 23% reduction in the risk of death (HR, 0.77; 95% CI, 0.71–0.83; $P < 0.0001$) in patients who received chemotherapy compared to best supportive care.[2] Hence, chemotherapy should be recommended to all fit patients (performance status ECOG 0-1) with advanced NSCLC. Older patients and patients with poor performance status (ECOG 2) are a particularly challenging group of patients and their management is discussed separately (Chapter 10).

Number of Agents
A meta-analysis of 65 trials ($n = 13,601$) found significantly better response rates (26% vs. 13%, $P < 0.001$) and 1-year survival (35% vs. 30%, $P < 0.001$) with chemotherapy doublets compared to single agents.[4] The addition of a third cytotoxic drug increased response rates, but there was no survival advantage and toxicity was increased.[4,5] Hence, doublet cytotoxic chemotherapy is considered the standard of care for most patients with good performance status.

Choice of Regimen
Platinum-based therapy is the mainstay of treatment of patients with metastatic NSCLC. Multiple studies have compared different platinum doublets. No single regimen has been consistently shown to be superior as first-line therapy of

advanced NSCLC (Table 9.1). In the United States, due to the lower toxicity seen with carboplatin-paclitaxel, this doublet was the most commonly used regimen in this setting for some time. That, however, may be changing with the advent of newer agents such as pemetrexed and bevacizumab.

Cisplatin versus Carboplatin

Two meta-analyses have suggested improved response rates with cisplatin.[6,7] However, the overall survival benefit with cisplatin was marginal and not statistically significant. Interestingly, patients who had a nonsquamous histology seemed to benefit more from cisplatin-based therapy (OR 1.58; 95% CI, 1.27–1.97).[7]

Cisplatin-based therapy was associated with more nausea, vomiting, and renal dysfunction, while carboplatin therapy was more commonly associated with thrombocytopenia. For patients with stage IV disease, where the main goal of therapy is palliation, avoidance of toxicity becomes important. Vomiting affects the quality of life to a much greater extent compared to thrombocytopenia, which is largely asymptomatic. Carboplatin is also logistically easier to administer. However, the improved response rates observed with cisplatin may be important for patients with symptoms secondary to their cancer and should be considered in specific settings.

Duration of Therapy

A meta-analysis of >3000 patients found that continuing chemotherapy beyond 4–6 cycles decreased the risk of progression by 25%.[8] However, the effect on overall survival was modest (HR, 0.92, 95% CI 0.86–0.99) and the incidence of adverse events was higher. Patient preferences, as well as the value of time off therapy, need to be considered while recommending prolonged therapy.[9] The role of maintenance therapy is discussed separately.

Role of Histology

Historically, histologic subtype of NSCLC was not considered in treatment selection. However, based on recent clinical trials, the antifolate agent pemetrexed and the anti-vascular endothelial growth factor (VEGF) antibody bevacizumab, are restricted to patients with nonsquamous histology due to efficacy and toxicity considerations, respectively.

A large phase III trial of 1725 chemotherapy-naïve stage IIIB/IV NSCLC patients comparing pemetrexed/cisplatin with gemcitabine/cisplatin showed that patients with nonsquamous cell histology responded better to pemetrexed/cisplatin.[10] The study analyzed treatment-by-histology interaction in a prespecified analysis. Overall survival was better with pemetrexed in patients with adenocarcinoma (n = 847; 12.6 vs. 10.9 months) and large-cell carcinoma (n = 153; 10.4 vs. 6.7 months). In contrast, overall survival was better with gemcitabine in patients with squamous cell carcinoma (n = 473; 10.8 vs. 9.4 months). The pemetrexed arm had lower myelosuppression, febrile neutropenia, and alopecia but higher grade 3 or 4 nausea.

This histology interaction has been demonstrated in all major pemetrexed trials (first line, maintenance, second line) conducted to date and thus pemetrexed is approved only for patients with nonsquamous histology.[11] It is hypothesized that differing thymidylate synthetase expression/activity between squamous and nonsquamous tumors may be responsible for this discordant activity.

Table 9.1 Selected First-Line Studies in Advanced Non–Small Cell Lung Cancer

Study	Regimen	RR (%)	Median OS (Months)	Comments
ECOG 1594[52]	Cisplatin/paclitaxel	21	7.4	No difference in outcomes with any of the regimens. Carboplatin/paclitaxel—lower rate of adverse events
	Cisplatin/gemcitabine	22	8.1	
	Cisplatin/docetaxel	17	7.8	
	Carboplatin/paclitaxel	17	8.1	
Italian Lung Cancer Project[53]	Cisplatin/gemcitabine	30	9.8	No difference in outcomes. Cisplatin-vinorelbine—more myelosuppression; carboplatin-paclitaxel—less blood transfusions
	Carboplatin/paclitaxel	32	9.9	
	Cisplatin/vinorelbine	30	9.5	
ECOG 4599[12]	Carboplatin/paclitaxel/bevacizumab	35	12.3*	More adverse events with bevacizumab
	Carboplatin/paclitaxel	15	10.3	
AVAiL[13]	Cisplatin/gemcitabine/bevacizumab (15 mg/kg)	35	13.4	Although response rates and progression-free survival were better with bevacizumab, there was no overall survival advantage.
	Cisplatin/gemcitabine/bevacizumab (7.5 mg/kg)	38	13.6	
	Cisplatin/gemcitabine	21.6	13.1	
Scagliotti et al.[10]	Cisplatin/gemcitabine	28.2	10.3	No difference in OS. Pemetrexed improved OS in nonsquamous histology; gemcitabine in squamous
	Cisplatin/pemetrexed	30.6	10.3	
FLEX[25]	Cisplatin/vinorelbine/cetuximab	36	11.3*	Inclusion criteria included IHC evidence of EGFR expression (≥1 positively stained tumor cell)
	Cisplatin/vinorelbine	29	10.1	
BMS 099[26]	Carboplatin/taxane#/cetuximab	26	9.7	No restrictions by histology or EGFR expression
	Carboplatin/taxane#	17	8.4	

*$p < 0.05$.

#Either paclitaxel or docetaxel based on investigator preference.

AVAiL, Avastin in Lung; BMS, Bristol Myers Squibb; ECOG, Eastern Cooperative Oncology Group; EGFR, epidermal growth factor receptor; FLEX, First-Line ErbituX in Lung Cancer; IHC, immunohistochemistry; OS, overall survival; RR, response rate.

CHAPTER 9 **Metastatic Non–Small Cell Lung Cancer**

Role of Bevacizumab

Bevacizumab is a monoclonal antibody that targets VEGF, thereby affecting angiogenesis.

- The Eastern Cooperative Oncology Group (ECOG) E4599 trial compared the effects of adding bevacizumab to carboplatin/paclitaxel.[12] This trial was limited to patients with nonsquamous histology, no history of brain metastasis, and no anticoagulation, based on concerns of increased hemorrhage seen in smaller phase II trials. The addition of bevacizumab improved response rate (35% vs. 15%) and overall survival (12.3 vs. 10.3 month; HR, 0.79; P = 0.003). There was increased toxicity with the addition of bevacizumab, especially myelosuppression and febrile neutropenia.

- The AVAiL (Avastin in Lung) study showed that the addition of bevacizumab to cisplatin-gemcitabine did not confer a survival advantage with either higher (15 mg/kg) or lower (7.5 mg/kg) doses of bevacizumab.[13] There was a small but statistically significant improvement in progression-free survival with bevacizumab.

Cost-Effectiveness

The data on cost-effectiveness of the various regimens are sparse. In a systematic review, Carlson et al. confirmed that chemotherapy improved health outcomes in advanced NSCLC over best supportive care at reasonable cost-effectiveness levels.[14] The SWOG S9509 study evaluated the resource utilization (mean overall costs over a 24-month period) between the two treatment groups (cisplatin/vinorelbine and carboplatin/paclitaxel).[15] The average overall cost for a patient who received vinorelbine and cisplatin was $40,292 compared with $48,940 for paclitaxel and carboplatin (P = 0.0004). A retrospective analysis of the costs of various platinum-based doublets found that gemcitabine and cisplatin had less direct patient treatment costs than other regimens (vinorelbine-cisplatin, paclitaxel-cisplatin, paclitaxel-carboplatin, and docetaxel-cisplatin).[16]

Epidermal Growth Factor Receptor Pathway in Advanced Non–Small Cell Lung Cancer

The epidermal growth factor receptor (EGFR) pathway plays a key role in the pathogenesis and progression of certain subsets of patients with NSCLC. Inhibition of the EGFR pathway has been used as a therapeutic strategy in NSCLC. The EGFR tyrosine kinase inhibitors (TKIs) erlotinib and gefitinib and the anti-EGFR monoclonal antibody cetuximab have been extensively studied in NSCLC.

Epidermal Growth Factor Receptor Molecular Mechanisms

The presence of somatic mutations in the tyrosine kinase domain of the EGFR gene appear to predict for response to EGFR TKIs at least in treatment-naïve patients.[17,18] It is now apparent that *EGFR* mutation–positive adenocarcinoma is a distinct subgroup of NSCLC that is particularly responsive to EGFR TKIs. Retrospective biomarker analyses in the initial studies using these agents in molecularly unselected populations (BR.21, ISEL, INTEREST, and SATURN studies[19–22]) have indicated that patients with *EGFR* mutations have a pronounced response to EGFR TKIs. In addition to predicting for response to EGFR TKIs, the presence of an *EGFR* mutation also confers an overall favorable prognosis.[23]

First-Line Therapy

The Iressa Pan-Asia Study (IPASS) trial randomly assigned treatment-naïve nonsmokers or former light smokers with advanced adenocarcinoma in East Asia to either gefitinib ($n = 609$) or carboplatin-paclitaxel ($n = 608$).[23] The PFS at 1 year was significantly better with gefitinib (24.9% vs. 6.7%). Response rates with gefitinib were dramatically higher in patients with tumors harboring EGFR mutations (71.2% vs. 1.1%). Patients with an EGFR mutation had a significantly longer PFS with gefitinib (HR 0.48; 95% CI, 0.36–0.64; $P <$ 0.001), while the results were opposite in patients without the mutation (HR with gefitinib, 2.85; 95% CI, 2.05–3.98; $P < 0.001$). However, even in the mutation-positive patients, gefitinib did not improve overall survival, probably due to the crossover nature of the study. These results have been replicated in multiple studies of mutation positive patients both in Asia and Europe (Table 9.2).

A weighted pooled analysis of studies of EGFR-mutated NSCLC treated with chemotherapy or EGFR TKIs showed that EGFR TKIs produced a longer median PFS versus chemotherapy, but there does not seem to be a beneficial effect on overall survival at this time, presumably due to the crossover design of these studies.[24] Based on these findings, EGFR TKIs appear to be the most effective initial treatment for patients with advanced EGFR-mutated NSCLC. Erlotinib was recently approved by the US FDA for first line therapy in patients with metastatic NSCLC, whose tumors have EGFR exon 19 deletions or exon 21 (L858R) substitution mutations.

Role of Cetuximab

Cetuximab is a chimeric monoclonal antibody that binds to EGFR and is currently approved for treatment of squamous cancer of the head and neck and KRAS wild-type metastatic colorectal cancer. The First-Line ErbituX in Lung Cancer (FLEX) trial randomly assigned chemotherapy-naïve patients with advanced EGFR-expressing (by immunohistochemistry) NSCLC to cisplatin/vinorelbine plus or minus cetuximab.[23] Patients randomized to cetuximab had a median OS of 11.3 months compared with 10.1 months for those who received chemotherapy alone (HR 0.871; $P = 0.044$). However, the BMS099 trial that evaluated the efficacy of cetuximab in combination with taxane/carboplatin chemotherapy did not show a benefit with cetuximab for either PFS or OS.[26] The role of cetuximab in the treatment of advanced NSCLC is unclear at this time.

Testing for Epidermal Growth Factor Receptor Mutations

A number of methods of testing for EGFR mutations are available.[27] Allele-specific mutation is a technique that uses polymerase chain reaction targeting specific mutations. The main advantage is efficiency, but this method is limited by low sensitivity. The amplification refractory mutation system (ARMS) requires a specially engineered primer for detection of a single mutation. The EGFR ScorpionsIM Kit (DxS, Manchester, United Kingdom) system is a commercialized kit that can detect 29 common EGFR mutations. The application is relatively easy and sensitivity is higher than that of standard sequencing.[28] Zhu et al. tested samples from BR.21, a randomized phase III study of erlotinib as second- or third-line therapy, with ARMS and found that 11 of the

Table 9.2 Trials of EGFR TKIs in *EGFR*-Mutation-Positive Patients

Study	Treatment	EGFR Testing	Median PFS (Months)	Median OS (Months)	Comments
IPASS[23,54]	Gefitinib[#]	Scorpion ARMS	HR for gefitinib: 0.48; 95% CI, 0.36 to 0.64*	21.6	The lack of OS benefit could be due to confounding by treatment received at progression
	Carboplatin + paclitaxel			21.9	
Maemondo et al., 2010[55]	Gefitinib	PNA-LNA clamping	10.8	30.5	Less hematologic and neurologic toxicity, but more interstitial lung disease with gefitinib
	Carboplatin + paclitaxel		5.4*	23.6	
WJTOG3405[56]	Gefitinib	Cycleave PCR	9.2	30.9	Chemotherapy—myelosuppression, alopecia, fatigue; erlotinib—skin toxicity, liver dysfunction
	Cispatin + docetaxel		6.3*	NR	
OPTIMAL[57]	Erlotinib	Cycleave PCR	13.1	NR	More grade 3–4 toxic effects, higher rate of dose reduction and discontinuation with chemotherapy
	Carboplatin + gemcitabine		4.6*		
EURTAC[58]	Erlotinib	Taqman PCR and fragment analysis	9.7	19.3	Non-Asian population. No increase in interstitial pneumonitis with erlotinib
	Chemotherapy**		5.2*	19.5	

*Statistically significant.

#Data for mutation positive patients only.

**Regimens included cisplatin-docetaxel; cisplatin-gemcitabine; carboplatin-docetaxel; and carboplatin-gemcitabine.

ARMS, Amplification Refractory Mutation System; EGFR, epidermal growth factor receptor; EURTAC, European Tarceva versus Chemotherapy; IPASS, Iressa Pan-Asia Study; NR, not reported; OS, overall survival; PCR, polymerase chain reaction; PNA-LNA, peptide nucleic acid–locked nucleic acid; TKI, tyrosine kinase inhibitor; WJTOG, West Japan Thoracic Oncology Group.

148 samples previously thought to be negative by direct sequencing had exon 19 deletion *EGFR* mutations.[19] The US FDA recently approved the cobas® EGFR mutation test as a companion diagnostic for patient selection. This was based on a retrospective evaluation of 134 specimens of patients enrolled in the EURTAC trial.[58] Analysis of the PFS of the 116 patients whose specimens were positive with this test, revealed a benefit consistent with the primary analysis in the trial.

Other Markers

The data on the ability of other markers, that is, immunohistochemical (IHC) assessment of EGFR expression, *EGFR* copy number by fluorescence *in situ* hybridization (FISH), and *KRAS* mutations are not as robust. Among the various molecular markers, *EGFR* mutation analysis most reliably identifies patients who would respond dramatically to EGFR TKIs. Current guidelines recommend testing specimens from all patients with advanced non-squamous NSCLC for *EGFR* mutations. However this practice has not been universally implemented.

Testing for *EGFR* mutations may be approached in a variety of ways. One approach may be to test for *KRAS* mutations and, if negative, to test for *EGFR* mutations and *ALK* fusions, as these three aberrations appear to be mutually exclusive.[29] The purpose of testing KRAS first is not to determine suitability for therapy but to halt further testing if positive.

Epidermal Growth Factor Receptor Testing Recommendations Summary

- If erlotinib is used as first-line therapy instead of chemotherapy, then the presence of an *EGFR* mutation must be documented.
- For erlotinib use in second- or third-line setting or for maintenance use, *EGFR* testing is not mandatory at the present time.
- The preferred method for predicting response to EGFR inhibitors is testing for *EGFR* mutations.

ALK-Positive Tumors

ALK gene rearrangements are seen in a specific subset of patients with NSCLC. As discussed in Chapter 3, the *EML4-ALK* fusion is formed by an inversion on the short arm of chromosome 2 that joins exons 1–13 of *EML4* to exons 20-29 of *ALK*.[30]

Crizotinib is an ALK inhibitor that has shown substantial activity in patients with NSCLC who harbor an *ALK* rearrangement. In a phase I trial of 82 patients with ALK positive NSCLC, the 1-year survival was 74% and the 2-year survival was 54%.[31] Crizotinib is well tolerated with grade 1-2 visual disturbances (e.g., floaters, flashing lights) being the major adverse events. In addition, crizotinib is associated with gastrointestinal complications such as nausea, vomiting, diarrhea, and liver enzyme abnormalities. Crizotinib may prolong the QT interval and should be stopped temporarily if QTc prolongation is noted. Crizotinib should be permanently discontinued if the QTc prolongation is accompanied by an arrhythmia, heart failure, hypotension, shock, syncope, or torsade de pointes.

Recommendations for Initial Treatment of Patients with Advanced Non–Small Cell Lung Cancer

- A platinum-pemetrexed regimen (cisplatin preferred, in patients able to tolerate it) or a combination of carboplatin, paclitaxel, and bevacizumab are suitable options in patients with nonsquamous NSCLC.
- Patients who have activating mutations of the EGFR gene should be treated with erlotinib monotherapy (gefitinib, in countries where it is approved).
- Crizotinib may be considered in patients with ALK positive NSCLC. It is currently approved for all lines of therapy in the United States, but is being studied in treatment-naïve patients in Europe and Asia.
- A platinum-based doublet is preferred for all other patients.

Commonly Used Platinum Doublets for Advanced Non–Small Cell Lung Cancer

- Carboplatin + paclitaxel: carboplatin AUC 5-6 IV day 1; paclitaxel 175–225 mg/m^2 IV over 3 hours day 1. Repeat every 3 weeks.
- Carboplatin + pemetrexed: carboplatin AUC 5 IV day 1; pemetrexed 500 mg/m^2 IV day 1. Repeat every 3 weeks.
- Cisplatin + pemetrexed: cisplatin 75 mg/m^2 IV day 1; pemetrexed 500 mg/m^2 IV day 1. Repeat every 3 weeks.
- Carboplatin + paclitaxel + bevacizumab: paclitaxel 200 mg/m^2 IV day 1; carboplatin AUC 6 IV day 1; bevacizumab 15 mg/kg IV day 1. Repeat every 3 weeks (carboplatin and paclitaxel for a maximum of six cycles and bevacizumab until progression).
- Carboplatin + docetaxel: carboplatin AUC 6 IV day 1; docetaxel 75 mg/m^2 IV day 1. Repeat every 3 weeks.
- Carboplatin + gemcitabine: carboplatin AUC 5 IV day 1; gemcitabine 1000–1250 mg/m^2 IV days 1, 8. Repeat every 3 weeks.
- Cisplatin + paclitaxel: cisplatin 70 mg/m^2 IV day 1; paclitaxel 175 mg/m^2 IV over 3 hours day 1. Repeat every 3 weeks.
- Cisplatin + gemcitabine: cisplatin 100 mg/m^2 IV day 1; gemcitabine 1000 mg/^{2} IV days 1, 8, 15. Repeat every 4 weeks.
- Cisplatin + docetaxel: cisplatin 75 mg/m^2 IV day 1; docetaxel 75 mg/m^2 IV day 1. Repeat every 3 weeks.
- Cisplatin + vinorelbine: cisplatin 100 mg/m^2 IV day 1 every 4 weeks; vinorelbine 25 mg/m^2 IV weekly.
- Carboplatin + vinorelbine: carboplatin AUC 5 IV day 1; vinorelbine 30 mg/m^2 IV day 1 and 8 every 3 weeks.
- Cisplatin + vinorelbine + cetuximab: cisplatin 80 mg/m^2 IV day 1; vinorelbine 25 mg/m^2 IV days 1 and 8; cisplatin and vinorelbine to be administered every 3 weeks for a maximum of six cycles; cetuximab 400 mg/m^2

IV loading, followed by 250 mg/m^2 IV weekly until progression or limiting toxicity.

Important Notes

- For pemetrexed: start vitamin supplements 1 week before initial dose of pemetrexed until 21 days after last dose of pemetrexed. Folic acid 350–1000 mcg PO qd. Vitamin B12 1000 mcg IM every 9 weeks. Dexamethasone 4 mg bid the day before, the day of, and the day after pemetrexed.
- For docetaxel: dexamethasone 8 mg bid the day before, the day of, and the day after docetaxel.
- For paclitaxel: dexamethasone 20 mg PO 12 hours, 6 hours, and 1 hour before chemotherapy; H-2 receptor antagonists (ranitidine)

Maintenance Therapy

The standard approach to the initial treatment of advanced NSCLC has been 4–6 cycles of platinum doublet therapy followed by second-line therapy at progression. Recent data suggest promising results with continuing therapy following completion of first-line therapy. Different approaches to "maintenance therapy" have been investigated, including "switch" maintenance (using an agent that the tumor was not exposed to during induction) and "continuation" maintenance (continuing an agent that has shown activity in the initial setting).

Clinical Trial Evidence

Across the studies summarized in Table 9.3, there is a consistent improvement in PFS with maintenance therapy. Effects on OS are mixed, with only pemetrexed and erlotinib maintenance showing a survival advantage.

The Sequential Tarceva in Unresectable NSCLC (SATURN) trial[32] demonstrated that maintenance erlotinib significantly improved both PFS (12.3 vs. 11.1 weeks; HR, 0.71; 95% CI, 0.62 to 0.82; $P < 0.0001$) and OS (12 vs. 11 months; $P = 0.0088$). However, the clinical significance of this improvement is debatable. Interestingly, this benefit was seen even in patients whose tumors did not harbor activating *EGFR* mutations (HR, 0.77; 95% CI 0.61–0.97; $P = 0.0243$). The recently reported PARAMOUNT trial of maintenance pemetrexed in patients who received four cycles of cisplatin-pemetrexed induction therapy found a 2.9-month significant survival benefit in patients randomized to maintenance therapy (16.9 vs. 14 months; $P = 0.0195$).[33]

Quality of Life

Very few studies have reported effects on quality of life, which is an important consideration when recommending long-term therapy to these patients.

- The INFORM trial of maintenance gefitinib[34] showed that in addition to an improvement in progression-free survival, gefitinib resulted in a prolonged time to worsening of lung cancer symptoms.

Table 9.3 Clinical Trials of Maintenance Therapy

Ref.	Initial Chemo-therapy	Maintenance	PFS (Months)	P-value/HR	OS (Months)	P-Value
Continuation maintenance						
39	Cisplatin + gemcitabine	Observation	6.6	<0.001	13	0.195
		Gemcitabine	5		11	
59	Carboplatin + gemcitabine	Observation	3.9	NS	9.3	NS
		Gemcitabine	3.8		8	
60*	Cisplatin + gemcitabine	Placebo	2.1	0.51 [0.39–0.66]	NA	
		Gemcitabine	3.7			
33	Cisplatin + pemetrexed	Observation	2.8	0.0002	16.9	0.0195
		Pemetrexed	4.1		14	
Switch maintenance						
32	Platinum-based	Placebo	11.1 weeks	<0.0001	12	0.0088
		Erlotinib	12.3 weeks	0.71 [0.62–0.82]	11	
61	Platinum based + bevacizumab	Bevacizumab	3.75	Significant	NA	
		Bevacizumab + erlotinib	4.76			
35	Carboplatin + gemcitabine	Observation	2.7	0.001	9.7	0.085
		Docetaxel	5.7		12.3	
37	Platinum doublet	Observation	2.6	<0.0001	10.6	0.012
		Pemetrexed	4.3		13.4	
34	Platinum doublet	Placebo	2.6	<0.0001	18.7	0.26
		Gefitinib	4.8		16.9	
60*	Cisplatin + gemcitabine	Placebo	2.1	0.83 [0.73–0.94]	NA	
		Erlotinib	2.8			

*This was a three-armed study comparing maintenance of gemcitabine and maintenance of erlotinib separately with placebo following induction chemotherapy with cisplatin and gemcitabine. The results with continuing maintenance (gemcitabine) and switch maintenance (erlotinib) have been presented separately in this table.

HR, hazard ratio; NA, not available; NS, not significant; OS, overall survival; PFS, progression-free survival.

- Docetaxel maintenance therapy was not associated with a difference in quality of life scores compared to observation.[35]
- Patients who received maintenance pemetrexed had increased time to worsening of pain symptoms and hemoptysis. However, there was also an increase in hospitalization for adverse events and an increase in loss of appetite with pemetrexed maintenance.[36]

Study Design

Several of the studies set PFS as the primary endpoint with overall survival (OS) as a secondary endpoint. It may be unreasonable to examine OS in light of the frequent crossover experienced in oncology trials; however, that raises the issue of whether improvement of PFS provides any clinical benefit to patients. It may be difficult to justify the use of maintenance therapy in the absence of any overall survival advantage or clinical symptom-related benefit to patients.

Predicting Role of Maintenance Therapy

A number of analyses have been performed to identify patient subsets most likely to benefit from maintenance chemotherapy. In switch maintenance trials with pemetrexed (JMEN) and erlotinib (SATURN), clinical benefit from maintenance therapy appeared to be limited to patients who had stable disease after induction therapy (in contrast to a radiographic response).[37,38] A subset analysis of the Central European Cooperative Oncology Group (CECOG) randomized trial of continuation gemcitabine maintenance showed a clinically relevant and statistically significant increase in OS among patients with Karnofsky Performance Status (KPS) greater than 80.[39]

Recommendations

- While continuing therapy with an agent used as part of the initial regimen, only pemetrexed has demonstrated a survival advantage.
- Maintenance therapy may be considered for patients with ECOG PS 0–1 as follows:
  - Pemetrexed may be appropriate for maintenance therapy in patients with nonsquamous histology.
  - Erlotinib is also approved as maintenance therapy, although the clinical significance of the 1-month survival advantage is unclear.
- Docetaxel and gemcitabine do not provide any survival advantage in the maintenance setting.
- The decision to recommend maintenance chemotherapy should be individualized and made after a detailed discussion of the risks and benefits with the patient.

Second-Line Therapy of Non–Small Cell Lung Cancer

Number of Agents and Choice of Regimen

For patients who have disease progression following initial therapy, currently three agents—docetaxel, erlotinib, and pemetrexed—are approved by the US Food and Drug Administration for second-line treatment (Table 9.4).[40]

Second-line treatment should be considered for patients with a good performance status, as it has been shown to improve survival. For patients who have received cytotoxic chemotherapy in the first-line setting, combination chemotherapy at relapse does not improve overall survival, even though response rates and progression-free survival are better.[41] Patients with specific mutations, who receive either erlotinib or crizotinib at diagnosis, often receive a platinum-doublet at the time of progression.

Docetaxel

Shepherd et al. compared two doses of docetaxel (75 mg/m² and 100 mg/m²) administered every 21 days, to best supportive care.[42] Time to progression was increased with docetaxel (10.6 vs. 6.7 weeks). Patients experienced significantly

Table 9.4 Selected Studies Comparing Second-Line Therapy

Ref.	Regimen	RR (%)	Median OS (Months)	1-Year Survival (%)	Toxicity
42	Docetaxel 75 mg/m² on day 1; q3 weeks	7.1	7.5	37	Neutropenia
	Placebo	0	4.6	12	
62	Docetaxel 75 mg/m² on day 1; q3 weeks	6.7	5.7	32	Neutropenia
	Docetaxel 100 mg/m² on day 1; q3 weeks	10.8	5.5	21	Neutropenia
	Vinorelbine (30 mg/m² on days 1, 8, 15 q3 weeks) OR Ifosfamide (2 mg/m²/d with mesna on days 1–3; q3 weeks)	0.8	5.6	19	Neutropenia
43	Erlotinib 150 mg PO daily	8.9	6.7	31	Rash, diarrhea
	Placebo	<1	4.7	22	
46	Pemetrexed 500 mg/m² on day 1; q3 weeks	9.1	8.3	29.7	Anemia
	Docetaxel 75 mg/m² on day 1; q3 weeks	8.8	7.9	29 7	Neutropenia
47	Topotecan 2.3 mg/m²/d on days 1–5; q3 weeks	5	27.9	25	Anemia, thrombocytopenia
	Docetaxel 75 mg/m² on day 1; q3 weeks	5	30.7	29	Neutropenia

OS, overall survival; RR, response rate.

more febrile neutropenia at the higher dose (22% vs. 1.8%), and hence the lower dose is routinely used in this setting.

Erlotinib

Shepherd et al. conducted a randomized, placebo-controlled, double-blind study (BR.21) of erlotinib in patients previously treated with platinum-based therapy.[43] Patients receiving erlotinib had improved median survival and 1-year survival. The erlotinib group experienced rash (12%) and diarrhea (5%).

Utility of testing for activating mutations of the EGFR gene in the second-line setting is more controversial than in the first-line setting. A multivariate analysis of the BR.21 study found that the status of EGFR expression, *EGFR* copy number, or *EGFR* mutation did not affect survival following erlotinib treatment.[44] Similarly in the INTEREST study,[45] the presence or absence of *EGFR* mutations did not seem to predict for outcomes following gefitinib. In all these analyses, while patients with tumors harboring *EGFR* mutations were more likely to respond to an EGFR TKI, those without the mutation also appeared to benefit.

Hence, it is likely that *EGFR* mutation status is a better predictor of response to EGFR-directed therapy in the first-line setting than in the relapsed setting.

Pemetrexed

In a phase III trial comparing pemetrexed to docetaxel in second-line NSCLC, Hanna et al. found similar progression-free survival (2.9 months) and 1-year survival rates (29.7%).[46] However, patients receiving docetaxel had a higher incidence of grade 3 or 4 neutropenia (40.2% vs. 5.3%). Pemetrexed also showed lower alopecia and treatment-related hospitalization rates. A subset analysis showed improved survival in patients with nonsquamous cell histology, especially large cell, with pemetrexed, while outcomes were inferior to docetaxel in squamous cell carcinoma.[11]

Topotecan

In the second-line setting, oral topotecan and docetaxel have equivalent response rates (5%).[47] The median overall survival and 1-year overall survival are not significantly different. Docetaxel has higher rates of neutropenia, while topotecan is associated with higher rates of anemia and thrombocytopenia.

Recommendations

- Second-line chemotherapy is recommended for fit patients.
  - Pemetrexed, if not previously administered, is recommended for non-squamous NSCLC.
  - Docetaxel, erlotinib and oral topotecan all appear to have similar efficacy with varying toxicities in this setting.

Specific Regimens Used in Patients with Relapsed Non–Small Cell Lung Cancer

- Pemetrexed 500 mg/m^2 IV on day 1. Repeat every 3 weeks.
- Docetaxel 75 mg/m^2 IV on day 1. Repeat every 3 weeks.
- Topotecan 2.3 mg/m^2/d PO days 1–5. Repeat every 3 weeks.
- Erlotinib 150 mg PO daily at least 1 hour before or 2 hours after a meal.

Note: Supplements and premedications are similar to those described earlier.

Treatment of Oligometastatic Disease

A subset of patients with NSCLC will either present with metastases that are limited in number or develop a limited number of metastases following potentially curative treatment of early stage disease.[48] It is believed that these patients with oligometastatic disease form a distinct group that may benefit from aggressive therapy directed towards the metastatic site(s).

Current evidence suggests that patients with isolated brain[49] and adrenal metastases[50] from NSCLC, whose primary site of cancer is well controlled, benefit from surgical resection of these lesions with 5-year survival rates of 12.5% and 25%, respectively. Multiple small series demonstrate that patients with limited metastatic disease (≤8 lesions) benefit from aggressive local therapy directed toward these lesions.[51] Prospective randomized studies are needed to confirm these findings, but available evidence suggests that carefully selected patients with limited metastases have the potential for prolonged survival with aggressive therapy.

References

1. Morgensztern D, Ng SH, Gao F, Govindan, R. Trends in stage distribution for patients with non-small cell lung cancer: a National Cancer Database survey. *J Thorac Oncol* 2010;5:29–33.

2. NSCLC Meta-Analyses Collaborative Group. Chemotherapy in addition to supportive care improves survival in advanced non-small-cell lung cancer: a systematic review and meta-analysis of individual patient data from 16 randomized controlled trials. *J Clin Oncol* 2008;26:4617–25.

3. Spiro SG, Rudd RM, Souhami RL, et al. Chemotherapy versus supportive care in advanced non-small cell lung cancer: improved survival without detriment to quality of life. *Thorax* 2004;59:828–36.

4. Delbaldo C, Michiels S, Syz N, Soria JC, Le Chevalier T, Pignon JP. Benefits of adding a drug to a single-agent or a 2-agent chemotherapy regimen in advanced non-small-cell lung cancer: a meta-analysis. *JAMA* 2004;292:470–84.

5. Azim HA Jr., Elattar I, Loberiza FR Jr, Azim H, Mok T, Ganti AK. Third generation triplet cytotoxic chemotherapy in advanced non-small cell lung cancer: a systematic overview. *Lung Cancer* 2009;64:194–8.

6. Hotta K, Matsuo K, Ueoka H, Kiura K, Tabata M, Tanimoto M. Meta-analysis of randomized clinical trials comparing Cisplatin to Carboplatin in patients with advanced non-small-cell lung cancer. *J Clin Oncol* 2004;22:3852–9.

7. Ardizzoni A, Boni L, Tiseo M, et al. Cisplatin- versus carboplatin-based chemotherapy in first-line treatment of advanced non-small-cell lung cancer: an individual patient data meta-analysis. *J Natl Cancer Inst* 2007;99:847–57.

8. Soon YY, Stockler MR, Askie LM, Boyer MJ. Duration of chemotherapy for advanced non-small-cell lung cancer: a systematic review and meta-analysis of randomized trials. *J Clin Oncol* 2009;27:3277–83.

9. Socinski MA. Re-evaluating duration of therapy in advanced non-small-cell lung cancer: is it really duration or is it more about timing and exposure? *J Clin Oncol* 2009;27:3268–70.

10. Scagliotti GV, Parikh P, von Pawel J, et al. Phase III study comparing cisplatin plus gemcitabine with cisplatin plus pemetrexed in chemotherapy-naïve patients with advanced-stage non-small-cell lung cancer. *J Clin Oncol* 2008;26:3543–51.

11. Scagliotti G, Hanna N, Fossella F, et al. The differential efficacy of pemetrexed according to NSCLC histology: a review of two Phase III studies. *Oncologist* 2009;14:253–63.

12. Sandler A, Gray R, Perry MC, et al. Paclitaxel-carboplatin alone or with bevacizumab for non-small-cell lung cancer. *N Engl J Med* 2006;355:2542–50.

13. Reck M, von Pawel J, Zatloukal P, et al. Overall survival with cisplatin-gemcitabine and bevacizumab or placebo as first-line therapy for nonsquamous non-small-cell lung cancer: results from a randomised phase III trial (AVAiL). *Ann Oncol* 2010;21:1804–9.

14. Carlson JJ, Veenstra DL, Ramsey SD. Pharmacoeconomic evaluations in the treatment of non-small cell lung cancer. *Drugs* 2008;68:1105–13.

15. Kelly K, Crowley J, Bunn PA Jr., et al. Randomized phase III trial of paclitaxel plus carboplatin versus vinorelbine plus cisplatin in the treatment of patients with advanced non-small-cell lung cancer: a Southwest Oncology Group trial. *J Clin Oncol* 2001;19:3210–8.

16. Schiller J, Tilden D, Aristides M, et al. Retrospective cost analysis of gemcitabine in combination with cisplatin in non-small cell lung cancer compared to other combination therapies in Europe. *Lung Cancer* 2004;43:101–12.

17. Lynch TJ, Bell DW, Sordella R, et al. Activating mutations in the epidermal growth factor receptor underlying responsiveness of non-small-cell lung cancer to gefitinib. *N Engl J Med* 2004;350:2129–39.

18. Bell DW, Lynch TJ, Haserlat SM, et al. Epidermal growth factor receptor mutations and gene amplification in non-small-cell lung cancer: molecular analysis of the IDEAL/INTACT gefitinib trials. *J Clin Oncol* 2005;23:8081–92.

19. Zhu CQ, da Cunha Santos G, Ding K, et al. Role of KRAS and EGFR as biomarkers of response to erlotinib in National Cancer Institute of Canada Clinical Trials Group Study BR.21. *J Clin Oncol* 2008;26:4268–75.

20. Hirsch FR, Varella-Garcia M, Bunn PA Jr., et al. Molecular predictors of outcome with gefitinib in a phase III placebo-controlled study in advanced non-small-cell lung cancer. *J Clin Oncol* 2006;24:5034–42.

21. Douillard JY, Shepherd FA, Hirsh V, et al. Molecular predictors of outcome with gefitinib and docetaxel in previously treated non-small-cell lung cancer: data from the randomized phase III INTEREST trial. *J Clin Oncol* 2010;28:744–52.

22. Brugger W, Triller N, Blasinska-Morawiec M, et al. Prospective biomarker analyses of EGFR and KRAS from a randomized, placebo-controlled study of erlotinib maintenance therapy in advanced non-small-cell lung cancer. *J Clin Oncol* 2011;29:4113–20.

23. Mok TS, Wu YL, Thongprasert S, et al. Gefitinib or carboplatin-paclitaxel in pulmonary adenocarcinoma. *N Engl J Med* 2009;361:947–57.

24. Paz-Ares L, Soulières D, Melezínek I, et al. Clinical outcomes in non-small-cell lung cancer patients with EGFR mutations: pooled analysis. *J Cell Mol Med* 2010;14:51–69.

25. Pirker R, Pereira JR, Szczesna A, et al. Cetuximab plus chemotherapy in patients with advanced non-small-cell lung cancer (FLEX): an open-label randomised phase III trial. *Lancet* 2009;373:1525–31.

26. Lynch TJ, Patel T, Dreisbach L, et al. Cetuximab and first-line taxane/carboplatin chemotherapy in advanced non-small-cell lung cancer: results of the randomized multicenter phase III trial BMS099. *J Clin Oncol* 2010;28:911–7.

27. Mok T, Wu YL, Zhang L. A small step towards personalized medicine for non-small cell lung cancer. *Discov Med* 2009;8:227–31.

28. Ellison G, Donald E, McWalter G, et al. A comparison of ARMS and DNA sequencing for mutation analysis in clinical biopsy samples. *J Exp Clin Cancer Res* 2010;29:132.

29. Zhang X, Zhang S, Yang X, et al. Fusion of EML4 and ALK is associated with development of lung adenocarcinomas lacking EGFR and KRAS mutations and is correlated with ALK expression. *Mol Cancer* 2010;9:188.

30. Soda M, Choi YL, Enomoto M, et al. Identification of the transforming EML4-ALK fusion gene in non-small-cell lung cancer. *Nature* 2007;448:561–6.

31. Shaw AT, Yeap BY, Solomon BJ, et al. Effect of crizotinib on overall survival in patients with advanced non-small-cell lung cancer harbouring ALK gene rearrangement: a retrospective analysis. *Lancet Oncol* 2011;12:1004–12.

32. Cappuzzo F, Ciuleanu T, Stelmakh L, et al. Erlotinib as maintenance treatment in advanced non-small-cell lung cancer: a multicentre, randomised, placebo-controlled phase 3 study. *Lancet Oncol* 2010;11:521–9.

33. Paz-Ares L, De Marinis F, Dediu M, et al. PARAMOUNT: final overall survival (OS) results of the phase III study of maintenance pemetrexed (pem) plus best supportive care (BSC) versus placebo (plb) plus BSC immediately following

induction treatment with pem plus cisplatin (cis) for advanced nonsquamous (NS) non-small cell lung cancer (NSCLC). *J Clin Oncol* 30, 2012 (suppl; abstr LBA7507).

34. Zhang L, Ma S, Song X, et al. Gefitinib versus placebo as maintenance therapy in patients with locally advanced or metastatic non-small-cell lung cancer (INFORM; C-TONG 0804): a multicentre, double-blind randomised phase 3 trial. *Lancet Oncol* 2012;13:466–75.

35. Fidias PM, Dakhil SR, Lyss AP, et al. Phase III study of immediate compared with delayed docetaxel after front-line therapy with gemcitabine plus carboplatin in advanced non-small-cell lung cancer. *J Clin Oncol* 2009;27:591–8.

36. Belani CP, Brodowicz T, Ciuleanu TE, et al. Quality of life in patients with advanced non-small-cell lung cancer given maintenance treatment with pemetrexed versus placebo (H3E-MC-JMEN): results from a randomised, double-blind, phase 3 study. *Lancet Oncol* 2012;13:292–9.

37. Ciuleanu T, Brodowicz T, Zielinski C, et al. Maintenance pemetrexed plus best supportive care versus placebo plus best supportive care for non-small-cell lung cancer: a randomised, double-blind, phase 3 study. *Lancet* 2009;374:1432–40.

38. Cappuzzo F, Ciuleanu T, Stelmakh L, et al. Erlotinib as maintenance treatment in advanced non-small-cell lung cancer: a multicentre, randomised, placebo-controlled phase 3 study. *Lancet Oncol* 2010;11:521–9.

39. Brodowicz T, Krzakowski M, Zwitter M, et al. Cisplatin and gemcitabine first-line chemotherapy followed by maintenance gemcitabine or best supportive care in advanced non-small cell lung cancer: a phase III trial. *Lung Cancer* 2006;52:155–63.

40. Ettinger DS, Akerley W, Borghaei H, et al. Non-small cell lung cancer. *J Natl Compr Canc Netw* 2012;8:740–801.

41. Di Maio M, Chiodini P, Georgoulias V, et al. Meta-analysis of single-agent chemotherapy compared with combination chemotherapy as second-line treatment of advanced non-small-cell lung cancer. *J Clin Oncol* 2009;27:1836–43.

42. Shepherd FA, Dancey J, Ramlau R, et al. Prospective randomized trial of docetaxel versus best supportive care in patients with non-small-cell lung cancer previously treated with platinum-based chemotherapy. *J Clin Oncol* 2000;18:2095–103.

43. Shepherd FA, Rodrigues Pereira J, Ciuleanu T, et al. Erlotinib in previously treated non-small-cell lung cancer. *N Engl J Med* 2005;353:123–32.

44. Tsao MS, Sakurada A, Cutz JC, et al. Erlotinib in lung cancer—molecular and clinical predictors of outcome. *N Engl J Med* 2005;353:133–44.

45. Kim ES, Hirsh V, Mok T, et al. Gefitinib versus docetaxel in previously treated non-small-cell lung cancer (INTEREST): a randomised phase III trial. *Lancet* 2008;372:1809–18.

46. Hanna N, Shepherd FA, Fossella FV, et al. Randomized phase III trial of pemetrexed versus docetaxel in patients with non-small-cell lung cancer previously treated with chemotherapy. *J Clin Oncol* 2004;22:1589–97.

47. Ramlau R, Gervais R, Krzakowski M, et al. Phase III study comparing oral topotecan to intravenous docetaxel in patients with pretreated advanced non-small-cell lung cancer. *J Clin Oncol* 2006;24:2800–7.

48. Mehta N, Mauer AM, Hellman S, et al. Analysis of further disease progression in metastatic non-small cell lung cancer: implications for locoregional treatment. *Int J Oncol* 2004;25:1677–83.

49. Wronski M, Arbit E, Burt M, Galicich JH. Survival after surgical treatment of brain metastases from lung cancer: a follow-up study of 231 patients treated between 1976 and 1991. *J Neurosurg* 1995;83:605–16.

50. Tanvetyanon T, Robinson LA, Schell MJ, et al. Outcomes of adrenalectomy for isolated synchronous versus metachronous adrenal metastases in non-small-cell lung cancer: a systematic review and pooled analysis. *J Clin Oncol* 2008;26:1142–7.

51. Patel PR, Yoo DS, Niibe Y, Urbanic JJ, Salama JK. A call for the aggressive treatment of oligometastatic and oligo-recurrent non-small cell lung cancer. *Pulm Med* 2012;2012:480961.

52. Schiller JH, Harrington D, Belani CP, et al. Comparison of four chemotherapy regimens for advanced non-small-cell lung cancer. *N Engl J Med* 2002;346:92–8.

53. Scagliotti GV, De Marinis F, Rinaldi M, et al. Phase III randomized trial comparing three platinum-based doublets in advanced non-small-cell lung cancer. *J Clin Oncol* 2002;20:4285–91.

54. Fukuoka M, Wu YL, Thongprasert S, et al. Biomarker analyses and final overall survival results from a phase III, randomized, open-label, first-line study of gefitinib versus carboplatin/paclitaxel in clinically selected patients with advanced non-small-cell lung cancer in Asia (IPASS). *J Clin Oncol* 2011;29:2866–74.

55. Maemondo M, Inoue A, Kobayashi K, et al. Gefitinib or chemotherapy for non-small-cell lung cancer with mutated EGFR. *N Engl J Med* 2010;362:2380–8.

56. Mitsudomi T, Morita S, Yatabe Y, et al. Gefitinib versus cisplatin plus docetaxel in patients with non-small-cell lung cancer harbouring mutations of the epidermal growth factor receptor (WJTOG3405): an open label, randomised phase 3 trial. *Lancet Oncol* 2010;11:121–8.

57. Zhou C, Wu YL, Chen G, et al. Erlotinib versus chemotherapy as first-line treatment for patients with advanced EGFR mutation-positive non-small-cell lung cancer (OPTIMAL, CTONG-0802): a multicentre, open-label, randomised, phase 3 study. *Lancet Oncol* 2011;12:735–42.

58. Rosell R, Carcereny E, Gervais R, et al. Erlotinib versus standard chemotherapy as first-line treatment for European patients with advanced EGFR mutation-positive non-small-cell lung cancer (EURTAC): a multicentre, open-label, randomised phase 3 trial. *Lancet Oncol* 2012;13:239–46.

59. Belani CP, Waterhouse DM, Ghazal H, et al. Phase III study of maintenance gemcitabine (G) and best supportive care (BSC) versus BSC, following standard combination therapy with gemcitabine-carboplatin (G Cb) for patients with advanced non-small cell lung cancer (NSCLC). *J Clin Oncol* 2010;28:15s (suppl; abstr 7506).

60. Perol M, Chouaid C, Pérol D, et al. Randomized, phase III study of gemcitabine or erlotinib maintenance therapy versus observation, with predefined second-line treatment, after cisplatin-gemciabine induction chemotherapy in advnaced non-small-cell lung cancer. *J Clin Oncol* 2012;30:3516–3524.

61. Miller VA, O'Connor P, Soh C, Kabbinavar F. A randomized, double-blind, placebo-controlled, phase IIIb trial (ATLAS) comparing bevacizumab (B) therapy with or without erlotinib (E) after completion of chemotherapy with B for first-line treatment of locally advanced, recurrent, or metastatic non-small cell lung cancer (NSCLC). *J Clin Oncol* 2009;27:407s (suppl; LBA8002).

62. Fossella FV, DeVore R, Kerr RN, et al. Randomized phase III trial of docetaxel versus vinorelbine or ifosfamide in patients with advanced non-small-cell lung cancer previously treated with platinum-containing chemotherapy regimens. The TAX 320 Non-Small Cell Lung Cancer Study Group. *J Clin Oncol* 2000;18:2354–62.

Chapter 10

Special Populations

Apar Kishor Ganti

This chapter will discuss the management of advanced non–small cell lung cancer (NSCLC) in two groups of patients for whom standard treatment approaches may not be recommended. These populations are older patients and patients with a marginal or poor performance status. Their age at diagnosis, altered physiology either due to age or comorbid conditions, and increased susceptibility to treatment-related toxicities make them a particularly difficult cohort of patients to treat. Despite this, they are two separate cohorts and should be approached distinctly. A common mistake made when developing clinical trials in the past was to group the two cohorts together, and this may have led to some of the confusion regarding their treatment.

Lung Cancer in the Older Patient

Introduction

The median age of diagnosis of NSCLC is 70 years.[1] Unfortunately, most clinical trials do not include enough older patients to make meaningful clinical decisions. Hence, management of older patients with NSCLC is extrapolated from data on younger patients.[2] Older patients are not often prescribed standard therapy, despite evidence that age does not predict for response.[3]

Geriatric Assessment

- Chronological age, functional status, co-morbid conditions, concurrent medications, nutritional status, and cognitive abilities should be taken into consideration while developing a management plan for older patients.
- Although multiple screening tools have been designed to assess patient fitness based on these parameters, there are no universally accepted and validated parameters to identify the fit older patient with lung cancer.
- The Comprehensive Geriatric Assessment (CGA) is a multidisciplinary approach aimed at assessing life expectancy and morbidity in older cancer patients.[4] This includes assessment of functional status (activities of daily living, instrumental activities of daily living, history of falls, gait speed, and performance status) and comorbid conditions (number and severity of various conditions that may affect lung cancer care).

Early-Stage Non–Small Cell Lung Cancer

Surgery

The evidence for the role of surgery in older patients comes from retrospective single-institution analyses from large centers with expertise in dealing with complex patients (see Table 10.1). Although older patients may have an increased risk of complications, the operative risk appears to be similar to younger individuals. However, older patients undergoing a pneumonectomy appear to have a higher

Table 10.1 Surgery for the Older Patient with Early-Stage Non–Small Cell Lung Cancer

Ref.	Treatment	Study Design	N	Outcomes
41	Lung resection for stages I and II	Single-institution report; 12% ($n = 34$) >70 years	70	No differences in postoperative mortality (3% vs. 4.8%) and stage-specific survival by age
42	Lung resection	Retrospective single-institution review of octogenarians	40	15% operative mortality. Increasing age predicted for mortality.
43	Surgery for lung cancer	Retrospective single-institution analysis	144 (70 were ≥ 70 years)	Older patients had fewer recognized postoperative complications; no difference in perioperative mortality and survival.
44	Curative pulmonary resection for NSCLC	Retrospective single-institution analysis	215 (85 > 70 years)	No differences in postoperative mortality, overall complications or long-term survival rates. Older patients—higher incidence of cardiovascular complications.
45	Resection for NSCLC	Single institution, single arm; age >70 years	185	Operative mortality—3%; mortality similar to younger patients.
5	Pneumonectomy for lung cancer	Single institution; age >70 years	122 (27 > 70 years)	Postoperative mortality higher in older patients (22.2 vs. 3.2%; $P < 0.005$)

NSCLC, non–small cell lung cancer.

Source: From Ganti AK, deShazo M, Weir AB 3rd, Hurria A. Treatment of non-small cell lung cancer in the older patient. *J Natl Compr Canc Netw.* 2012;10:230–9. Reprinted with permission from *JNCCN—Journal of the National Comprehensive Cancer Network.*

mortality.[5] These single-institution trials magnify the risk of selection bias, making it difficult for clinicians to apply these results directly to the elderly patient at hand.

Adjuvant Chemotherapy

Adjuvant chemotherapy following resection is the standard of care for patients with stages II and IIIA and selected patients with stage I (large tumor size) NSCLC.[6] The data supporting the use of adjuvant chemotherapy in older patients are retrospective. In the retrospective analysis of the JBR.10 study (adjuvant cisplatin + vinorelbine following resection of stage IB and II NSCLC), while older patients received lower cumulative doses due to adverse effects, the extent of benefit was similar to younger patients.[7] A recent SEER-Medicare database analysis shows similar findings.[8] In this analysis of 3759 patients >65 years, the patients who received adjuvant chemotherapy had a significantly better overall survival (hazard ratio, 0.80; 95% CI, 0.72 to 0.89) compared to those who did not receive adjuvant therapy.

In summary, the available retrospective evidence suggests that while older patients tolerate surgery well, these procedures should be performed only by thoracic surgeons who have special expertise in this population. Older patients appear to benefit from adjuvant chemotherapy, and recommendations should be based on the patient's functional status, rather than chronological age.

Locally Advanced Non–Small Cell Lung Cancer

Patients with locally advanced NSCLC are a heterogeneous group of patients and many of these patients are treated using a multimodality approach. Unfortunately, many trials of combined modality therapy included patients with stages I–III disease and the lack of statistical power makes the treatment decisions in older patients challenging (see Table 10.2).

- Initial studies suggested that in older patients (≥70 years) the addition of chemotherapy to radiation did not provide any benefit but did increase toxicity.[9,10]
- Retrospective analyses of Radiation Therapy Oncology Group (RTOG) and North Central Cancer Treatment Group (NCCTG) studies have suggested that, as compared to younger patients, older patients had a greater incidence of both hematologic and nonhematologic toxicities (esophagitis, pneumonia).[11–13] Despite this, the incidence of long-term adverse effects and overall survival did not appear to differ by age.

In summary, older patients appear to respond to combined modality therapy as well as younger patients. However, they have an increased incidence of acute side effects, which may necessitate the need for closer monitoring and aggressive, early intervention, should these appear.

Advanced/Metastatic Non–Small Cell Lung Cancer

The data on the treatment of advanced NSCLC in the elderly come from two main sources: retrospective subset analyses of clinical trials that did not discriminate by age and prospective trials specific for older patients.

Retrospective Analyses of Non-Age-Specific Trials

Platinum-based doublet therapy is the standard of care in advanced NSCLC, but most of the evidence supporting its use in older patients is derived from

Table 10.2 Combined Modality Therapy in the Older Patient with Locally Advanced Non–Small Cell Lung Cancer

Ref.	Treatment	Study Design	N	Median Survival (Months)		Toxicity, Quality of Life
				Young	Elderly	
9	Various modalities for Stage II–IIIB	Retrospective analysis of patients enrolled on six RTOG phase II/III trials	979 (144 > 70 years)	NR	NR	Patients <70 years—improved survival with multimodality therapy; older patients—best quality-adjusted survival with RT alone as opposed to multi-modality therapy
10	Various modalities; Stage II-IIIB	Retrospective analysis of nine RTOG trials	1999 (429 ≥ 70 years)	11.4	7.6	Increased age associated with a poor outcome only in patients with KPS <90
11	Cisplatin + vinblastine + sequential RT	Retrospective analysis of RTOG 9410	595 (104 ≥ 70 years)	15.7	10.8	Esophagitis and neutropenia more common in older patients treated with concurrent chemoRT. Survival better with concurrent therapy.
	Cisplatin + vinblastine + concurrent RT			15.5	22.4	
	Cisplatin + etoposide with twice daily RT			16	16.4	
12	Cisplatin + etoposide + daily RT	Retrospective analysis of an NCCTG trial	246 (63 ≥ 70 years)	39%*	36%*	Myelosuppression, pneumonitis—more pronounced in older patients
	Cisplatin + etoposide + split course twice daily RT					
46	Cisplatin-vinorelbine followed by RT	Retrospective analysis of CALGB 9130	250 (54 ≥ 70 years)	NR	NR	Increased myelosuppression and renal failure during induction with increasing age. No difference in treatment completion rates, response rates, and overall survival
	Cisplatin-vinorelbine followed by concurrent carboplatin-RT					
13	RT	Retrospective analysis of patients ≥65 years enrolled on NCCTG 9024–51 and 9024-52	166	–	10.5	Increased weight loss and toxicity (both hematologic and nonhematologic) in patients receiving combined modality therapy
	RT + chemotherapy			–	13.7**	

*2-year survival.

**Statistically significant.

CALGB, Cancer and Leukemia Group B; KPS, Karnofsky Performance Status; NCCTG, North Central Cancer Treatment Group; NR, not reported; RTOG, Radiation Therapy Oncology Group; RT, radiation therapy.

Source: From Ganti AK, deShazo M, Weir AB 3rd, Hurria A. Treatment of non-small cell lung cancer in the older patient. *J Natl Compr Canc Netw.* 2012;10:230–9. Reprinted with permission from *JNCCN—Journal of the National Comprehensive Cancer Network.*

retrospective analyses of non-age-specific trials (Table 10.3). The results consistently demonstrate that older patients had outcomes similar to younger patients, but often at the expense of increased toxicity. Hence, although standard therapy may be appropriate in some older patients, it cannot be routinely recommended to the entire population.

Elderly-Specific Trials

Single Agent Therapy

- The Elderly Lung Cancer Vinorelbine Italian Study (ELVIS) study found that single-agent vinorelbine improved median survival compared to best supportive care (28 vs. 21 weeks) in patients ≥70 years of age.[14]
- The West Japan Thoracic Oncology Group (WJTOG) found an improvement in progression-free survival, response rate, symptom control, and a nonsignificant improvement in survival with docetaxel compared to vinorelbine.[15]

Combination versus Single Agent Therapy

- The Southern Italy Cooperative Oncology Group (SICOG) found that a combination of gemcitabine and vinorelbine improved survival compared to vinorelbine in patients ≥70 years of age.[16]
- The larger Multicenter Italian Lung Cancer in the Elderly Study (MILES) study found that either gemcitabine or vinorelbine was as effective as their combination,[17] but with less toxicity.
- The Intergroupe Francophone de Cancérologie Thoracique (IFCT)-0501 trial compared a combination of carboplatin and paclitaxel with single-agent chemotherapy (either gemcitabine or vinorelbine) in patients between the age of 70 and 89 years.[18] In this study, median overall survival was better in the doublet arm (6.2 vs. 10.3 months; $P = 0.0001$).

Despite the relative safety of the aforementioned chemotherapy agents (also see Table 10.4), toxicity remains a major concern in this population with a significant proportion of patients developing grade 3-4 myelosuppression. In the IFCT study, despite the survival advantage, there were more toxic deaths in the combination arm (23.7% vs. 16.6%).[18]

Targeted Therapies

Targeted therapies affect specific molecules or pathways that are critical in tumor growth and progression.[19–21] It is widely believed that they have a broader therapeutic index and are potentially less toxic than cytotoxic chemotherapeutic agents.[22] Three such agents—erlotinib, crizotinib, and bevacizumab—are currently approved by the US Food and Drug Administration for the treatment of NSCLC.

Erlotinib, a small-molecule epidermal growth factor receptor (EGFR) tyrosine kinase inhibitor, is approved for patients with advanced NSCLC who had failed prior chemotherapy. A subgroup analysis of the older patients (≥70 years) in this trial,[23] found no significant differences in survival or quality of life between older and young patients who received erlotinib. However, older patients had more grade ≥3 toxicities and were more likely to discontinue the drug due to adverse effects.

Table 10.3 Advanced Disease: Subset Analyses of Non-Age-Specific Trials

Ref.	Regimen	Study Design	N	Response Rate (%)		Median Survival (Months)		Toxicity, Quality of Life
				Young	Elderly	Young	Elderly	
47	Paclitaxel + carboplatin Vinorelbine + cisplatin Cisplatin	Combined retrospective analysis of two phase III trials	608 (117 ≥70 years)	NR	NR	8.6	6.9	Nonsignificant higher hematologic toxicity in older patients
48	Etoposide + cisplatin Paclitaxel + carboplatin Paclitaxel + carboplatin + G-CSF	Retrospective subset analysis. 15% ≥70 years	200 198 201	22	23	9.1	8.5	Older males—more leucopenia, neuropsychiatric toxicity. Older women—more weight loss.
49	Cisplatin + paclitaxel Cisplatin + gemcitabine Cisplatin + docetaxel Carboplatin + paclitaxel	Unplanned subset analysis. 20% ≥70 years	1139	22.1	24.5	8.15	8.25	Similar grade 4 or higher toxicity
50	Paclitaxel Carboplatin + paclitaxel	Prespecified subset analysis of a phase III trial (N = 561)	78 77	15 28	21 36	6.8 9	5.8 8	NR
25	Carboplatin + paclitaxel Carboplatin + paclitaxel + bevacizumab	Retrospective subset analysis (N = 878)	113 111	15 35	28.7 17.3	10.3 12.3*	12.1 11.3	More neutropenia in the elderly on the triplet arm; no difference with doublet

*All patients enrolled.

NR, not reported.

Source: From Ganti AK, deShazo M, Weir AB 3rd, Hurria A. Treatment of non-small cell lung cancer in the older patient. *J Natl Compr Canc Netw.* 2012;10:230–9. Reprinted with permission from *JNCCN—Journal of the National Comprehensive Cancer Network.*

Table 10.4 Advanced Non–Small Cell Lung Cancer: Randomized Phase III Trials in Older Patients

Ref.	Treatment	N	Response Rate (%)	Median Survival (Weeks)	Toxicity, Quality of Life
14	Vinorelbine	76	19.7	28*	Vinorelbine better in overall health status, quality of life; measures of cognitive, social, and physical function; less dyspnea, hemoptysis, pain, cough
	Best supportive care	78	NR	21	
16	Gemcitabine + vinorelbine	60	22	29	Combination therapy—delayed symptom and quality of life deterioration; but increased grade 3/4 neutropenia, thrombocytopenia, severe emesis
	Vinorelbine	60	15	18	
17	Gemcitabine + vinorelbine	236	21	30	Combination therapy—more thrombocytopenia, hepatic toxicity than vinorelbine; more neutropenia, vomiting, fatigue, cardiac toxicity, constipation than gemcitabine
	Vinorelbine	236	18	36	
	Gemcitabine	235	16	28	
15	Vinorelbine	92	9.9	9.9 months	Global quality of life—no difference. Docetaxel—more neutropenia, alopecia, but better improvement in overall symptom score.
	Docetaxel	90	22.7*	14.3 months	
10	Gemcitabine or vinorelbine	225	10.9	6.2 months	More myelosuppression and toxic deaths with doublet; but fewer early deaths
	Carboplatin + weekly paclitaxel	226	29	10.3 months*	
51	Weekly cisplatin + docetaxel	139	NR	13.3 months	Increased neutropenia/febrile neutropenia with docetaxel but better quality of life
	Docetaxel	137	NR	17.3 months	

*$P < 0.05$.

Source: From Ganti AK, deShazo M, Weir AB 3rd, Hurria A. Treatment of non-small cell lung cancer in the older patient. *J Natl Compr Canc Netw.* 2012;10:230–9. Reprinted with permission from *JNCCN—Journal of the National Comprehensive Cancer Network.*

Bevacizumab, a monoclonal antibody targeting vascular endothelial growth factor (VEGF), is approved for patients with metastatic nonsquamous NSCLC in combination with carboplatin-paclitaxel.[24]

- An unplanned subgroup analysis of older patients (≥70 years) demonstrated higher toxicity with bevacizumab, but no survival benefit (OS: 11.3 [with bevacizumab] vs. 12.1 months [without bevacizumab]; $P = 0.4$).[25]

- Similar findings were seen in a retrospective review of Medicare patients. In this analysis, the addition of bevacizumab to carboplatin-paclitaxel did not improve overall survival in patients >65 years.[26] Although retrospective, this study provides a more real-world view of the impact of bevacizumab in advanced NSCLC.

Thus, the use of bevacizumab in the older patient should be evaluated on an individual benefit given the lack of a significant survival advantage and the increased incidence of adverse events.

Summary

- Chemotherapy is associated with an improved quality of life even in the older population.
- Emerging data suggest that doublet therapy may confer a survival advantage over single-agent therapy, but toxicity, especially myelosuppression, may prevent routine use of doublets in this cohort of patients.
- Individuals treated with doublet therapy should be offered more aggressive supportive care, including more liberal use of myeloid growth factors and closer monitoring.

Patients with Poor Performance Status

Performance status (PS) is determined with the help of two major scoring systems; the Eastern Oncology Cooperative Group (ECOG) score[27] and the Karnofsky Performance Status (KPS)[28] (Table 10.5). Patients who are able to care for themselves but are not able to carry out most work-related activities, that is, ECOG ≥2 or KPS ≤70%, are considered as having a poor PS. There appear to be two major subsets of patients who can be included in this group:

- Those who are in poor health and develop lung cancer
- Those previously in good health who experienced a decline in performance status as a result of the malignancy.

Since most trials do not distinguish between these two groups, it is unclear whether they are physiologically similar. However, these patients comprise almost 30%–40% of all patients with advanced NSCLC.[29] These patients have poorer outcomes compared to patients with a good PS[30,31] and generally have been excluded from clinical trials.

In an attempt to determine the predictors for outcomes in this diverse patient population, Lilenbaum et al. analyzed using data from two large randomized phase III trials conducted in poor PS patients.[32] The two trials included in this analysis were Selective Targeting for Efficacy in Lung Cancer, Lower Adverse Reaction (STELLAR)-3 (carboplatin/paclitaxel vs. carboplatin/paclitaxel poliglumex)[33] and STELLAR-4 (paclitaxel poliglumex vs. either gemcitabine or vinorelbine).[34] This secondary analysis identified four factors that predicted for worse outcomes:

- Serum albumin ≤3.5 g/dL
- Serum LDH >200 IU/L
- Extra-thoracic metastases
- Presence of two or more comorbid conditions[32]

Table 10.5 Assessment of Performance Status

Score	Description
Eastern Cooperative Oncology Group (ECOG) Performance Status[27]	
0	Fully active, able to carry on all predisease performance without restriction
1	Restricted in physically strenuous activity but ambulatory and able to carry out work of a light or sedentary nature, e.g., light house work, office work
2	Ambulatory and capable of all self-care but unable to carry out any work activities. Up and about more than 50% of waking hours
3	Capable of only limited self-care; confined to bed or chair more than 50% of waking hours
4	Completely disabled. Cannot carry on any self-care. Totally confined to bed or chair
5	Dead
Karnofsky Performance Status (KPS)[28]	
100	Normal, no complaints; no evidence of disease
90	Able to carry on normal activity; minor signs or symptoms of disease
80	Normal activity with effort; some signs or symptoms of disease
70	Cares for self; unable to carry on normal activity or to do active work
60	Requires occasional assistance but is able to care for most of his or her personal needs
50	Requires considerable assistance and frequent medical care
40	Disabled; requires special care and assistance
30	Severely disabled; hospital admission is indicated although death not imminent
20	Very sick; hospital admission necessary; active supportive treatment necessary
10	Moribund; fatal processes progressing rapidly
0	Dead

Standard Chemotherapy

While older studies suggested that poor PS patients do not tolerate cytotoxic chemotherapy well and have inferior outcomes,[31] more recent evidence suggests that at least a subset of these patients derive clinical benefit (Table 10.6).

- A retrospective analysis of two multicenter trials conducted by the Lineberger Comprehensive Cancer Center found that although patients with poor PS had worse survival compared to those with a good performance status, they had similar response rates and toxicities following the same chemotherapy.[35]

- A secondary analysis of the STELLAR-3 and STELLAR-4 trials found that combination chemotherapy increased response rates and time to progression. Although chemotherapy-related adverse effects were increased, this did not affect overall survival.[32]

Table 10.6 Trials for Stage IV Non–Small Cell Lung Cancer Patients with a Poor Performance Status

Ref.	Regimen	N	Response Rate (%)	Median Survival (Months)	1-Year Survival (%)	Comments
52	Carboplatin + paclitaxel	54	14	4.8	19.6	More neutropenia and neuropathy with carboplatin-paclitaxel; more nausea, vomiting, and thrombocytopenia with cisplatin-gemcitabine
	Cisplatin + gemcitabine	49	23	4.2	25.5	
53	Gemcitabine 1000 mg/m^2 3 weeks of 4	87	6	83 days	9	No difference in quality of life improvement. Significant early attrition in both arms due to death/progression
	Gemcitabine 1500 mg/m^2 2 weeks of 3	87	10	65 days	13	
50*	Paclitaxel	50	10	2.4	10	Combination chemotherapy improved survival, without increased toxicity
	Carboplatin + paclitaxel	49	24	4.7	18	
54*	Docetaxel	57	NR	2.9	NR	No improvement in survival with the doublet. Both groups had worse than expected results
	Docetaxel + gemcitabine	65	NR	3.8	NR	
33	Carboplatin + paclitaxel	201	36	5.8	31	No difference in quality of life. Paclitaxel—more cardiac and musculoskeletal toxicity; PPX—increased nausea and vomiting
	Carboplatin + PPX	199	21	7.2	31	
34	Gemcitabine or vinorelbine	190	15	6.6	26	No difference in quality of life. PPX—lesser gastrointestinal and hematological toxicity but more neuropathy
	PPX	191	11	7.3	26	
36	Pemetrexed	102	10	5.6	22	Increased anemia and neutropenia with doublet
	Carboplatin + pemetrexed	103	24	9.1	39	

*Only data on PS 2 patients shown.

NR, not reported; PPX, paclitaxel poliglumex.

- Similar results were seen in a recent Brazilian trial comparing pemetrexed with carboplatin-pemetrexed.[36]

Because there has not been a benefit demonstrated consistently for combination therapy in this population, the trend has been to treat these patients with single-agent chemotherapy. The National Comprehensive Cancer Network recommends either single-agent therapy or platinum-based combinations for this population.[6] A trial comparing single-agent and combination chemotherapy in these patients is warranted.

Targeted Agents

It is widely believed that targeted agents provide effective and less toxic therapy while at the same time allowing patients to maintain their functional independence.[22] Thus, there has been great interest in targeted agents in patients with poor PS.

- Data from two trials suggest that erlotinib and gefitinib do not have a role in poor PS patients without activating *EGFR* mutations. In one trial of 103 patients, carboplatin-paclitaxel was associated with better response rates, progression-free and overall survival compared to erlotinib.[37] In another larger trial, gefitinib was not superior to placebo in terms of response rates or overall survival.[38]
- In contrast, patients with an activating *EGFR* mutation appear to tolerate and benefit from EGFR tyrosine kinase inhibitors. In a Japanese study of 30 patients with an *EGFR* mutation and poor PS, the response rate was 66% and approximately 80% patients had an improvement in their PS.[39]
- Anaplastic lymphoma kinase (ALK) positive NSCLC patients have an excellent response to the ALK inhibitor crizotinib. Crizotinib has been evaluated in patients with PS 0-3 in clinical trials. It is reasonable to administer crizotinib to patients with *ALK* rearrangements regardless of their functional status.
- In the FLEX study (cisplatin-vinorelbine with/without cetuximab in patients with advanced NSCLC) approximately 18% of patients had a PS of 2.[40] Cetuximab was associated with a decreased risk of death in this cohort (HR, 0.74; 95% CI 0.55–1.01).
- There is currently no evidence for using bevacizumab in poor PS patients. The results of the ToPPS trial (pemetrexed vs. pemetrexed-bevacizumab vs. pemetrexed-carboplatin-bevacizumab; NCT00892710) should help answer this question.

Summary

- The treatment of poor PS patients with advanced NSCLC is challenging.
- While some of these patients tolerate standard platinum-based doublets and benefit from them, identifying these individuals is difficult.

- The decision to offer doublet therapy should be made on an individualized basis.
- If doublet therapy is recommended to these patients, they should be monitored closely for signs of intolerance.

References

1. Avery EJ, Kessinger A, Ganti AK. Therapeutic options for elderly patients with advanced non-small cell lung cancer. *Cancer Treat Rev* 2009;35:340–4.

2. Hutchins LF, Unger JM, Crowley JJ, Coltman CA, Jr, Albain KS. Underrepresentation of patients 65 years of age or older in cancer-treatment trials. *N Engl J Med* 1999;341:2061–7.

3. Earle CC, Venditti LN, Neumann PJ, et al. Who gets chemotherapy for metastatic lung cancer? *Chest* 2000;117:1239–46.

4. Extermann M, Hurria A. Comprehensive geriatric assessment for older patients with cancer. *J Clin Oncol* 2007;25:1824–31.

5. Mizushima Y, Noto H, Sugiyama S, et al. Survival and prognosis after pneumonectomy for lung cancer in the elderly. *Ann Thorac Surg* 1997;64:193–8.

6. Ettinger DS, Akerley W, Bepler G, et al. Non-small cell lung cancer. *J Natl Compr Canc Netw* 2010;8:740–801.

7. Pepe C, Hasan B, Winton TL, et al. Adjuvant vinorelbine and cisplatin in elderly patients: National Cancer Institute of Canada and Intergroup Study JBR.10. *J Clin Oncol* 2007;25:1553–61.

8. Wisnivesky JP, Smith CB, Packer S, et al. Survival and risk of adverse events in older patients receiving postoperative adjuvant chemotherapy for resected stages II-IIIA lung cancer: observational cohort study. *BMJ* 2011;343:d4013.

9. Movsas B, Scott C, Sause W, et al. The benefit of treatment intensification is age and histology-dependent in patients with locally advanced non-small cell lung cancer (NSCLC): a quality-adjusted survival analysis of radiation therapy oncology group (RTOG) chemoradiation studies. *Int J Radiat Oncol Biol Phys* 1999;45:1143–9.

10. Werner-Wasik M, Scott C, Cox JD, et al. Recursive partitioning analysis of 1999 Radiation Therapy Oncology Group (RTOG) patients with locally-advanced non-small-cell lung cancer (LA-NSCLC): identification of five groups with different survival. *Int J Radiat Oncol Biol Phys* 2000;48:1475–82.

11. Langer CJ, Hsu C, Curran WJ, et al. Elderly patients (pts) with locally advanced non-small cell lung cancer (LA-NSCLC) benefit from combined modality therapy: secondary analysis of Radiation Therapy Oncology Group (RTOG) 94-10. *Proc Am Soc Clin Oncol* 2002;21 (abstr 1193).

12. Schild SE, Stella PJ, Geyer SM, et al. The outcome of combined-modality therapy for stage III non-small-cell lung cancer in the elderly. *J Clin Oncol* 2003;21:3201–6.

13. Schild SE, Mandrekar SJ, Jatoi A, et al. The value of combined-modality therapy in elderly patients with stage III nonsmall cell lung cancer. *Cancer* 2007;110:363–8.

14. Gridelli C. The ELVIS trial: a phase III study of single-agent vinorelbine as first-line treatment in elderly patients with advanced non-small cell lung cancer. Elderly Lung Cancer Vinorelbine Italian Study. *Oncologist* 2001;6(Suppl 1):4–7.

15. Kudoh S, Takeda K, Nakagawa K, et al. Phase III study of docetaxel compared with vinorelbine in elderly patients with advanced non-small-cell lung cancer: results of the West Japan Thoracic Oncology Group Trial (WJTOG 9904). *J Clin Oncol* 2006;24:3657–63.

16. Frasci G, Lorusso V, Panza N, et al. Gemcitabine plus vinorelbine yields bet-ter survival outcome than vinorelbine alone in elderly patients with advanced non-small cell lung cancer. A Southern Italy Cooperative Oncology Group (SICOG) phase III trial. *Lung Cancer* 2001;34(Suppl 4):S65–9.

17. Gridelli C, Perrone F, Gallo C, et al. Chemotherapy for elderly patients with advanced non-small-cell lung cancer: the Multicenter Italian Lung Cancer in the Elderly Study (MILES) phase III randomized trial. *J Natl Cancer Inst* 2003;95:362–72.

18. Quoix E, Zalcman G, Oster JP, et al. Carboplatin and weekly paclitaxel doublet chemotherapy compared with monotherapy in elderly patients with advanced non-small-cell lung cancer: IFCT-0501 randomised, phase 3 trial. *Lancet* 2011;378:1079–88.

19. Tsuruo T, Naito M, Tomida A, et al. Molecular targeting therapy of cancer: drug resistance, apoptosis and survival signal. *Cancer Sci* 2003;94:15–21.

20. Weiner LM, Dhodapkar MV, Ferrone S. Monoclonal antibodies for cancer immunotherapy. *Lancet* 2009;373:1033–40.

21. Zhang J, Yang PL, Gray NS. Targeting cancer with small molecule kinase inhibi-tors. *Nat Rev Cancer* 2009;9:28–39.

22. Gonsalves W, Ganti AK. Targeted anti-cancer therapy in the elderly. *Crit Rev Oncol Hematol* 2011;78:227–42.

23. Wheatley-Price P, Ding K, Seymour L, Clark GM, Shepherd FA. Erlotinib for advanced non-small-cell lung cancer in the elderly: an analysis of the National Cancer Institute of Canada Clinical Trials Group Study BR.21. *J Clin Oncol* 2008;26:2350–7.

24. Sandler A, Gray R, Perry MC, et al. Paclitaxel-carboplatin alone or with bevaci-zumab for non-small-cell lung cancer. *N Engl J Med* 2006;355:2542–50.

25. Ramalingam SS, Dahlberg SE, Langer CJ, et al. Outcomes for elderly, advanced-stage non small-cell lung cancer patients treated with bevacizumab in combination with carboplatin and paclitaxel: analysis of Eastern Cooperative Oncology Group Trial 4599. *J Clin Oncol* 2008;26:60–5.

26. Zhu J, Sharma DB, Gray SW, Chen AB, Weeks JC, Schrag D. Carboplatin and paclitaxel with vs without bevacizumab in older patients with advanced non small cell lung cancer. *JAMA* 2012;307.1593–1601.

27. Oken MM, Creech RH, Tormey DC, et al. Toxicity and response criteria of the Eastern Cooperative Oncology Group. *Am J Clin Oncol* 1982;5:649–55.

28. Schag CC, Heinrich RL, Ganz PA. Karnofsky performance status revisited: reli-ability, validity, and guidelines. *J Clin Oncol* 1984;2:187–93.

29. Lilenbaum RC, Cashy J, Hensing TA, Young S, Cella D. Prevalence of poor per-formance status in lung cancer patients: implications for research. *J Thorac Oncol* 2008;3:125–9.

30. Albain KS, Crowley JJ, LeBlanc M, Livingston RB. Survival determinants in extensive-stage non-small-cell lung cancer: the Southwest Oncology Group experience. *J Clin Oncol* 1991;9:1618–26.

31. Sweeney CJ, Zhu J, Sandler AB, et al. Outcome of patients with a perfor-mance status of 2 in Eastern Cooperative Oncology Group Study E1594: a Phase II trial in patients with metastatic nonsmall cell lung carcinoma. *Cancer* 2001;92:2639–47.

32. Lilenbaum R, Villaflor VM, Langer C, et al. Single-agent versus combination che-motherapy in patients with advanced non-small cell lung cancer and a perfor-mance status of 2: prognostic factors and treatment selection based on two large randomized clinical trials. *J Thorac Oncol* 2009;4:869–74.

33. Langer CJ, O'Byrne KJ, Socinski MA, et al. Phase III trial comparing paclitaxel poliglumex (CT-2103, PPX) in combination with carboplatin versus standard paclitaxel and carboplatin in the treatment of PS 2 patients with chemotherapy-naive advanced non-small cell lung cancer. *J Thorac Oncol* 2008;3:623–30.

34. O'Brien ME, Socinski MA, Popovich AY, et al. Randomized phase III trial comparing single-agent paclitaxel Poliglumex (CT-2103, PPX) with single-agent gemcitabine or vinorelbine for the treatment of PS 2 patients with chemotherapy-naive advanced non-small cell lung cancer. *J Thorac Oncol* 2008;3:728–34.

35. Stinchcombe TE, Choi J, Schell MJ, et al. Carboplatin-based chemotherapy in patients with advanced non-small cell lung cancer and a poor performance status. *Lung Cancer* 2006;51:237–43.

36. Lilenbaum R, Zukin M, Pereira JR, et al. A randomized phase III trial of single-agent pemetrexed (P) versus carboplatin and pemetrexed (CP) in patients with advanced non-small cell lung cancer (NSCLC) and performance status (PS) of 2. *J Clin Oncol* 2012;30 (suppl; abstr 7506).

37. Lilenbaum R, Axelrod R, Thomas S, et al. Randomized phase II trial of erlotinib or standard chemotherapy in patients with advanced non-small-cell lung cancer and a performance status of 2. *J Clin Oncol* 2008;26:863–9.

38. Goss G, Ferry D, Wierzbicki R, et al. Randomized phase II study of gefitinib compared with placebo in chemotherapy-naive patients with advanced non-small-cell lung cancer and poor performance status. *J Clin Oncol* 2009;27:2253–60.

39. Inoue A, Kobayashi K, Usui K, et al. First-line gefitinib for patients with advanced non-small-cell lung cancer harboring epidermal growth factor receptor mutations without indication for chemotherapy. *J Clin Oncol* 2009;27:1394–1400.

40. Pirker R, Pereira JR, Szczesna A, et al. Cetuximab plus chemotherapy in patients with advanced non-small-cell lung cancer (FLEX): an open-label randomised phase III trial. *Lancet* 2009;373:1525–31.

41. Cangemi V, Volpino P, D'Andrea N, et al. Lung cancer surgery in elderly patients. *Tumori* 1996;82:237–41.

42. Naunheim KS, Kesler KA, D'Orazio SA, Fiore AC, Judd DR. Lung cancer surgery in the octogenarian. *Eur J Cardiothorac Surg* 1994;8:453–6.

43. Jack CI, Lye M, Lesley F, Wilson G, Donnelly RJ, Hind CR. Surgery for lung cancer: age alone is not a contraindication. *Int J Clin Pract* 1997;51:423–6.

44. Morandi U, Stefani A, Golinelli M, et al. Results of surgical resection in patients over the age of 70 years with non small-cell lung cancer. *Eur J Cardiothorac Surg* 1997;11:432–9.

45. Ishida T, Yokoyama H, Kaneko S, Sugio K, Sugimachi K. Long-term results of operation for non-small cell lung cancer in the elderly. *Ann Thorac Surg* 1990;50:919–22.

46. Rocha Lima CM, Herndon JE, II, Kosty M, Clamon G, Green MR. Therapy choices among older patients with lung carcinoma: an evaluation of two trials of the Cancer and Leukemia Group B. *Cancer* 2002;94:181–7.

47. Branchard EM, Moon J, Kesketh PJ, et al. Comparison of platinum-based chemotherapy in patients older and younger than 70 years: an analysis of Southwest Oncology Group Trials 9308 and 9509. *J Thorac Oncol* 2011;6:115–20.

48. Langer CJ, Manola J, Bernardo P, et al. Cisplatin-based therapy for elderly patients with advanced non-small-cell lung cancer: implications of Eastern Cooperative Oncology Group 5592, a randomized trial. *J Natl Cancer Inst* 2002;94:173–81.

49. Langer CJ, Vangel M, Schiller J, et al. Age-specific subanalysis of ECOG 1594: fit elderly patients (70–80 YRS) with NSCLC do as well as younger pts (<70). *Proc Am Soc Clin Oncol* 2003;22 (abstr 2571).

50. Lilenbaum RC, Herndon JE, II, List MA, et al. Single-agent versus combination chemotherapy in advanced non-small-cell lung cancer: the cancer and leukemia group B (study 9730). *J Clin Oncol* 2005;23:190–6.

51. Abe T, Yokoyama A, Takeda K, et al. Randomized phase III trial comparing weekly docetaxel (D)-cisplatin (P) combination with triweekly D alone in elderly patients (pts) with advanced non-small cell lung cancer (NSCLC): an intergroup trial of JCOG0803/WJOG4307L. *J Clin Oncol* 2011;29 (suppl; abstr 7509).

52. Langer C, Li S, Schiller J, et al. Randomized phase II trial of paclitaxel plus carboplatin or gemcitabine plus cisplatin in Eastern Cooperative Oncology Group performance status 2 non-small-cell lung cancer patients: ECOG 1599. *J Clin Oncol* 2007;25:418–23.

53. Baka S, Ashcroft L, Anderson H, et al. Randomized phase II study of two gemcitabine schedules for patients with impaired performance status (Karnofsky performance status </= 70) and advanced non-small-cell lung cancer. *J Clin Oncol* 2005;23:2136–44.

54. Hainsworth JD, Spigel DR, Farley C, et al. Weekly docetaxel versus docetaxel/gemcitabine in the treatment of elderly or poor performance status patients with advanced nonsmall cell lung cancer: a randomized phase 3 trial of the Minnie Pearl Cancer Research Network. *Cancer* 2007;110:2027–34.

Chapter 11

Small Cell Lung Cancer

Apar Kishor Ganti

Small cell lung cancer (SCLC) has a behavior distinct from its more common counterpart, non–small cell lung cancer (NSCLC).[1] The incidence of SCLC is decreasing in the United States from approximately 25% of all lung cancers in 1993 to about 13% in a recent Surveillance Epidemiology and End Results (SEER) database analysis.[2] The reasons for this decline in incidence are likely multifactorial.[3] The disease occurs almost exclusively in smokers, and smoking habits have changed in the past few decades. The advent of filtered cigarettes may also contribute to this trend. Nonetheless, SCLC continues to be a major clinical problem, with an aggressive clinical course and short disease-free duration after initial therapy.

Pathology

The biology and pathology of SCLC are covered in detail in Chapters 2 and 3. An interesting, recently reported phenomenon is the development of SCLC as a mechanism of acquired resistance in patients with epidermal growth factor receptor (EGFR) mutation positive lung cancer who have been treated with an EGFR tyrosine kinase inhibitor.[4]

Staging

Two systems are currently used to stage SCLC: the American Joint Committee on Cancer's tumor-node-metastasis (TNM) classification[5] and the Veterans Affairs Lung Study Group (VALSG) system.[6] While the TNM classification is the same for both NSCLC and SCLC, the VA classification subdivides SCLC into limited stage disease and extensive stage disease. Limited stage disease is confined to the ipsilateral hemithorax and within a single radiation port (TNM stages I through IIIB), while extensive stage disease includes metastatic disease outside the ipsilateral hemithorax. The recent International Association for the Study of Lung Cancer (IASLC) classification project analyzed 8088 cases of SCLC[7] and found that survival was directly correlated to both T and N category; hence, it is recommended that this system be adopted in the future.[8]

Goals of Therapy

SCLC is an aggressive disease and in the absence of treatment, survival is measured in months. Systemic chemotherapy is the mainstay of the treatment of SCLC as it improves survival for all stages.[9] Despite a high likelihood of response to initial therapy, relapses are common and remissions usually last for only 6–8 months. The goals of therapy depend on the stage of the disease and the patient's performance status.

- About 10%–15% of patients with limited stage disease survive for ≥5 years with combined modality therapy (chemotherapy and thoracic radiation),[10] and hence long-term survival should be the goal for patients with a good performance status.
- Patients with extensive stage disease have a high likelihood of response to initial therapy, but subsequent disease progression often occurs rapidly, with a 5-year survival rate of ≈2%.
- Patients who have relapsed disease have a poor prognosis, and treatment should be geared toward symptom palliation.

Cytotoxic Chemotherapy

SCLC is highly chemosensitive (response rates of ≈65%), and multiple agents have shown activity, including platinums (cisplatin, carboplatin), camptothecins (topotecan, irinotecan), podophyllotoxins (etoposide), anthracyclines (doxorubicin, epirubicin, amrubicin), alkylating agents (cyclophosphamide, ifosfamide), taxanes (paclitaxel, docetaxel), and vinca alkaloids (vincristine).

- Initial trials found high response rates with cyclophosphamide, doxorubicin/epirubicin, and vincristine (CAV/CEV).[11,12]
- Combination of etoposide with cisplatin (EP) demonstrated superior response rates compared to CAV.[13,14] Also, EP was better tolerated and is thus the regimen of choice for initial treatment of SCLC.
- A Japan Clinical Oncology Group trial (JCOG 9511) of patients with extensive stage SCLC found higher response rates (84% vs. 68%) and median survival (12.8 vs. 9.4 months) with cisplatin-irinotecan compared to EP.[15] Irinotecan had lower hematologic side effects but increased diarrhea compared to etoposide.
- However, multiple trials outside Japan did not find any differences in outcomes between platinum-etoposide and platinum-irinotecan.[16–19] These discrepancies may be due to pharmacogenomic differences between Japanese and Western populations.

Cisplatin versus Carboplatin

- Cisplatin and carboplatin appear to have comparable efficacy in the first-line treatment of SCLC, both limited stage disease and extensive stage disease.[20] Hematologic toxicity is higher with carboplatin and non-hematologic toxicity is higher with cisplatin.
- In the setting of limited stage SCLC, where the goal of treatment is cure, cisplatin may be preferable to carboplatin.

Duration of Therapy

- Two randomized trials conducted to evaluate the role of additional cycles of therapy following four cycles of platinum-etoposide in patients with extensive stage SCLC[21,22] showed that while extending the duration of therapy improved progression-free survival, there was no overall survival benefit.

- A meta-analysis of 14 trials and 2550 patients suggested that maintenance or consolidation chemotherapy following initial treatment of SCLC was associated with a 33% decreased risk of death at 1 and 2 years.[23] However, only one trial used modern chemotherapy regimens in both induction and consolidation phases. Hence, maintenance therapy for SCLC cannot be considered standard at this time.

Thoracic Radiation

Two meta-analyses found that combining thoracic radiation therapy (TRT) and chemotherapy produced a small but definite improvement in survival albeit at the expense of a small but significant increase in mortality.[24,25] Hence, concurrent TRT and combination chemotherapy is currently the standard of care in patients with limited stage SCLC. However, a number of issues associated with TRT remain unresolved.

Dose

- A National Cancer Institute-Canada (NCI-C) trial found that patients receiving a higher dose (37.5 vs. 25 Gy) had better local control.[26]
- Arriagada et al. analyzed the data from patients enrolled in three consecutive chemoradiation trials (45, 55, 65 Gy).[27] They found similar local control and overall survival.

Fractionation

- Currently utilized standard fractionation schedules involve single daily treatments of 1.8 to 2.0 Gy, five times per week, over 5 to 6 weeks for total radiation doses ranging from 45 to 60 Gy.
- Hyperfractionated radiotherapy (twice daily radiation with lower treatment fractions) has been developed to improve local control and possibly survival. In a randomized phase III study,[28] patients receiving the hyperfractionated schedule (1.5 Gy/fraction BID x 15 days over 3 weeks) significantly improved survival (23 vs. 19 months) compared to a once-a-day schedule (1.8 Gy per fraction QD x 5 weeks). Esophagitis necessitating feeding tube placement was significantly higher in the twice daily arm.
- The two radiation doses used in the above study are not biologically equivalent. The equivalent dose for 45 Gy BID when using conventional fractionation, would be 70 Gy.[29]

Timing of Radiation

The issue of early (i.e., initiation of TRT with first cycle of chemotherapy) versus late (i.e., initiation of TRT with subsequent cycle of chemotherapy of after chemotherapy completed) administration of radiation in conjunction with chemotherapy has been highly controversial. The results of studies comparing early with late radiation are conflicting (Table 11.1). Two trials show a benefit for early radiation,[30,31]

Table 11.1 Timing of Thoracic Radiation Therapy

Ref.	Chemotherapy: Radiation Regimen	N Early	N Late	XRT Early	XRT Late	Median OS (Months) Early	Median OS (Months) Late	Comments
53	CAVE: 40 Gy in 4 weeks, followed by a 10 Gy "boost" to residual disease	125	145	Day 1	Day 64	13.0	14.5	No difference in outcomes
54	CAV EP (RT with EP): 40 Gy; protocol amended to 54 Gy	99	100	Day 1	Week 18	10.7	12.9	No difference in in-field recurrence, CNS recurrence, or OS
55	Carb/E: 1.5 Gy fractions twice daily to 45 Gy	42	39	Cycle 1	Cycle 4	17.5	17	Distant relapses more with late TRT
30	CAV/EP: 40 Gy in 15 fractions	155	153	Week 3	Week 15	21.2*	16	Increased incidence of brain metastases in the late TRT arm
31	Carb/E (RT) + EP: 54 Gy in 1.5 Gy fractions twice daily	52	51	Week 1–4	Week 6–9	34*	26	Better local control with early TRT
56	EP: 45 Gy over 3 weeks (1.5 Gy twice daily)	114	114	Day 2	After cycle 4	27.2	19.7	Hazard ratio for death lower with early TRT – 0.70 (95% CI, 0.52 to 0.94, $P = 0.02$), but more hematologic toxicity
57	CAV/EP: 40 Gy in 15 fractions using cobalt-60 or a linear accelerator	159	166	Cycle 2	Cycle 6	13.5	15.1	No survival benefit, but delivery of chemotherapy optimal with early TRT

*Statistically significant.

Carb/E, carboplatin, etoposide; CAV, cyclophosphamide, doxorubicin, vincristine; CAVE, cyclophosphamide, doxorubicin, vincristine, etoposide; CNS, central nervous system; EP, etoposide, cisplatin; Gy, gray; OS, overall survival; TRT thoracic radiation therapy.

while others do not, suggesting that either approach may be valid. A meta-analysis[32] suggested that there was no difference in overall survival. However, when only trials using platinum-based chemotherapy concurrently with radiation were considered, there was a significantly higher 5-year survival with early TRT.

Surgery

SCLC has for long been considered a systemic disease without a role for surgery. However, the role of surgery in the management of SCLC is evolving.

Peripheral Small Cell Lung Cancer

This represents a very small subpopulation of patients with limited stage SCLC, with most estimates placing this group at 5% of all cases.[33] These patients are usually asymptomatic and diagnosed incidentally. If a preoperative tissue diagnosis suggests SCLC, surgical staging of the mediastinum is recommended, as positive N2 or N3 nodes significantly decrease the benefits of resection.

- For those patients proceeding to surgery, a lobectomy and mediastinal lymph node dissection is recommended. Patients who have pathologic Stage I disease have a reported 5-year survival of 25%.
- Patients requiring a pneumonectomy appear to have much lower survival than those with tumors amenable to a lobectomy, and hence a non-surgical treatment strategy may be appropriate in this setting.[34]
- Given the high risk of recurrence, consideration of postoperative therapy appears desirable. Current recommendations are for using chemotherapy alone for node-negative disease and concurrent chemoradiation for node-positive disease.

Thus, while the majority of patients diagnosed with SCLC will not be surgical candidates, surgery does have the potential to provide an impact on survival in a small, select group of patients with SCLC.[35]

Prophylactic Cranial Irradiation

The central nervous system (CNS) is a common site of metastasis in patients with SCLC. Of all the patients who achieve a complete response with initial therapy, approximately 45% present with CNS-only relapse within 2 years.[36,37] CNS relapse is associated with considerable morbidity and functional decline. Therefore, prevention of CNS relapse would be beneficial.

- In a meta-analysis of 12 trials (1547 patients; limited stage and extensive stage), Meert et al. found that prophylactic cranial irradiation (PCI) decreased the incidence of brain metastases by 52%,[38] with an 18% improvement of survival in patients who received PCI while in a complete response.
- In another meta-analysis, Auperin et al. included those studies where patients had achieved a complete response to initial therapy (7 trials, 984 patients; limited stage and extensive stage disease).[39] There was a 16% decrease in relative risk of death (5.4% increase in 3-year survival) with PCI.

- In a randomized phase III trial in patients with extensive stage SCLC who had not progressed following initial therapy, PCI decreased both the incidence of brain metastases (14.6% vs. 40.4%) and improved overall survival (5.4 vs. 6.7 months).[40]

Dose

The current recommendations are doses between 25 and 36 Gy, given in one of the following schedules: 25 Gy in 10 fractions, 30 Gy in 15 fractions, or 36 Gy in 18 fractions.[41]

Toxicity

The major factor limiting the widespread use of PCI has been the concern for long-term neurotoxicity. Patients who receive PCI tend to live longer and thus are at greater risk of developing chronic neurotoxicity. Despite these concerns, a small retrospective analysis of 98 patients who received PCI showed a significant improvement in mean Q-TWiST (quality time without symptoms and toxicity) survival.[42]

Relapsed Small Cell Lung Cancer

Relapsed SCLC is much less chemosensitive than treatment-naïve SCLC. Factors predicting response to second-line treatment include performance status, chemosensitive (relapse >3 months after initial therapy) versus refractory (relapse within 3 months following initial therapy) disease, and extent of tumor (limited vs. extensive stage).[43,44]

Chemotherapy Regimens for Relapsed/Refractory Small Cell Lung Cancer

Repeating the Initial Regimen

In patients with chemosensitive disease, repeating the original regimen may be effective in achieving a second remission,[45–47] especially if the initial duration of response was ≥6 months.

CAV

In a trial of 29 patients, half of whom had a chemosensitive relapse, Shepherd et al.[48] reported a 28% response rate and a median survival of 4 months. Given this modest activity and considerable toxicity, CAV is not a preferred salvage regimen.

Topotecan

Topotecan is a water-soluble, semisynthetic derivative of camptothecin that has demonstrated antitumor activity in relapsed/refractory SCLC.[49]

- A randomized phase III study of 210 patients with sensitive relapse showed similar response rates, time to progression, and median survival with CAV and topotecan.[49]
- Patients randomized to topotecan experienced greater symptom control and decreased interference with daily activities. Severe neutropenia was

significantly less common with topotecan, but severe thrombocytopenia and anemia were more common.

- Oral and intravenous topotecan have similar response rates (18% vs. 22%), median survival (33 vs. 35 weeks), and 1-year survival rates (33% vs. 29%) in patients with a chemosensitive relapse.[50]

Amrubicin

Amrubicin is a synthetic 9-amino anthracycline with minimal cardiotoxicity. It inhibits topoisomerase II and has shown promising activity in SCLC.[51]

- Preliminary results of a phase III trial comparing amrubicin to topotecan in 637 patients[52] suggest that survival was similar in the two groups. In the subset of patients with refractory disease, amrubicin was associated with a better median survival (6.2 vs. 5.7 months, $P = 0.047$).
- Patients treated with amrubicin had significant improvement in appetite, cough, and dyspnea but had increased febrile neutropenia.

Other Agents

Multiple other agents have been studied with modest activity in relapsed/refractory SCLC. These include paclitaxel, docetaxel, irinotecan, oral etoposide, vinorelbine, and gemcitabine. In addition, multiple combinations of these agents have been studied, but none of them is consistently superior to single-agent regimens.

Commonly Used Chemotherapy Regimens

First-Line Therapy

Cisplatin + etoposide:
- Cisplatin 60 mg/m² IV day 1; etoposide 120 mg/m² per day IV days 1–3. Repeat every 3 weeks.
- Cisplatin 80 mg/m² IV day 1; etoposide 100 mg/m² per day IV days 1–3. Repeat every 3–4 weeks.
- Cisplatin 80 mg/m² IV day 1; etoposide 80 mg/m² per day IV days 1–3. Repeat every 3 weeks.
- Cisplatin 25 mg/m² IV days 1–3; etoposide 80 mg/m² per day IV days 1–3. Repeat every 3–4 weeks.

Carboplatin + etoposide:
- Carboplatin AUC 5 IV day 1; etoposide 100 mg/m² per day IV days 1–3. Repeat every 4 weeks.
- Carboplatin AUC 5 IV day 1; etoposide 80 mg/m² per day IV days 1–3. Repeat every 3–4 weeks.

Cisplatin + irinotecan:
- Cisplatin 60 mg/m² IV day 1; irinotecan 60 mg/m² IV days 1, 8, and 15. Repeat every 4 weeks.
- Cisplatin 30 mg/m² IV days 1, 8; irinotecan 60 mg/m² IV days 1, 8, and 15. Repeat every 3 weeks.

Carboplatin + irinotecan:
- Carboplatin AUC 5 IV day 1; irinotecan 50 mg/m² IV days 1, 8, and 15. Repeat every 4 weeks.
- Carboplatin AUC 5 IV day 1; irinotecan 175 mg/m² IV day 1. Repeat every 3 weeks.

Relapsed Disease

Topotecan:
- Topotecan 2.3 mg/m² per day PO on days 1–5*. Repeat every 3 weeks.
- Topotecan 1.5 mg/m² per day IV on days 1–5. Repeat every 3 weeks.

Amrubicin 40 mg/m² per day IV on days 1–3. Repeat every 3 weeks.

Paclitaxel:
- Paclitaxel 80 mg/m² IV weekly for 6 weeks. Repeat every 8 weeks.
- Paclitaxel 175 mg/m² IV day 1. Repeat every 3 weeks.

Etoposide 50 mg/m² PO daily x 21 days.* Repeat every 4 weeks.

Docetaxel 100 mg IV day 1. Repeat every 3 weeks.

Temozolomide 75 mg/m² PO daily for 21 days.* Repeat every 4 weeks.

(*Note:* *Oral topotecan doses should be rounded to the nearest 0.25 mg while oral etoposide doses should be rounded to the nearest 50 mg dose.)

Commonly Used Radiation Schedules

Thoracic Radiation Therapy

- 1.5 Gy twice daily (at least 6 hours apart) over 3 weeks for a total dose of 45 Gy
- 1.8 Gy daily over 6.5 weeks to a total dose of at least 60 Gy

Prophylactic Cranial Irradiation

- 25 Gy in 10 daily fractions
- 30 Gy in 10–15 daily fractions
- 24 Gy in 8 daily fractions

References

1. Cohen MH, Matthews MJ. Small cell bronchogenic carcinoma: a distinct clinico-pathologic entity. *Semin Oncol* 1978;5:234–43.

2. Govindan R, Page N, Morgensztern D, et al. Changing epidemiology of small-cell lung cancer in the United States over the last 30 years: analysis of the surveillance, epidemiologic, and end results database. *J Clin Oncol* 2006;24:4539–44.

3. Ettinger DS, Aisner J. Changing face of small-cell lung cancer: real and artifact. *J Clin Oncol* 2006;24:4526–7.

4. Sequist LV, Waltman BA, Dias-Santagata D, et al. Genotypic and histological evolution of lung cancers acquiring resistance to EGFR inhibitors. *Sci Translational Med* 2011;3:75ra26.

5. Mountain CF. Revisions in the International System for Staging Lung Cancer. *Chest* 1997;111:1710–7.

6. Argiris A, Murren JR. Staging and clinical prognostic factors for small-cell lung cancer. *Cancer J* 2001;7:437–47.

7. Shepherd FA, Crowley J, Van Houtte P, et al. The International Association for the Study of Lung Cancer lung cancer staging project: proposals regarding the clinical staging of small cell lung cancer in the forthcoming (seventh) edition of the tumor, node, metastasis classification for lung cancer. *J Thorac Oncol* 2007;2:1067–77.

8. Vallieres E, Shepherd FA, Crowley J, et al. The IASLC Lung Cancer Staging Project: proposals regarding the relevance of TNM in the pathologic staging of small cell lung cancer in the forthcoming (seventh) edition of the TNM classification for lung cancer. *J Thorac Oncol* 2009;4:1049–59.

9. Agra Y, Pelayo M, Sacristan M, Sacristán A, Serra C, Bonfill X. Chemotherapy versus best supportive care for extensive small cell lung cancer. *Cochrane Database Syst Rev* 2003;4:CD001990.

10. Gaspar LE, Gay EG, Crawford J, Putnam JB, Herbst RS, Bonner JA. Limited-stage small-cell lung cancer (stages I-III): observations from the National Cancer Data Base. *Clin Lung Cancer* 2005;6:355–60.

11. Livingston RB, Moore TN, Heilbrun L, et al. Small-cell carcinoma of the lung: combined chemotherapy and radiation: a Southwest Oncology Group study. *Ann Intern Med* 1978;88:194–9.

12. Feld R, Evans WK, DeBoer G, et al. Combined modality induction therapy without maintenance chemotherapy for small cell carcinoma of the lung. *J Clin Oncol* 1984;2:294–304.

13. Sierocki JS, Hilaris BS, Hopfan S, et al. cis-Dichlorodiammineplatinum(II) and VP-16-213: an active induction regimen for small cell carcinoma of the lung. *Cancer Treat Rep* 1979;63:1593–7.

14. Evans WK, Shepherd FA, Feld R, Osoba D, Dang P, Deboer G. VP-16 and cisplatin as first-line therapy for small-cell lung cancer. *J Clin Oncol* 1985;3:1471–7.

15. Noda K, Nishiwaki Y, Kawahara M, et al. Irinotecan plus cisplatin compared with etoposide plus cisplatin for extensive small-cell lung cancer. *N Engl J Med* 2002;346:85–91.

16. Hanna N, Bunn PA Jr, Langer C, et al. Randomized phase III trial comparing irinotecan/cisplatin with etoposide/cisplatin in patients with previously untreated extensive-stage disease small-cell lung cancer. *J Clin Oncol* 2006;24:2038–43.

17. Lara PN, Jr., Natale R, Crowley J, et al. Phase III trial of irinotecan/cisplatin compared with etoposide/cisplatin in extensive-stage small-cell lung cancer: clinical and pharmacogenomic results from SWOG S0124. *J Clin Oncol* 2009;27:2530–5.

18. Zatloukal P, Cardenal F, Szczesna A, et al. A multicenter international randomized phase III study comparing cisplatin in combination with irinotecan or etoposide in previously untreated small-cell lung cancer patients with extensive disease. *Ann Oncol* 2010;21:1810–6.

19. Schmittel A, Sebastian M, Fischer von Weikersthal L, et al. A German multicenter, randomized phase III trial comparing irinotecan-carboplatin with etoposide-carboplatin as first-line therapy for extensive-disease small-cell lung cancer. *Ann Oncol* 2011;22:1798–1804.

20. Rossi A, Di Maio M, Chiodini P, et al. Carboplatin- or Cisplatin-based chemotherapy in first-line treatment of small-cell lung cancer: the COCIS meta-analysis of individual patient data. *J Clin Oncol* 2012;30:1692–8.

21. Schiller JH, Adak S, Cella D, DeVore RF, 3rd, Johnson DH. Topotecan versus observation after cisplatin plus etoposide in extensive-stage small-cell lung cancer: E7593—a phase III trial of the Eastern Cooperative Oncology Group. *J Clin Oncol* 2001;19:2114–22.

22. Hanna NH, Sandler AB, Loehrer PJ Sr, et al. Maintenance daily oral etoposide versus no further therapy following induction chemotherapy with etoposide plus ifosfamide plus cisplatin in extensive small-cell lung cancer: a Hoosier Oncology Group randomized study. *Ann Oncol* 2002;13:95–102.

23. Bozcuk H, Artac M, Ozdogan M, Savas B. Does maintenance/consolidation chemotherapy have a role in the management of small cell lung cancer (SCLC)? A metaanalysis of the published controlled trials. *Cancer* 2005;104:2650–7.

24. Pignon JP, Arriagada R, Ihde DC, et al. A meta-analysis of thoracic radiotherapy for small-cell lung cancer. *N Engl J Med* 1992;327:1618–24.

25. Warde P, Payne D. Does thoracic irradiation improve survival and local control in limited-stage small-cell carcinoma of the lung? A meta-analysis. *J Clin Oncol* 1992;10:890–5.

26. Coy P, Hodson I, Payne DG, et al. The effect of dose of thoracic irradiation on recurrence in patients with limited stage small cell lung cancer. Initial results of a Canadian Multicenter Randomized Trial. *Int J Radiat Oncol Biol Phys* 1988;14:219–26.

27. Arriagada R, le Chevalier T, Ruffie P, et al. Alternating radiotherapy and chemotherapy in 173 consecutive patients with limited small cell lung carcinoma. GROP and the French Cancer Center's Lung Group. *Int J Radiat Oncol Biol Phys* 1990;19:1135–8.

28. Turrisi AT, Kim K, Blum R, et al. Twice-daily compared with once-daily thoracic radiotherapy in limited small-cell lung cancer treated concurrently with cisplatin and etoposide. *N Engl J Med* 1999;340:265–71.

29. Choi NC, Herndon J, Rosenman J, et al. Long term survival data from CALGB 8837: radiation dose escalation and concurrent chemotherapy (CT) in limited stage small cell lung cancer (LD-SCLC). Possible radiation dose-survival relationship. *Proc Am Soc Clin Oncol* 2002;21 (abstr 1190).

30. Murray N, Coy P, Pater JL, et al. Importance of timing for thoracic irradiation in the combined modality treatment of limited-stage small-cell lung cancer. The National Cancer Institute of Canada Clinical Trials Group. *J Clin Oncol* 1993;11:336–44.

31. Jeremic B, Shibamoto Y, Acimovic L, Milisavljevic S. Initial versus delayed accelerated hyperfractionated radiation therapy and concurrent chemotherapy in limited small-cell lung cancer: a randomized study. *J Clin Oncol* 1997;15:893–900.

32. De Ruysscher D, Pijls-Johannesma M, Vansteenkiste J, Kester A, Rutten I, Lambin P. Systematic review and meta-analysis of randomised, controlled trials of the timing of chest radiotherapy in patients with limited-stage, small-cell lung cancer. *Ann Oncol* 2006;17:543–52.

33. Quoix E, Fraser R, Wolkove N, Finkelstein H, Kreisman H. Small cell lung cancer presenting as a solitary pulmonary nodule. *Cancer* 1990;66:577–82.

34. Muller LC, Salzer GM, Huber H, et al. Multimodal therapy of small cell lung cancer in TNM stages I through IIIa. *Ann Thorac Surg* 1992;54:493–7.

35. Brock MV, Hooker CM, Syphard JE, et al. Surgical resection of limited disease small cell lung cancer in the new era of platinum chemotherapy: Its time has come. *J Thorac Cardiovasc Surg* 2005;129:64–72.

36. Arriagada R, Le Chevalier T, Borie F, et al. Prophylactic cranial irradiation for patients with small-cell lung cancer in complete remission. *J Natl Cancer Inst* 1995;87:183–90.

37. Ball DL, Matthews JP. Prophylactic cranial irradiation: more questions than answers. *Sem Radiat Oncol* 1995;5:61–8.

38. Meert AP, Paesmans M, Berghmans T, et al. Prophylactic cranial irradiation in small cell lung cancer: a systematic review of the literature with meta-analysis. *BMC Cancer* 2001;1:5.

39. Auperin A, Arriagada R, Pignon JP, et al. Prophylactic cranial irradiation for patients with small-cell lung cancer in complete remission. Prophylactic Cranial Irradiation Overview Collaborative Group. *N Engl J Med* 1999;341:476–84.

40. Slotman B, Faivre-Finn C, Kramer G, et al. Prophylactic cranial irradiation in extensive small-cell lung cancer. *N Engl J Med* 2007;357:664–72.

41. Johnson BE, Crawford J, Downey RJ, et al. Small cell lung cancer clinical practice guidelines in oncology. *J Natl Compr Canc Netw* 2006;4:602–22.

42. Tai TH, Yu E, Dickof P, et al. Prophylactic cranial irradiation revisited: cost-effectiveness and quality of life in small-cell lung cancer. *Int J Radiat Oncol Biol Phys* 2002;52:68–74.

43. Albain KS, Crowley JJ, Hutchins L, et al. Predictors of survival following relapse or progression of small cell lung cancer. Southwest Oncology Group Study 8605 report and analysis of recurrent disease data base. *Cancer* 1993;72:1184–91.

44. Seifter EJ, Ihde DC. Therapy of small cell lung cancer: a perspective on two decades of clinical research. *Semin Oncol* 1988;15:278–99.

45. Batist G, Ihde DC, Zabell A, et al. Small-cell carcinoma of lung: reinduction therapy after late relapse. *Ann Intern Med* 1983;98:472–4.

46. Giaccone G, Ferrati P, Donadio M, Testore F, Calciati A. Reinduction chemotherapy in small cell lung cancer. *Eur J Cancer Clin Oncol* 1987;23:1697–9.

47. Collard P, Weynants P, Francis C, Rodenstein DO. Treatment of relapse of small cell lung cancer in selected patients with the initial combination chemotherapy carboplatin, etoposide, and epirubicin. *Thorax* 1992;47:369–71.

48. Shepherd FA, Evans WK, MacCormick R, Feld R, Yau JC. Cyclophosphamide, doxorubicin, and vincristine in etoposide- and cisplatin-resistant small cell lung cancer. *Cancer Treat Rep* 1987;71:941–4.

49. von Pawel J, Schiller JH, Shepherd FA, et al. Topotecan versus cyclophosphamide, doxorubicin, and vincristine for the treatment of recurrent small-cell lung cancer. *J Clin Oncol* 1999;17:658–67.

50. Eckardt JR, von Pawel J, Pujol JL, et al. Phase III study of oral compared with intravenous topotecan as second-line therapy in small-cell lung cancer. *J Clin Oncol* 2007;25:2086–92.

51. Inoue A, Sugawara S, Yamazaki K, et al. Randomized phase II trial comparing amrubicin with topotecan in patients with previously treated small-cell lung cancer: North Japan Lung Cancer Study Group Trial 0402. *J Clin Oncol* 2008;26:5401–6.

52. Jotte R, Jones J, Hartwell D, et al. Randomized phase III trial of amrubicin versus topotecan (Topo) as second-line treatment for small cell lung cancer (SCLC). *J Clin Oncol* 2011;29 (suppl; abstr 7000).

53. Perry MC, Herndon JE, III, Eaton WL, Green MR. Thoracic radiation therapy added to chemotherapy for small-cell lung cancer: an update of Cancer and Leukemia Group B Study 8083. *J Clin Oncol* 1998;16:2466–7.

54. Work E, Nielsen OS, Bentzen SM, Fode K, Palshof T. Randomized study of initial versus late chest irradiation combined with chemotherapy in limited-stage small-cell lung cancer. Aarhus Lung Cancer Group. *J Clin Oncol* 1997;15:3030–7.

55. Skarlos DV, Samantas E, Briassoulis E, et al. Randomized comparison of early versus late hyperfractionated thoracic irradiation concurrently with chemotherapy

in limited disease small-cell lung cancer: a randomized phase II study of the Hellenic Cooperative Oncology Group (HeCOG). *Ann Oncol* 2001;12:1231–8.

56. Takada M, Fukuoka M, Kawahara M, et al. Phase III study of concurrent versus sequential thoracic radiotherapy in combination with cisplatin and etoposide for limited-stage small-cell lung cancer: results of the Japan Clinical Oncology Group Study 9104. *J Clin Oncol* 2002;20:3054–60.

57. Spiro SG, James LE, Rudd RM, et al. Early compared with late radiotherapy in combined modality treatment for limited disease small-cell lung cancer: a London Lung Cancer Group multicenter randomized clinical trial and meta-analysis. *J Clin Oncol* 2006;24:3823–30.

Chapter 12

Pulmonary Neuroendocrine Tumors

Apar Kishor Ganti

The spectrum of neuroendocrine malignancies of the lung extends from the poorly differentiated small cell lung cancer at one end to the well-differentiated carcinoids at the other. In contrast to small cell lung cancer, bronchial carcinoids are relatively rare (≈1% of lung tumors) and have a much more indolent course. Nevertheless, they have the potential to metastasize.

Epidemiology

Carcinoids originating from the bronchopulmonary system account for almost 25% of all neuroendocrine tumors, with most of the remaining cases arising from the gastrointestinal tract.[1] Carcinoids of the lung tend to occur at a younger age as compared to other lung tumors with a median age at diagnosis of 50–56 years.[2,3] Patients with typical carcinoid are about 10 years younger than those with atypical carcinoids.[4] In contrast to other lung tumors (more common in males) and other neuroendocrine tumors (no gender preponderance), bronchial carcinoids demonstrate a female preponderance.[2,3]

The association of smoking with the development of carcinoids is not as clear as that seen with lung cancer. Patients with atypical carcinoids appear to be more likely to have a history of smoking as compared to those with typical carcinoids.[2,5]

Pathology

The pathology of bronchopulmonary neuroendocrine tumors is discussed in detail in Chapter 3. In brief, neuroendocrine tumors of the lung may be conceptualized in three different categories:

- Low grade (typical carcinoid): Prominent neuroendocrine growth patterns, low-grade cytology, minimal mitotic activity, no evidence of necrosis.
- Intermediate grade (atypical carcinoid): Prominent neuroendocrine growth pattern; increased mitotic figures (2–10 mitoses/2 mm^2) and/or focal necrosis.

- High grade (large cell neuroendocrine carcinoma [LCNEC] and small cell lung cancer [SCLC]): High-grade cytology, extensive necrosis, and substantial mitotic activity (60–80 mitoses/2 mm²). The management of SCLC is discussed elsewhere (Chapter 11), while current guidelines recommend following the non–small cell lung cancer paradigm for LCNEC.

The following discussion will be limited to typical and atypical carcinoids.

Clinical Features

Almost 25% of patients with carcinoid are asymptomatic at presentation and are diagnosed incidentally.[6,7] The most common presentation in symptomatic patients appears to be obstruction of the central airways leading to atelectasis or obstructive pneumonia. This may lead to multiple unsuccessful courses of antibiotics before a diagnosis of carcinoid is made. Occasionally patients may present with hemoptysis, reflecting local trauma to these hypervascular tumors. Although wheezing may be commonly seen in these patients, it is more often due to obstruction of the airways, rather than an effect of a carcinoid syndrome caused by the release of active amines by the tumor.[8,9] In fact, carcinoid syndrome is seen in less than 5% of patients with bronchopulmonary carcinoid. A primary reason for this appears to be the relative rarity of liver metastases. Carcinoid syndrome occurs when hepatic involvement results in a concentration of bioactive tumor products that exceeds the ability of the liver to degrade them.[10]

Diagnosis and Staging

Laboratory Investigations

Approximately 75% of patients with bronchopulmonary carcinoids have elevated plasma chromogranin A concentrations. Chromogranin A levels may be falsely elevated in renal failure, atrophic gastritis, and during proton-pump inhibitor therapy. Other markers that may be positive in carcinoids include serotonin, urinary 5-hydroxy indole acetic acid (5-HIAA), adrenocorticotrophic hormone (ACTH), cortisol, and insulin-like growth factor-1 (IGF-1).

Imaging Studies

Carcinoid tumors usually appear as round or oval lesions on a chest X-ray, with sharp borders. They are often associated with stigmata of airway compression (atelectasis, air trapping, obstructive pneumonia, and mucoid impaction). Hilar and mediastinal lymphadenopathy are rare.[11,12] Atypical carcinoids are more likely to present as peripheral lesions.

Carcinoids have a characteristic appearance on computed tomography (CT) scan; they appear as well-defined centrally located tumors that have diffuse or punctate calcification.[12] In addition, a triphasic contrast enhanced CT scan of the abdomen is useful in evaluating for liver metastases in patients with suspected extrathoracic disease. A triphasic CT scan shows three different stages of contrast dye uptake: (1) before the injection of the dye (pre-contrast); (2) when the dye is in the arteries, approximately 20 seconds after injection (arterial phase); and (3) when the dye has reached the veins a few minutes later (venous phase). However, only about 2% of patients with typical carcinoids and 20% of patients with atypical carcinoids will have metastatic disease at presentation.[2]

Fluorodeoxyglucose (FDG) positron emission tomography (PET) scanning is not recommended for the evaluation of carcinoid tumors due to the low metabolic activity of these tumors.[13] However, it may be used to differentiate carcinoids from more aggressive diseases such as non–small cell and small cell lung cancer prior to a tissue diagnosis. Alternate tracers such as ^{11}C-L-DOPA and ^{11}C-5-hydroxytryptophan (11C-5-HT) are currently being evaluated for their ability to detect carcinoid tumors accurately.

The majority of bronchopulmonary carcinoids express somatostatin receptors. This allows the use of somatostatin receptor scintigraphy (SRS; octreotide scan) using somatostatin analogs such as ^{111}In-octreotide and ^{111}In-lanreotide in the staging of carcinoid tumors.[14] However, given the rarity of distant metastases with bronchial carcinoids and improvements in other imaging modalities, the role of SRS in the staging of these tumors is being re-evaluated.[15]

The staging of carcinoid tumors follows the American Joint Committee on Cancer's *Cancer Staging Manual*, seventh edition, classification of lung tumors (described in Chapter 6). Typical carcinoids often present at an early stage (>85% stage I); in contrast, atypical carcinoids often spread to locoregional lymph nodes and less than half are stage I at presentation.[2]

Treatment

Localized Disease

Surgical resection is the mainstay of therapy for nonmetastatic carcinoid tumors. Given the relatively indolent nature of these tumors, especially typical carcinoids, emphasis is placed upon a complete resection with negative margins, but preservation of as much lung function as possible.[16] The National Comprehensive Cancer Network (NCCN) guidelines recommend a lobectomy or other anatomic resection with mediastinal lymph node dissection or systematic sampling for all patients with carcinoid tumors,[17] but lung-sparing surgery may be considered in patients with small peripheral low-grade tumors. Patients who are not candidates for surgical resection due to medical causes should be offered radiation therapy.

The role of adjuvant therapy in patients with resected carcinoids has not been well evaluated and current evidence comes from small single-institution retrospective analyses. The available data do not suggest a benefit to either adjuvant radiation or chemotherapy in patients with locally advanced carcinoid tumors, both typical and atypical. However, consensus guidelines from the NCCN recommend the use of adjuvant chemotherapy (cisplatin + etoposide) with or without radiation for patients with resected stage II and III atypical carcinoids (see Fig. 12.1).[17]

Since many of these tumors present in central airways, bronchoscopic resection with a Neodymium Yttrium Aluminum Garnet (Nd:YAG) laser may be possible in patients whose tumors are completely intraluminal. Given the

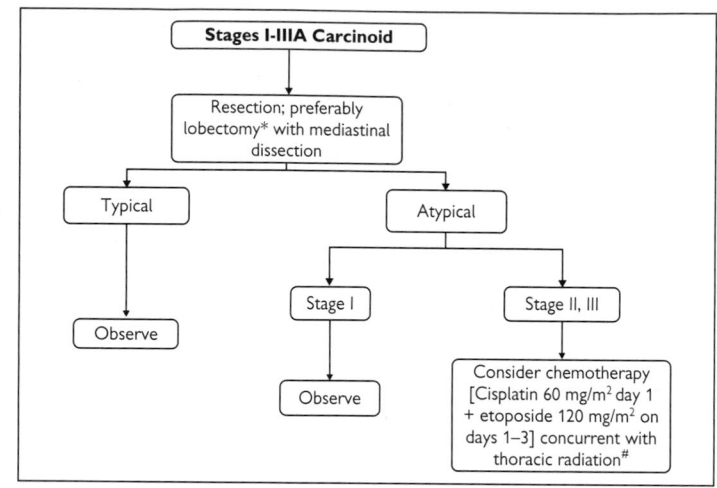

Figure 12.1 Schematic for management of early-stage carcinoid tumors.
* Lesser resection, i.e. wedge resection may be appropriate in small, peripheral typical carcinoid.
# Thoracic radiation may be considered if: positive margins, multiple lymph nodes involved.

uncertainty regarding the completeness of such a resection, this approach should be limited to patients who are not surgical candidates. This approach may be a useful palliative tool in patients with large obstructing central lesions[18] and may also help the surgeon better plan definitive resection following the removal of the endobronchial component of the tumor.[19]

Posttreatment Surveillance

The optimal posttreatment surveillance strategy for carcinoid tumors is not well defined. Even though these tumors have low malignant potential, they may recur and even develop metastases years after initial presentation. Annual history and physical examination combined with CT scans may be an optimal approach for patients with locally advanced atypical carcinoids.

Metastatic Disease

The role of chemotherapy in the management of metastatic carcinoid is unclear. The response rates with systemic cytotoxic agents are not consistent, and hence there is no single recommended regimen for these patients.[20] The most commonly utilized regimen is a combination of a platinum agent and etoposide or single-agent temozolomide.

Since the most common site of metastasis is the liver, localized therapies may be utilized. The goal of these approaches is to decrease symptoms associated with hormone hypersecretion and to prolong survival. These include the following:

- *Limited resection.* Helps with debulking and may be associated with a good biochemical response and an excellent 5-year survival.
- *Transarterial embolization.* This procedure is based on the principle that liver tumors derive most of their blood supply from the hepatic artery, whereas normal hepatocytes are supplied by the portal vein. Hence,

hepatic artery embolization (HAE) could selectively affect the tumor, while sparing normal liver. It is contraindicated in the setting of portal vein thrombosis. In this procedure, gel foam powder is infused into the hepatic artery through an angiography catheter (bland embolization) or in conjunction with chemotherapy, most commonly doxorubicin or cisplatin or drug-eluting beads (chemoembolization). In another approach, radioactive isotopes (for example, yttrium-90) tagged to glass or resin microspheres are delivered selectively to the tumor via the hepatic artery. Carcinoid crisis (profound circulatory collapse, respiratory failure secondary to bronchoconstriction, diarrhea, flushing, acidosis, and renal failure) is a rare but serious complication of hepatic artery embolization. It is due to massive systemic release of serotonin and other vasoactive peptides upon tumor necrosis. Premedication with somatostatin analogs and symptomatic treatment are recommended in patients undergoing HAE.

- *Radiofrequency ablation (RFA) and cryoablation.* RFA is more commonly used than cryoablation. These procedures can be performed either percutaneously or laparoscopically. They are less morbid than either surgery or HAE. However, they are effective only for lesions <3 cm in diameter.

Another alternative is to use somatostatin analogs such as octreotide to palliate symptoms associated with the secretion of bioactive amines or peptides. Radiographic responses with this approach are rare, although the disease can be controlled for an extended period of time.

Recent studies have suggested that the mammalian target of rapamycin (mTOR) inhibitor everolimus may have some activity in these tumors. A phase III trial comparing the combination of everolimus and octreotide with octreotide alone in patients with neuroendocrine tumors (including bronchial carcinoid) suggested a modest improvement in progression-free survival with the combination (16.4 vs. 11.3 months; multivariate HR, 0.62; 95% CI, 0.51–0.87; $P = 0.003$).[21] Studies using this and other targeted agents such as sunitinib and bevacizumab are currently under way.

Prognosis

The prognosis for completely resected typical carcinoids is excellent, with 5-year survival of 87%–100% and 10-year survival of 87%–93%. The corresponding values for atypical carcinoids (40%–59% and 31%–59%, respectively), though not as good, are still better than those seen with lung cancer.[6,9] Patients with metastatic disease have a 5-year survival of 15%–25%, which is also superior to advanced lung cancer.[1]

References

1. Modlin IM, Lye KD, Kidd M. A 5-decade analysis of 13,715 carcinoid tumors. *Cancer* 2003;97:934–59.

2. Fink G, Krelbaum T, Yellin A, et al. Pulmonary carcinoid: presentation, diagnosis, and outcome in 142 cases in Israel and review of 640 cases from the literature. *Chest* 2001;119:1647–51.

3. Quaedvlieg PF, Visser O, Lamers CB, Janssen-Heijen ML, Taal BG. Epidemiology and survival in patients with carcinoid disease in The Netherlands. An epidemiological study with 2391 patients. *Ann Oncol* 2001;12:1295–1300.

4. Froudarakis M, Fournel P, Burgard G,, et al. Bronchial carcinoids. A review of 22 cases. *Oncology* 1996;53:153–8.

5. Kayser K, Kayser C, Rahn W, Bovin NV, Gabius HJ. Carcinoid tumors of the lung: immuno- and ligandohistochemistry, analysis of integrated optical density, syntactic structure analysis, clinical data, and prognosis of patients treated surgically. *J Surg Oncol* 1996;63:99–106.

6. Cerilli LA, Ritter JH, Mills SE, Wick MR. Neuroendocrine neoplasms of the lung. *Am J Clin Pathol* 2001;116(Suppl):S65–S96.

7. Chong S, Lee KS, Chung MJ, Han J, Kwon OJ, Kim TS. Neuroendocrine tumors of the lung: clinical, pathologic, and imaging findings. *Radiographics* 2006;26:41–57; discussion 57–8.

8. Bertino EM, Confer PD, Colonna JE, Ross P, Otterson GA. Pulmonary neuroendocrine/carcinoid tumors: a review article. *Cancer* 2009;115:4434–41.

9. Skuladottir H, Hirsch FR, Hansen HH, Olsen JH. Pulmonary neuroendocrine tumors: incidence and prognosis of histological subtypes. A population-based study in Denmark. *Lung Cancer* 2002;37:127–35.

10. Gustafsson BI, Kidd M, Chan A, Malfertheiner MV, Modlin IM. Bronchopulmonary neuroendocrine tumors. *Cancer* 2008;113:5–21.

11. Nessi R, Basso Ricci P, Basso Ricci S, Bosco M, Blanc M, Uslenghi C. Bronchial carcinoid tumors: radiologic observations in 49 cases. *J Thorac Imag* 1991;6:47–53.

12. Jeung MY, Gasser B, Gangi A, et al. Bronchial carcinoid tumors of the thorax: spectrum of radiologic findings. *Radiographics* 2002;22:351–65.

13. Daniels CE, Lowe VJ, Aubry MC, Allen MS, Jett JR. The utility of fluorodeoxyglucose positron emission tomography in the evaluation of carcinoid tumors presenting as pulmonary nodules. *Chest* 2007;131:255–60.

14. Granberg D, Sundin A, Janson ET, Oberg K, Skogseid B, Westlin JE. Octreoscan in patients with bronchial carcinoid tumours. *Clin Endocrinol* 2003;59:793–9.

15. Reidy-Lagunes DL, Gollub MJ, Saltz LB. Addition of octreotide functional imaging to cross-sectional computed tomography or magnetic resonance imaging for the detection of neuroendocrine tumors: added value or an anachronism? *J Clin Oncol* 2011;29:e74–5.

16. Filosso PL, Rena O, Donati G, et al. Bronchial carcinoid tumors: surgical management and long-term outcome. *J Thorac Cardiovasc Surg* 2002;123:303–9.

17. Kalemkerian GP, Akerley W, Bogner P, et al. Small cell lung cancer. *J Natl Compr Canc Netw* 2011;9:1086–113.

18. Diaz-Jimenez JP, Canela-Cardona M, Maestre-Alcacer J. Nd:YAG laser photoresection of low-grade malignant tumors of the tracheobronchial tree. *Chest* 1990;97:920–2.

19. Schreurs AJ, Westermann CJ, van den Bosch JM, et al. A twenty-five-year follow-up of ninety-three resected typical carcinoid tumors of the lung. *J Thorac Cardiovasc Surg* 1992;104:1470–5.

20. Beasley MB, Thunnissen FB, Brambilla E, et al. Pulmonary atypical carcinoid: predictors of survival in 106 cases. *Hum Pathol* 2000;31:1255–65.

21. Yao JC, Hainsworth JD, Woliln EM, et al. Multivariate analysis including biomarkers in the phase III RADIANT-2 study of octreotide LAR plus everolimus (E+O) or placebo (P+O) among patients with advanced neuroendocrine tumors (NET). *J Clin Oncol* 2012;30 (suppl; abstr 4014).

Chapter 13

Mesothelioma

Jonathan E. Dowell

Malignant pleural mesothelioma is an uncommon, but deadly, malignancy arising from the mesothelial cells of the pleura. The vast majority of cases occur in patients with prior exposure to asbestos, but other etiologic agents, such as previous radiotherapy, may play a role in selected cases.[1] A description of asbestos and its uses can be found in Chapter 1.

The incidence of mesothelioma varies considerably in different countries around the world, presumably secondary to differences in asbestos utilization. In the United States, there are approximately 2500 new cases annually (roughly 6 per million inhabitants), and it is estimated that the incidence peaked in 2005 and will continue to decline gradually. Conversely, in Europe and Australia the incidences are 20 per million and 40 per million, respectively, with the peaks not expected to occur until 2015–2025.[2] Given that the latency period between exposure to asbestos and the development of mesothelioma can be as long as 70 years,[1] the disease will remain a significant worldwide health problem for many years to come.

Clinical Presentation

Patients with malignant pleural mesothelioma most commonly present with the following triad:
- Pleural effusion
- Dyspnea
- Chest wall pain

Each of these symptoms occurs in greater than 60% of patients.[2,3] Dyspnea may be due to the accumulation of pleural fluid or encasement of the lung by tumor, which can also predispose these patients to pneumonia due to the inability to adequately expand the chest wall on the affected side.

Complications due to local invasion within the chest are relatively common and may include:
- Superior vena cava syndrome
- Spinal cord compression
- Horner's syndrome (ipsilateral miosis, ptosis, and hemifacial anhidrosis due to direct invasion of the stellate ganglion of the sympathetic chain)
- Dysphagia due to esophageal compression
- Cardiac tamponade

- Paralysis of the recurrent laryngeal or phrenic nerves with resultant hoarseness or diaphragmatic dysfunction, respectively

In addition, spread across the diaphragm into the abdominal cavity can lead to ascites and even bowel obstruction. Subcutaneous masses can also occur as a result of direct extension of tumor through the chest wall or, more commonly, at sites of prior instrumentation.

While hematogenous metastases to virtually any organ have been reported, they are typically a late feature of the disease, as are constitutional symptoms such as fevers, night sweats, weight loss, and fatigue.[2,3]

Diagnosis

A variety of options are available to obtain a diagnosis of malignant pleural mesothelioma.

Radiographic Findings

Radiographic findings are nonspecific (typically pleural effusion with or without pleural thickening and/or pleural based masses) and are insufficient to confirm the diagnosis. Nevertheless, certain radiographic features heighten the suspicion for malignancy (see Figs. 13.1a–b and 13.2a–c).

Chest X-Ray

- Small hemithorax
- Circumferential nodular pleural thickening

Computed Tomography

- Circumferential pleural thickening
- Involvement of mediastinal pleura
- Nodular thickening of pleura
- Pleural thickening greater than 1 cm

The role of these and other specific radiographic studies is discussed in the "Pretreatment Evaluation" section.

Pathologic Evaluation

There are several approaches to pathologic evaluation:

- *Pleural fluid cytology*: utility and accuracy are debated, with diagnostic yield ranging widely from 4% to 76%.[4,5] Immunohistochemical staining has improved sensitivity.
- *Blind pleural biopsy*: performed with an Abrams needle; reported diagnostic rates for mesothelioma of 21%–71%.[4,5]
- *Needle biopsy under computed tomography (CT) guidance*: diagnostic yield is 83%–88%[4]
- *Thoracosopy*: employed as a diagnostic tool in suspected malignant effusion with reported sensitivities of 94%–98%.[4,5] Given the higher yield of this procedure and its ability to provide additional staging information, in many centers thoracoscopy has become a preferred approach when a diagnosis of mesothelioma is suspected

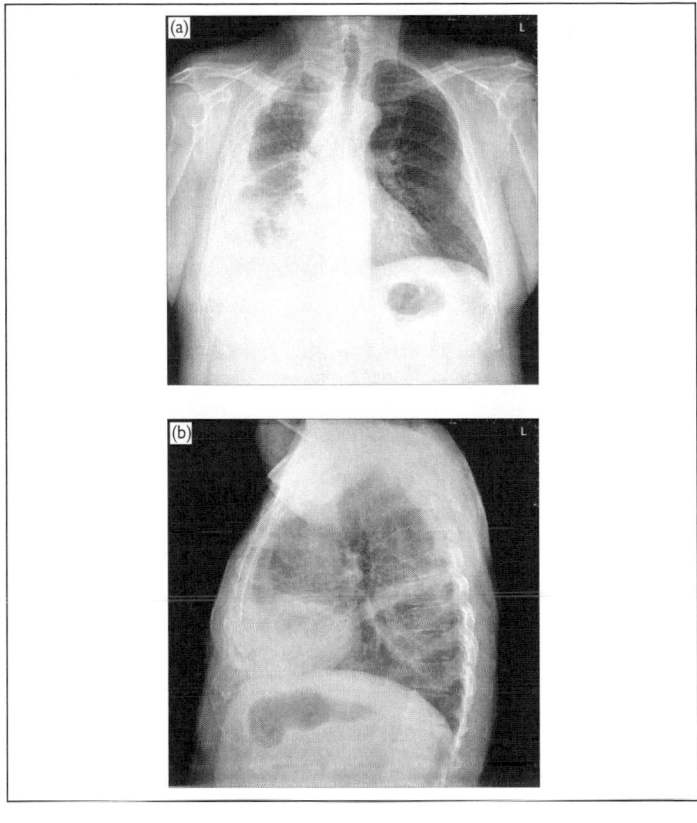

Figure 13.1 Postero-anterior (PA) (*a*) and lateral (*b*) chest X ray (CXR) images of mesothelioma. (Images courtesy of Matthew J. DeVries, MD.)

Serum Tumor Markers

Serum mesothelin has been evaluated as a possible diagnostic tool for mesothelioma. Depending on the threshold chosen, sensitivity ranges from 19% to 68% and specificity ranges from 88% to 100%.[6] Low sensitivity limits the use of serum mesothelin as a diagnostic tool. However, because serum mesothelin levels fall predictably with response to treatment, it may be employed as an indicator of disease course.

Staging

Mesothelioma is currently staged with the International Mesothelioma Interest Group (IMIG) Staging System for Diffuse Malignant Pleural Mesothelioma, which has been adopted by both the American Joint Committee on Cancer (AJCC) and the International Union for Cancer Control (UICC). As shown in Table 13.1, tumor (T) stage is determined by the local extent and invasion of

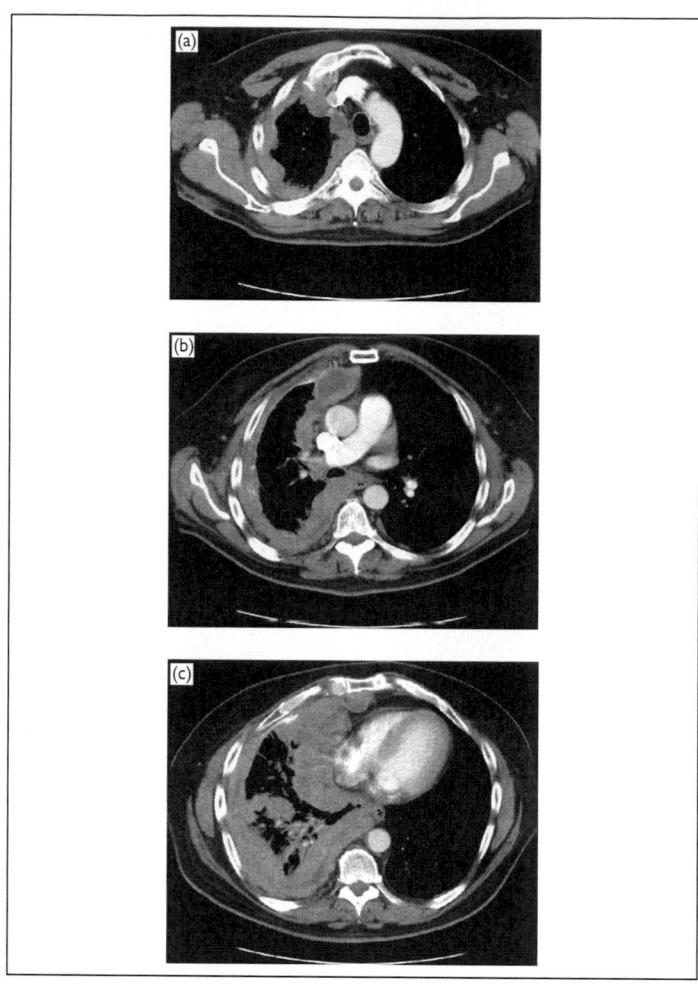

Figure 13.2 Computed tomography (CT) images of mesothelioma in upper (a), middle (b), and lower (c) right hemothorax. (Images courtesy of Matthew J. DeVries, MD.)

the primary, and the nodal (N) staging is virtually identical to that utilized in lung cancer.

Pathology

There are three primary histologic subtypes of malignant pleural mesothelioma:

- Epithelioid: 50%–70% of cases (Fig. 13.3)
- Sarcomatoid: 10%–20% of cases (Fig. 13.4)

Table 13.1 AJCC/UICC Staging Classification of Malignant Pleural Mesothelioma

T1a	Involvement of ipsilateral parietal pleura with or without mediastinal or diaphragmatic involvement but without involvement of the visceral pleura	**N0**	No lymph node involvement
		N1	Involvement of ipsilateral broncho-pulmonary, hilar lymph nodes
T1b	Involvement of ipsilateral parietal pleura, with focal involvement of the visceral pleura	**N2**	Involvement of ipsilateral mediastinal and/or internal mammary and/or peri-diaphragmatic lymph nodes
T2	Involvement of any of the ipsilateral pleural surfaces (peritoneal, mediastinal, diaphragmatic) with at least one of the following: • Involvement of diaphragmatic muscle • And/or invasion from visceral pleura into underlying lung parenchyma	**N3**	Involvement of any contralateral mediastinal and/or internal mammary and/or supraclavicular lymph nodes
T3	Involvement of all of the ipsilateral pleural surfaces, with at least one of the following: • Invasion of the endothoracic fascia • Extension into mediastinal fat • Solitary focus of tumor invading the soft tissues of the chest wall • Nontransmural involvement of the pericardium	**M0**	No extrathoracic metastasis
		M1	Extrathoracic metastasis, hematogenous or in nonregional lymph nodes
T4	Involvement of all of the ipsilateral pleural surfaces with at least one of the following: • Extension to the internal surface of the pericardium with or without effusion peritoneum, mediastinal structures, contralateral pleura, spine • Diffuse extension or multifocal masses in chest wall with or without rib destruction	**Stage I**	T1a N0 (IA); T1b N0 (IB)
		Stage II	T2N0
		Stage III	Any T3, any N1 or any N2
		Stage IV	Any T4, any N3 or any M1

Source: Adapted from van Meerbeeck JP, Scherpereel A, Surmont VF, Baas P. Malignant pleural mesothelioma: the standard of care and challenges for future management. *Critical reviews in oncology/hematology* 2011;78:92–111, with permission from Elsevier.

- Mixed variant (a combination of epithelioid and sarcomatoid histologies): 10%–30% of cases

Rare histologic variants, such as desmoplastic, make up the remainder of cases.[1,7]

The pathologic diagnosis of malignant mesothelioma can be challenging. Difficulties arise both in distinguishing benign from malignant mesothelial proliferations, as well as with differentiating the specific subtypes of mesothelioma from other malignancies. Accordingly, the IMIG has recommended the following[8]:

- Cases with cytologic suspicion for mesothelioma should be confirmed with tissue biopsy because cytology alone may be insufficient to diagnose malignant mesothelioma definitively.

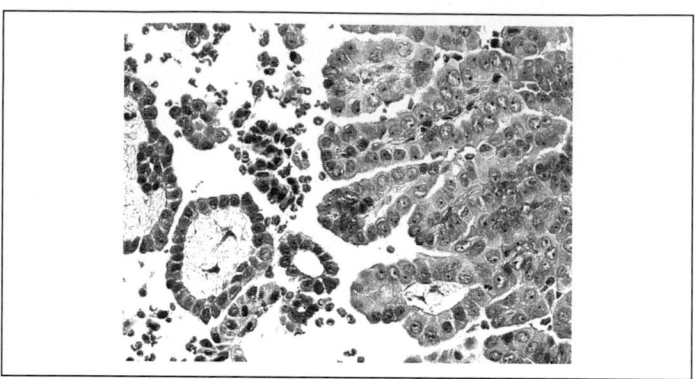

Figure 13.3 Malignant mesothelioma, epithelial type, tubulo-papillary pattern. This pleural tumor showed foci of chest wall invasion in other microscopic slides to confirm malignancy (hematoxylin & eosin, 400× original magnification). (Image courtesy of William W. West, MD.)

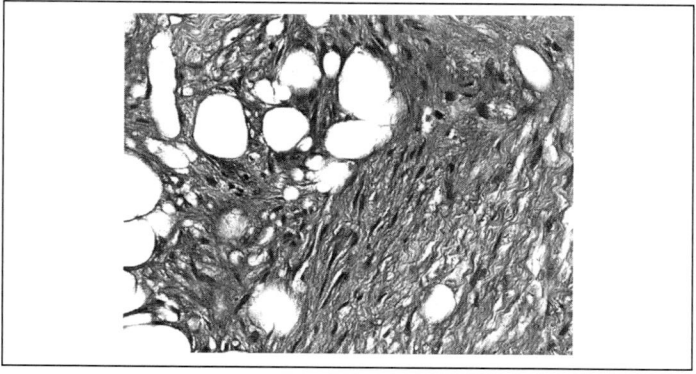

Figure 13.4 Malignant mesothelioma, sarcomatoid type, desmoplastic pattern. This pleural tumor is shown invading fat of the chest wall but consists of spindle cells with only mild cytologic atypia (hematoxylin & eosin, 400× original magnification). (Image courtesy of William W. West, MD.)

- At least two mesothelial immunohistochemical markers and two carcinoma immunohistochemical markers should be used when differentiating between mesothelioma and carcinoma (especially lung) (Table 13.2).
- Pathologists should not rely on a patient's history of exposure to asbestos when making a diagnosis of malignant mesothelioma, as this malignancy can be seen in patients without an obvious prior exposure and other malignancies involving the pleura may occur in patients with prior exposure. Instead, a diagnosis of malignant mesothelioma should be based on the pathologic features (along with relevant clinical and radiologic data).

Table 13.2 Immunohiostochemical Markers to Distinguish Epithelioid Mesothelioma from Lung Adenocarcinoma and Squamous Cell Carcinoma

Marker	Epithelioid Mesothelioma	Lung Adenocarcinoma	Lung Squamous Cell Carcinoma
Calretinin	90%–100%	5%–10%[*]	40%[*]
WT-1	43%–93%	Negative	Negative
Podoplanin (D2–40)	86%–100%	0–7%	50%
Keratin 5/6	75%–100%	2%–19%[*]	100%
TTF-1	Negative	70%–85%	Negative
p63	7%[*]	NR	100% (diffuse)
MOC-31	2%–10%[*]	95%–100%	97%–100%
BG8 (Lewis[y])	3%–7%[*]	89%–100%	80%
Ber-EP4	0–20%[*]	95%–100%	87%–100%
CEA	0–5%[*]	50%–90%	NR

Note: Immunohistochemical markers are not typically used to differentiate sarcomatoid mesothelioma from lung cancer.

[*]Focally positive.

BG8, blood group 8; CEA, carcinoembryonic antigen; NR, not reported; TTF-1, thyroid transcription factor-1; WT-1, Wilm's tumor-1.

Source: Adapted from Husain AN, Colby TV, Ordonez NG. Guidelines for pathologic diagnosis of malignant mesothelioma, a consensus statement from the International Mesothelioma Interest Group. *Arch Pathol Lab Med.* 2009;133:1317–1331.

Pretreatment Evaluation

Radiographic Studies

- *CT of the chest and abdomen*: provides an initial assessment of the extent of disease.

Additional radiologic studies may be performed in selected patients being considered for aggressive surgery.

- *Magnetic resonance imaging (MRI) of the chest*: can be performed to evaluate patients with suspected vascular, diaphragmatic, or spine invasion.
- *Positron emission tomography (PET)*: most useful for detecting extrathoracic spread. Importantly, if pleurodesis is planned, it is recommended that PET be performed first, as pleurodesis will result in diffuse pleural uptake of fluoro-deoxyglucose glucose (FDG) and a resultant inability to assess accurately the local extent of disease.

Invasive Staging Procedures

In those patients considered for aggressive surgery, additional surgical interventions are often performed to determine the extent of local spread as well as to evaluate for the presence or absence of extrathoracic disease.

- *Mediastinal lymph node sampling*: via either mediastinoscopy or endo-bronchial/esophageal ultrasound.
- *Video-assisted thoracoscopy (VATS)*: to evaluate the extent of pleural and diaphragmatic involvement, and contralateral VATS to exclude extension into the contralateral lung.
- *Laparoscopy*: to exclude transdiaphragmatic extension into the peritoneal cavity, which is found incidentally in approximately 10% of patients.[9]

Prognosis

Malignant pleural mesothelioma confers a poor prognosis with reported median survivals of 6–12 months and fewer than 5% of patients surviving beyond 5 years.[2,3]

The European Organization for the Research and Treatment of Cancer (EORTC) and the Cancer and Leukemia Group B (CALGB) have published prognostic scoring systems for this disease.[10,11]

The CALGB identified the following as independent predictors of poor outcome:

- Pleural (as opposed to peritoneal) primary site
- Lactate dehydrogenase (LDH) >500 IU/L
- ECOG performance status greater than 0
- Platelet count >400,000/μL
- Nonepithelial histology
- Age >75 years.

The EORTC identified the following predictors of poor outcome:

- ECOG performance status greater than 0
- Sarcomatoid histology
- Elevated white blood cell count
- Male gender
- Possible/probable diagnosis of mesothelioma (as opposed to a definite diagnosis)

Utilizing these prognostic factors, the EORTC created a complex model that classifies patients into two groups: a low-risk group with a median survival of 10.8 months and a high-risk group with a median survival of 5.5 months.

In addition to the clinical factors reviewed earlier, multiple groups have attempted to identify prognostic molecular markers, including gene expression analyses. However, to date, none have shown sufficient promise to be incorporated into routine clinical care.

Treatment

Chemotherapy

The majority of patients with malignant pleural mesothelioma are not candidates for aggressive surgery. In those patients unable or unwilling to have surgery, and with an adequate performance status, chemotherapy is a reasonable treatment option. Platinum analogues, selected antimetabolites (pemetrexed, raltitrexed, methotrexate), gemcitabine, vinorelbine, and doxorubicin have demonstrated activity in mesothelioma with reported single agent response rates of 7%–20%.[12]

Combination chemotherapy has also been extensively evaluated in this setting. The largest phase III trial ever conducted in untreated patients with malignant pleural mesothelioma established the standard of care in the United States. Vogelzang and colleagues randomized 456 chemonaïve patients to cisplatin and pemetrexed or cisplatin alone. The primary endpoint of median overall survival was significantly longer in the cisplatin and pemetrexed arm (12.1 months versus 9.3 months, $P = 0.02$).[13]

A similar trial conducted in Europe compared the combination of cisplatin and raltitrexed with cisplatin alone. Overall survival was the primary endpoint, and again a statistically significant improvement in median overall survival was seen in the combination arm (11.4 months versus 8.8 months, $P = .048$).[14]

Many patients with mesothelioma are elderly and/or have comorbidities that preclude the use of cisplatin. Although no randomized comparisons of cisplatin versus carboplatin have been conducted, available data suggest carboplatin in combination with pemetrexed has acceptable antitumor activity. In addition, the combination of a platinum analog and gemcitabine may be utilized in those patients unable to receive pemetrexed.[12]

The impact of second-line chemotherapy on survival has been examined in a single phase III trial. Jassem and colleagues randomized 243 patients with previously treated malignant pleural mesothelioma who had not received prior pemetrexed to pemetrexed or best supportive care. They reported a significant improvement in median time to progression in the pemetrexed arm (3.7 months versus 1.5 months, $P = .0002$) but no difference in overall survival or mean change in quality of life.[15] Additional second-line options are limited but both gemcitabine and vinorelbine have activity in this setting.

Specific Chemotherapy Regimens

Single Agent

Pemetrexed 500 mg/m^2 day 1 every 21 days
Gemcitabine 1000–1250 mg/m^2 day 1, 8, 15 every 28 days
Vinorelbine 25–30 mg/m^2 weekly

Combination

Cisplatin 75 mg/m^2 + pemetrexed 500 mg/m^2 day 1 every 21 days
Carboplatin AUC 5 + pemetrexed 500 mg/m^2 day 1 every 21 days
Cisplatin 80–100 mg/m^2 day 1 + gemcitabine 1000–1250 mg/m^2 days 1, 8, 15 every 21–28 days

Radiation

The use of radiotherapy in the multimodality treatment of malignant pleural mesothelioma is discussed later in this chapter. In the palliative setting, radiation can be utilized to treat chest wall pain as well as subcutaneous extensions from mesothelioma. At some centers, prophylactic radiation is used to prevent seeding of surgical incisions and port sites. However, a recent systematic review of the literature on this topic concluded that the available evidence does not support the routine use of prophylactic radiation.[16]

Surgery

Aggressive surgical options for malignant pleural mesothelioma include either pleurectomy/decortication (P/D) or extrapleural pneumonectomy (EPP).

- *Pleurectomy/decortication (P/D)*: complete visceral and parietal pleurectomy with the goal of removal of all gross disease. Removal of the ipsilateral diaphragm and/or pericardium may be included when those areas are involved.

- *Extrapleural pneumonectomy (EPP)*: en bloc resection of the lung, visceral and parietal pleura, diaphragm, and adjacent pericardium.

The true value of these procedures in mesothelioma is debated extensively in the literature for several reasons:

- There have been no definitive comparisons of EPP and P/D or comparisons of these procedures against nonsurgical treatment of mesothelioma.

- Both procedures have substantial associated morbidity and mortality.

- Neither EPP nor P/D results in a complete R0 resection. They are, therefore, not curative as a single modality.

Median survival following EPP ranges 9.4 to 27.5 months, with reported 5-year survival rates ranging from 0 to 24%.[17] Perioperative mortality rates range from 0 to 11.8% with major morbidity seen in 12.5%–48% of patients. The most common complications are atrial arrhythmias, respiratory infections, respiratory failure, pulmonary embolus, and myocardial infarction. Nonepithelioid histology and N2 nodal involvement consistently predict for poor outcome and are often considered contraindications to EPP.[18]

For patients undergoing complete P/D, a recent comprehensive review reports that median survival ranges 11.5–18.1 months, with 5-year survival rates from 0 to 23%.[19] Operative mortality rates range from 0 to 6%, and morbidity rates were not consistently stated.

Flores and colleagues reviewed 663 consecutive patients at three institutions who underwent EPP or P/D for malignant pleural mesothelioma[20]:

- Operative mortality was 7% for EPP and 4% for P/D.

- Severe or life-threatening (grade 3–5) respiratory complications occurred in 10% of EPP patients and 6.4% of P/D patients.

- In a multivariate analysis of prognostic variables that controlled for stage, histology (epithelioid versus nonepithelioid), gender, and multimodality therapy, EPP had a hazard ratio of 1.4 compared with P/D ($P < 0.001$), indicating a worse overall survival for the group that received EPP.

The authors concluded from this nonrandomized comparison of EPP and P/D that the available evidence does not provide a strong rationale to support one surgical procedure over the other.

Although there is no consensus on the role of aggressive surgery in mesothelioma or the most appropriate surgical procedure, there is general agreement on the following points:

- Patients considered for these procedures require rigorous staging (see earlier) to determine nodal status and to exclude extrathoracic spread.
- Extensive cardiac and pulmonary evaluation is necessary to ensure patient fitness for surgery.
- Patients with proven N2 disease or nonepithelioid histology do not appear to benefit from EPP.
- These procedures should be restricted to centers with extensive experience in the management of this disease.

Multimodality Therapy

High rates of both local and distant recurrence following either EPP or P/D provide a rationale for the evaluation of adjuvant therapies.[21]

Adjuvant Radiation Therapy

Rusch and colleagues reported a single institution experience of 57 patients who received postoperative hemithoracic radiation to 54 Gray following EPP. The approach appeared to be feasible and to reduce local recurrence when compared to historical controls.[21]

Adjuvant Chemotherapy

The largest series of adjuvant chemotherapy includes 183 patients who underwent EPP at a single institution between 1980 and 1997.[22] Postoperatively they received a variety of different chemotherapy regimens (doxorubicin and cyclophosphamide with or without cisplatin or carboplatin and paclitaxel) followed by radiation therapy. For the 176 patients who survived EPP, median survival was an encouraging 19 months.

Trimodality Therapy

Several groups have evaluated the feasibility of neoadjuvant chemotherapy followed by EPP followed by postoperative hemithoracic radiation. Across studies, 37%–71% of patients successfully completed all therapy. Median survivals ranged from 14 to 25.5 months. While these outcomes appear superior to those of patients receiving either surgery or chemotherapy alone, patient selection is likely influencing these results substantially.

The issue of patient selection is well illustrated by the Mesothelioma and Radical Surgery (MARS) randomized feasibility study.[23] In this trial, patients deemed medically fit and eligible for EPP after extensive evaluation received three cycles of platinum-based chemotherapy. Patients who completed chemotherapy and were deemed still to be surgical candidates following restaging were randomized to EPP followed by radiation or no EPP. After an initial 50 patients were enrolled in a feasibility portion of the study, median survival was 14.4 months in the EPP arm and 19.5 months in the no-EPP arm. The hazard ratio for overall survival in the EPP group versus the no-EPP group was 1.9 ($P = 0.082$). When one considers that overall survival in this trial was measured from the time of randomization (following completion of chemotherapy), the median survivals in the no-EPP arm are comparable to those observed in numerous phase II trials of trimodality therapy. This again argues that patient selection heavily influences the survivals reported in multimodality trials and that definitive randomized trials will be necessary to define the role of multimodality therapy in this disease.

References

1. Carbone M, Ly BH, Dodson RF, et al. Malignant mesothelioma: facts, myths, and hypotheses. *J Cell Physiol* 2012;227:44–58.

2. Robinson BW, Lake RA. Advances in malignant mesothelioma. *N Engl J Med* 2005;353:1591–603.

3. van Meerbeeck JP, Scherpereel A, Surmont VF, Baas P. Malignant pleural mesothelioma: the standard of care and challenges for future management. *Crit Rev Oncol/Hematol* 2011;78:92–111.

4. Adams RF, Gray W, Davies RJ, Gleeson FV. Percutaneous image-guided cutting needle biopsy of the pleura in the diagnosis of malignant mesothelioma. *Chest* 2001;120:1798–802.

5. Boutin C, Rey F, Gouvernet J, Viallat JR, Astoul P, Ledoray V. Thoracoscopy in pleural malignant mesothelioma: a prospective study of 188 consecutive patients. Part 2: prognosis and staging. *Cancer* 1993;72:394–404.

6. Hollevoet K, Reitsma JB, Creaney J, et al. Serum mesothelin for diagnosing malignant pleural mesothelioma: an individual patient data meta-analysis. *J Clin Oncol* 2012;30:1541–9.

7. Goldberg M, Imbernon E, Rolland P, et al. The French National Mesothelioma Surveillance Program. *Occup Environ Med* 2006;63:390–5.

8. Husain AN, Colby TV, Ordonez NG, et al. Guidelines for pathologic diagnosis of malignant mesothelioma: a consensus statement from the International Mesothelioma Interest Group. *Arch Pathol Lab Med* 2009;133:1317–31.

9. Rice DC, Erasmus JJ, Stevens CW, et al. Extended surgical staging for potentially resectable malignant pleural mesothelioma. *Ann Thorac Surg* 2005;80:1988–92; discussion 92-3.

10. Curran D, Sahmoud T, Therasse P, van Meerbeeck J, Postmus PE, Giaccone G. Prognostic factors in patients with pleural mesothelioma: the European Organization for Research and Treatment of Cancer experience. *J Clin Oncol* 1998;16:145–52.

11. Herndon JE, Green MR, Chahinian AP, Corson JM, Suzuki Y, Vogelzang NJ. Factors predictive of survival among 337 patients with mesothelioma treated between 1984 and 1994 by the Cancer and Leukemia Group B. *Chest* 1998;113:723–31.

12. Tsao AS, Wistuba I, Roth JA, Kindler HL. Malignant pleural mesothelioma. *J Clin Oncol* 2009;27:2081–90.

13. Vogelzang NJ, Rusthoven JJ, Symanowski J, et al. Phase III study of pemetrexed in combination with cisplatin versus cisplatin alone in patients with malignant pleural mesothelioma. *J Clin Oncol* 2003;21:2636–44.

14. van Meerbeeck JP, Gaafar R, Manegold C, et al. Randomized phase III study of cisplatin with or without raltitrexed in patients with malignant pleural mesothelioma: an intergroup study of the European Organisation for Research and Treatment of Cancer Lung Cancer Group and the National Cancer Institute of Canada. *J Clin Oncol* 2005;23:6881–9.

15. Jassem J, Ramlau R, Santoro A, et al. Phase III trial of pemetrexed plus best supportive care compared with best supportive care in previously treated patients with advanced malignant pleural mesothelioma. *J Clin Oncol* 2008;26:1698–704.

16. Nagendran M, Pallis A, Patel K, Scarci M. Should all patients who have mesothelioma diagnosed by video-assisted thoracoscopic surgery have their intervention sites irradiated? *Interact Cardiovasc Thorac Surg* 2011;13:66–9.

17. Cao CQ, Yan TD, Bannon PG, McCaughan BC. A systematic review of extrapleural pneumonectomy for malignant pleural mesothelioma. *J Thorac Oncol* 2010;5:1692–703.

18. Cao C, Yan TD, Bannon PG, McCaughan BC. Summary of prognostic factors and patient selection for extrapleural pneumonectomy in the treatment of malignant pleural mesothelioma. *Ann Surg Oncol* 2011;18:2973–9.

19. Teh E, Fiorentino F, Tan C, Treasure T. A systematic review of lung-sparing extirpative surgery for pleural mesothelioma. *J Royal Soc Med* 2011;104:69–80.

20. Flores RM, Pass HI, Seshan VE, et al. Extrapleural pneumonectomy versus pleurectomy/decortication in the surgical management of malignant pleural mesothelioma: results in 663 patients. *J Thorac Cardiovasc Surg* 2008;135:620–6.

21. Rusch VW, Piantadosi S, Holmes EC. The role of extrapleural pneumonectomy in malignant pleural mesothelioma. A Lung Cancer Study Group trial. *J Thorac Cardiovasc Surg* 1991;102:1–9.

22. Sugarbaker DJ, Flores RM, Jaklitsch MT, et al. Resection margins, extrapleural nodal status, and cell type determine postoperative long-term survival in trimodality therapy of malignant pleural mesothelioma: results in 183 patients. *J Thorac Cardiovasc Surg* 1999;117:54–63.

23. Treasure T, Lang-Lazdunski L, Waller D, et al. Extra-pleural pneumonectomy versus no extra-pleural pneumonectomy for patients with malignant pleural mesothelioma: clinical outcomes of the Mesothelioma and Radical Surgery (MARS) randomised feasibility study. *Lancet Oncol* 2011;12:763–72.

200

Chapter 14

Supportive Care in Lung Cancer

Daniel H. Ahn and David E. Gerber

Supportive care is a key component to the management of patients with lung cancer. The underlying malignancy may cause multiple complications, including pain, airway obstruction, pleural and pericardial effusions, cough, hemoptysis, skeletal fractures, spinal cord compression, and neurologic symptoms from brain metastases. Additionally, lung cancer treatments may lead to numerous complications, among them pulmonary toxicities, cytopenias, nausea and vomiting, peripheral neuropathy, and rash.

This chapter reviews the management of these and other complications experienced by patients with lung cancer.

Disease-Related Complications

Cancer-Associated Pain

Cancer-associated pain may affect an individual's physical functioning, daily activity, psychological and emotional status, and overall quality of life. Often, a patient's signs and symptoms may suggest a specific cancer pain syndrome. Commonly seen pain syndromes in this population are as follows:

1. *Pain directly related to the tumor/tumor-related somatic pain syndromes.* Pleuritic pain or chest discomfort may result from direct chest wall invasion from the primary tumor. However, most primary lung tumors are not associated with pain or discomfort, which is one reason for late stage at diagnosis. Another less common example is adrenal pain syndrome. This occurs in lung cancer metastatic to one or both adrenal glands. Patients present with unilateral flank discomfort, which may radiate to the ipsilateral upper and lower quadrants of the abdomen, or acute severe pain due to adrenal hemorrhage.

2. *Bone pain.* Osseous metastases are a common cause of chronic pain in cancer patients. Up to 40% of patients with advanced lung cancer will develop bone metastases, with the thoracic spine being the most common site of involvement, followed by the pelvis and lumbar spine.[1, 2] The pain associated with bone metastases may be due to direct invasion, pathologic fracture, or damage to adjacent structures. The mechanism of pain is multifocal, including direct nociception receptor activation, mechanical distortion, and release of growth factors.

3. *Tumor-related neuropathic pain.* Radiculopathy may be caused by direct neoplastic invasion into the spinal cord, nerve roots, plexuses, or peripheral nerves. This phenomenon is relatively common: up to 40% of patients with chronic cancer-related pain may have a neuropathic component to their symptoms.[3]

Pain Evaluation

Cancer-associated pain results from complex interactions among biologic, psychological, and social factors.[4] Effective management is based on a multidimensional evaluation, which includes a thorough history and physical examination, as well as objective testing.

During the medical history, clinicians should elicit the following pain characteristics:

- Intensity
- Location
- Radiation
- Quality
- Onset

In some cases, pain may indicate an oncologic urgency, such as new metastatic disease or a pathologic fracture, prompting further investigation with appropriate laboratory and imaging studies in addition to analgesic and condition-specific treatments.

In the evaluation, clinicians should consider and address other comorbidities that can alter pain, such as anxiety and depression. Additionally, patient self-reporting tools are available to facilitate the assessment of cancer-associated pain. Pain rating scales provide information about pain intensity at any specific point in time as well as average and worst pain levels. However, these tools do not address the full psychosocial nature of pain. Multidimensional tools assess a variety of parameters related to a patient's pain. The McGill Pain Questionnaire examines pain quality, intensity, and location, while the Brief Pain Inventory takes into account the effect of pain on a patient's quality of life, sleep, mood, and interpersonal relationships.[5]

In certain patient populations, special considerations must be taken into account in the evaluation and treatment of pain. For example, the use of nonsteroidal anti-inflammatory drugs should be used cautiously in the elderly and avoided in those with a history of gastrointestinal events or renal dysfunction.

Treatment

Pharmacologic Therapy

Opioids are a mainstay in the treatment of cancer-associated pain. Although the original analgesic ladder from the World Health Organization recommends the use of codeine for moderate pain with morphine for more severe pain, there is no pharmacologic or clinical rationale for following these opioid-specific regimens. Due to inter- and intraindividual variability in clinical responses to analgesics, it is not possible to predict the most favorable opioid for a given cancer patient. Furthermore, opioids are available in different formulations and may be administered by different routes, each with its own unique set of risks and benefits. Appropriate and effective use of opioids requires an understanding of pharmacologic profiles, routes of administration, dosing guidelines, and adverse effects.

Pharmacology

The μ-opioid receptor is responsible for analgesia. Various medications affect the receptor, including full receptor agonists, partial agonists, and antagonists. Initial medication selection should be based on the patient's previous response to opioids, if available. Medical comorbidity, drug metabolism, and potential drug–drug interactions should be taken into consideration.

Cytochrome P450 (CYP) and uridine 5′-diphospho-glucuronosyltransferases (UGTs) are two enzymes that are involved in opioid metabolism.[6]

- Morphine, hydromorphone, and oxymorphone are transformed via glucuronidation.
- The CYP system is responsible for the metabolism of oxycodone, fentanyl, hydrocodone, and methadone.

Genetic polymorphisms in genes encoding these enzymes contribute to variable clinical responses to opioids.[6] Medications, supplements, and dietary components interact with CYP and must be taken into consideration. Additionally, because morphine metabolites are excreted by the kidney, this agent should be used with caution in patients with renal dysfunction.

Among opioids, the use of methadone may present particular challenges for clinicians. Methadone acts as an N-methyl-d-aspartate (NMDA) receptor antagonist that can reverse opioid tolerance. This effect, in addition to its variable pharmacokinetics and potential for QT interval prolongation, requires initiation at low doses and use by an experienced physician.[7]

Administration and Formulations

It is preferred that opioids be given via the least invasive routes. Therefore, oral and transdermal formulations are preferred over subcutaneous or intravenous dosing. These formulations are classified as short-acting opioids (SAOs) or long-acting opioids (LAOs) based on their duration of action (see Table 14.1).

- SAOs have rapid onset of action but a short half-life. They are used for breakthrough pain and to titrate dosage. Patients may then be transitioned to LAOs, such as sustained-release morphine or transdermal fentanyl patch.
- LAOs require less frequent dosing and are believed to improve adherence in patients requiring continuous analgesic therapy.[8,9] Also, pain prevention is generally more successful than pain management. Therefore, in patients with persistent pain, scheduled dosing is preferred to relying solely on as-needed dosing to provide consistent analgesia.

When titrating LAOs, sufficient time should be allowed for plasma concentrations to reach a steady state[10]:

- 2–3 days for modified-release oral formulations
- 3–5 days for transdermal fentanyl patch
- 3–5 days for methadone

Alternative routes, such as subcutaneous or intravenous administration, are used for specific situations. They provide rapid analgesia and are often used in the inpatient setting and in patients unable to tolerate oral medications.[9] In

Table 14.1 Opioid Dosing

Drug	Approximate Opioid Equianalgesic Dose		Duration (Oral Formulation) (Hours)	Starting Dose for Opioid Naïve Patients (for Adults)	
	IV (mg)	Oral (mg)		IV (mg)	Oral (mg)
Morphine (IR)	10	30	3–4	2	5 mg Q4 hr
Morphine (SR)	N/A	30	8–12	N/A	15 mg Q12 hr
Hydromorphone	1.5	6	3–4	0.5	2 mg Q4 hr
Codeine	130	200	3–4	N/A	30 mg Q4 hr
Oxycodone	N/A	20	3–4	N/A	5 mg Q4 hr
Oxycodone (SR)	N/A	20	8–12	N/A	10 mg Q12 hr
Hydrocodone	N/A	30	3–4	N/A	5 mg Q4 hr
Methadone (see Table 14.3)	10		8–12	N/A	see Table 14.3
Fentanyl (see Table 14.2)	0.1		1 hr	0.1–0.2	see Table 14.2
Meperidine	75–100	300	2–3 hr	25 mg	N/A

IR, instant release; SR, sustained release.

situations where patients are unable to tolerate the systemic side effects of opioids at analgesic doses, administration of opioids through alternative delivery systems such as an intraspinal infusion may be beneficial.

Table 14.1 provides an overview of opioid agents, including dosing and duration. Table 14.2 provides information on fentanyl administration. Table 14.3 provides information on methadone administration.

Opioid Rotation

Often there is substantial variability in patients' responses to opioids. Despite individualized dosing and scheduling, certain patients may still respond poorly to opioids. For example, medical comorbidities may predispose individuals to certain opioid-related toxicities, pain may be unresponsive to opioids, or renal impairment may lead to accumulation of active metabolites and the associated side effects.

Patients who develop tolerance in response to long-term therapy with a given opioid will generally show incomplete cross-tolerance to the effects of other opioids.[11] When the degree of tolerance is greater for the adverse effects of an opioid than for the analgesic effects, administration of an alternative opioid may enhance pain relief without a concurrent increase in toxicity. This clinical strategy is known as "opioid rotation."[11]

Opioid rotation may be helpful for certain clinical situations, including the following[11]:

• Poor analgesic effect after aggressive dose titration
• Intolerable adverse effects (somnolence, nausea)
• Drug–drug interactions

Table 14.2 Fentanyl Dosing

24-Hour Oral Morphine Equivalent (mg/day)	Fentanyl Transdermal Patch Dose (mcg/hour)
60–130	25
130–220	50
220–300	75
300–400	100
400–490	125
490–580	150
580–670	175
670–760	200
760–850	225
850–940	250
940–1030	275
1030–1120	300

Table 14.3 Methadone Conversion

24-Hour Oral Morphine Equivalent Dose (mg/day)	Methadone Conversion Rate (Morphine to Methadone Ratio)
30–90	4:1
90–300	8:1
301–600	12:1
601–800	15:1
>800	20:1

Note: Methadone's duration and half-life will increase with repeat use due to cumulative effect. Titrate dose every 48–72 hours. The total dose of methadone can be divided into every 8 or 12 hours. Monitor for drug–drug interactions (especially cardiac medications, as methadone prolongs QT interval). Check electrocardiogram in patients >50 years of age and in those with cardiac conditions. Avoid in patients with QTc >500 ms.

Source: Reprinted from Portenoy RK, Treatment of cancer pain. The Lancet. 2011;377:2236–2247, with permission from Elsevier.

- Need for a different route of administration (i.e., transdermal instead of oral)
- Concern about drug abuse
- Drug availability
- Opiod-induced hyperalgesia (discussed below)

Opioid-Related Toxicities

An understanding of the incidence, severity, and management of opioid-related side effects is essential to optimize pain control. Common side effects of opioid administration include constipation, nausea and vomiting, sedation, respiratory depression, delirium, pruritis, and secondary hypogonadism (leading to diminished libido, fatigue, and loss of muscle mass).[12]

Constipation

Constipation occurs in up to 50% of patients and is the most common adverse effect associated with chronic opioid use.[13] Patients should be educated to maintain hydration, increase fiber intake, and, if feasible, exercise on a regular basis.

The medical management of opioid-induced constipation is described in Table 14.4.

- A combination of laxatives (e.g., bisacodyl, senna, lactulose) and stool softeners (e.g., docusate), which address decreased bowel motility and increased water resorption, should be used.

- For prolonged cases, laxatives (magnesium citrate), bowel prep solutions (polyethylene glycol-electrolyte solution), enemas (tap water, mineral oil, Colace) or suppositories (bisacodyl) are effective for immediate relief.

- In severe cases where constipation does not respond to laxative therapy, methylnaltrexone, a peripherally acting μ-opioid antagonist, is specifically approved for opioid-induced constipation.

Although constipation is often induced from chronic opioid use, other pharmacologic causes, such as antiemetics, steroids, antidepressants, antacids, and diuretics should be taken into consideration. Importantly, unlike other opioid-induced side effects, gastrointestinal dysfunction does not improve with tolerance and patients should be started prophylactically on a bowel regimen (e.g., the stool softener docusate and the laxative senna) at the time of opioid initiation.

Nausea and Vomiting

Although not as prevalent as constipation, nausea and vomiting are distressing adverse effects associated with opioid use. However, nausea often lessens with

Table 14.4 Medical Management of Constipation

Medication	Onset of Action (Hours)	Starting Dose	Site and Mechanism of Action
Osmotic laxatives			
Polyethylene glycol	48–96	17 g in 8 oz water PO	GI tract; osmotic effect
Lactulose	24–48	15–30 mL PO Q12–24h	Colon; osmotic effect
Magnesium citrate	0.5–3	120–240 mL PO x 1	Small and large bowel; attracts water and retains in bowel
Magnesium hydroxide	0.5–3	30 mL PO Q12–24h	Colon; osmotic effect
Stimulant laxatives			
Bisacodyl	6–10	5 mg PO x 1	Colon; increase peristalsis
Senna	6–10	2 tabs PO QHS	Colon; increase peristalsis
Surface laxatives			
Docusate	24–72	100 mg PO Q12h	Small and large bowel; detergent activity

long-term opioid use and may be prevented by slow dose escalation. Persistent nausea may require a period of scheduled antiemetic dosing or the use of a 5-HT$_3$-receptor antagonist, such as ondansetron. Other potentially effective agents include scopolamine, prochlorperazine, and droperidol.[14]

Respiratory Depression

Respiratory depression is the most feared adverse effect of opioid use. Evidence suggests that in non-oxygen-dependent cancer patients, appropriately titrated opioids will not induce hypoventilation.[15] However, many patients with lung cancer also have pulmonary comorbid conditions (such as chronic obstructive pulmonary disease) and may be susceptible to respiratory depression. If a patient experiences an acute respiratory problem due to opioids, naloxone may be administered to reverse the respiratory depression. Patients should receive 0.4 to 2 mg subcutaneously, intramuscularly, or intravenously up to every 3–5 minutes as needed. If the patient is responsive but is requiring frequent dosing, a continuous infusion may be necessary to assist in the patient's respiration. Administration of naloxone may also reduce analgesia, inducing a pain crisis.

Sedation

Sedation is a common side effect in patients taking opioids, particularly at the time of initiation or after a significant dose escalation. It is usually temporary and subsides quickly. Patients should be educated about the likelihood of this short-term symptom to prevent motor vehicle accidents or work-related incidents. If sedation is persistent and remains an issue, caffeine or psychostimulants (e.g., methylphenidate, starting dose 2 mg orally every 12 hours) may be considered to ameliorate this effect.

Opioid-Induced Hyperalgesia

This is a condition in which patients who are on chronic opioids actually become more sensitive to pain stimuli and increasing the opioid dose may actually worsen their pain symptoms. Diffuse or worsening pain, associated with tremulousness and confusion with increased analgesic dose should alert the clinician to the possibility of opioid-induced hyperalgesia. Opioid rotation or treatment with a non-opioid approach may help treat this condition.

Multimodality Treatment Strategies for Cancer Pain

Radiation Therapy

External beam radiation therapy is highly effective for the treatment of localized sites of pain. It is particularly useful in addressing skeletal lesions, where it may also be used to prevent complications such as pathologic fracture or spinal cord compression. Because reirradiation of anatomic sites may convey substantial toxicity, this treatment modality is generally reserved for cases that are refractory to medical management or at risk for complications.

Interventional Modalities in Pain Management

Table 14.5 lists common interventional procedures available for the management of cancer pain. Patients considered for these modalities require input from a multidisciplinary team that may include interventional radiologists, anesthesiologists, and neurosurgeons.

Table 14.5 Interventional Procedures for Pain Management

Procedure	Indications	Mechanism	Complications
Implanted neuraxial infusion	Intractable, focal isolated pain	Delivery of either opioids or anesthetics to spinal opioid receptors via epidural or intrathecal infusion by indwelling catheter	Infection, bleeding, respiratory depression (from cephalad spread of opioid); mechanical failure
Implanted neurostim-ulator	Intractable, focal, isolated pain of neuropathic origin	Alters local neurochemistry in dorsal horn ($\uparrow$ GABA, serotonin; $\downarrow$ glutamate, aspartate), suppressing neuronal hyperexcitability	Lead migration or breakage, infection, cerebrospinal fluid leak, transient paraplegia
Radio frequency ablation (RFA)	Refractory chest pain, dyspnea, cough, or hemoptysis from large lung tumors. Refractory pain from osseous metastasis	Placement of an electrode into the site of disease to cause focal tissue destruction with thermal energy	Pneumothorax, bronchopleural fistula, tumor tract seeding, bleeding
Nerve blocks (myofascial injections, intercostal blocks, neurolysis)	Localized areas of refractory pain	Anesthetizing or destroying neural pathways or sympathetic structures involved in pain transmission via surgery, cryotherapy, radiofrequency thermal coagulation, or injection of neurolytic agent (e.g., phenol)	"Deafferentation" pain syndrome (pain due to loss of sensory input into CNS), collateral normal tissue damage
Vetebroplasty	Intractable pain from vertebral fractures caused by spinal metastases	Introduction of inflatable balloon into the vertebral body to restore its height followed by injection of radiopaque polymethylmethacrylate cement with image guidance into a painful compressed vertebra	Spinal cord compression (epidural involvement by the spinal metastasis is generally considered a contraindication), paraplegia
Kyphoplasty	Intractable pain from vertebral fractures caused by spinal metastases	Percutaneous injection of radiopaque polymethylmethacrylate cement with image guidance into a painful compressed vertebra	Paraplegia, intradural cement leakage, spinal cord compression, pulmonary embolism
Surgical fixation	Metastasis to long and/or weight-bearing bones causing refractory pain or at risk for fracture	Includes internal fixation and osteosynthesis, resection of joint and joint replacement, segmental resection of a large tract of bone and prosthetic replacement, and arthroplasty	Postoperative pain, infection, bleeding, recovery time

CNS, central nervous system; GABA, gamma-aminobutyric acid.

Cardiopulmonary Complications

Among patients with lung cancer, respiratory symptoms (such as dyspnea, cough, and hemoptysis) are prevalent and potentially highly distressful. Dyspnea may be due to a variety of etiologies:

- Direct involvement of the cardiopulmonary system by the cancer
- Indirect respiratory complications caused by lung cancer (e.g., postobstructive pneumonia, effusions)
- Treatment-induced respiratory complications (e.g., surgery induced, chemotherapy induced, or radiation induced)
- Medical comorbidities (e.g., chronic obstructive pulmonary disease, chronic heart failure)

Central Airway Obstruction

Central airway obstruction may arise from extrinsic tumor compression, endobronchial involvement, or both. Obstruction and the resulting airflow limitation may lead to dyspnea, atelectasis, and postobstructive pneumonia.

Several techniques are available to manage central airway obstruction, including bronchoscopy with airway dilation and/or stenting, ablation techniques, radiation therapy, and surgery.

Bronchoscopy

Bronchoscopy allows for visualization of the obstructing lesion, the ability to determine the extent of luminal narrowing and whether the obstruction is due to an intra- or extraluminal process.

The choice of bronchoscope, either flexible or rigid, is an important consideration. The rigid bronchoscope does not occlude the airway lumen and allows for better airway protection and ventilation. It allows for suctioning of secretions and blood, as well as passage of instruments (such as lasers, cautery devices, and stents). Rigid bronchoscopy requires general anesthesia. Flexible bronchoscopy offers the advantage that it can be performed under conscious sedation but is limited in the amount of interventional procedures that can be performed.

Endobronchial Balloon Dilatation

Endobronchial balloon dilatation has a limited role as sole treatment of central airway obstruction. Its principal use is preparing an obstructed airway for the placement of stents.

Endobronchial Laser Therapy

Endobronchial laser therapy is useful in relieving intraluminal bronchial obstruction. It can be performed by either rigid or flexible bronchoscopy. Various types of laser therapy are available such as potassium triphosphate and carbon dioxide. The effect is immediate, and up to 90% of patients experience relief of symptoms. Complications include hemorrhage, pneumothorax, and pneumomediastinum. Its use is limited by requirements for special training and equipment.

Cryotherapy

Cryotherapy employs cryoprobes that apply frigid temperatures to tumor tissue. Malignant cells are killed by repeated cycles of cold application followed by thawing. Nitrous oxide and liquid nitrogen are commonly used to achieve temperatures below −80 degrees Celsius. The use of cryotherapy is limited to intraluminal lesions. Compared to laser therapy, cryotherapy is considered somewhat less effective but involves equipment that is less expensive and easier to use. The principal disadvantage of this technique is the time required to treat large tumors; consequently, it is not employed as a first-line therapy.

Airway Stents

Airway stents are employed to relieve intra- or extraluminal airway obstruction caused by a malignant tumor. Stent placement is generally restricted to the trachea and mainstem bronchi. They are often used after other therapeutic interventions to maintain airway patency. Complications include stent migration and promotion of granulation tissue.

Radiation Therapy

Radiotherapy plays an integral role in the management of central airway obstruction. However, a prolonged time course, typically greater than 2 weeks, is required to achieve the desired effect, which may not be adequate if the patient's symptoms require immediate relief. Radiation treatment can be administered as external beam radiation therapy (EBRT) or as brachytherapy delivered through a bronchoscope catheter. The main advantage of brachytherapy is the ability to limit radiation exposure to adjacent healthy tissue. Thus, brachytherapy may be considered for palliation of airway obstruction in patients who have already received a maximum dose of EBRT. Brachytherapy may be used as a stand-alone treatment or in conjunction with EBRT, stent placement, or other debulking procedures (e.g., laser, surgical resection). Complications of radiation therapy include fistula and stricture formation, bronchitis, hemoptysis, esophagitis, and pneumonitis.

Surgery

Surgical resection is considered when unusual types of central tumors amenable to resection are encountered. These include carcinoid, cylindroma, and mucoepidermoid tumors.[16] The involved segment of trachea or major bronchus should be short enough to permit the surgeon to resect the tumor with an anastomosis site free of malignant cells.

Pleural Effusions

Malignant fluid collections within the pleura and/or pericardium occur commonly in lung cancer. Approximately one-third of malignant pleural effusions are related to lung cancer. Up to 50% of patients with advanced disease develop a pleural effusion during the course of their disease.[17]

Symptomatic malignant effusions typically present with dyspnea on exertion, which is progressive as the effusion enlarges. Evaluation entails obtaining a chest X-ray with decubitus films to access the amount of pleural fluid and to ensure that it is free flowing and not loculated.

For patients with poor prognosis and effusions that may reaccumulate slowly, the initial approach is a therapeutic thoracentesis, which can be repeated as needed. Generally, no more than 1.5 L is removed at a time to prevent re-expansion pulmonary edema.

For patients with longer anticipated survival, more definite therapies are chosen. Pleurodesis, a medical procedure in which the pleural space is artificially obliterated, reduces effusion recurrence with up to a 90% success rate. Chemicals, such as bleomycin, talc, tetracycline, and povidone iodine, are introduced into the pleural space, causing irritation between the parietal and visceral layers of the pleura. This closes the space between them, preventing further fluid accumulation.[18] Long-term indwelling pleural catheters/peritoneal draining systems, variably known as Pleur(x) or pigtail catheters, are equally effective and can be placed in the ambulatory care setting. Recent studies suggest that catheter drainage may be more successful than pleurodesis at achieving lung re-expansion and preventing fluid reaccumulation.[19]

Pericardial Effusions

Malignant pericardial effusions confer a poor prognosis in lung cancer.[20] Pericardial effusions are associated with the following clinical features:

- Central chest pain relieved with sitting up
- Dyspnea
- Pericardial friction rub
- Distant heart sounds with a quiet precordium
- Presence of pulsus paradoxus (a decrease in systolic pressure more than 10mm Hg during inspiration)

The principal tool in the evaluation of a pericardial effusion is an echocardiogram. It establishes the presence and quantity of the effusion and determines its hemodynamic impact. It also provides a means to monitor changes in effusion size and hemodynamic status over time. Findings on electrocardiogram (ECG) include low voltage with electrical alternans (alternation of the amplitude of the QRS complex between beats, usually seen with large pericardial effusions) and evidence of pericarditis (diffuse ST segment elevations with reciprocal PR segment depression and T wave inversions). Chest radiographs may show cardiomegaly with the appearance of a "water-bottle" heart and epicardial halo.

Management goals are symptom relief and prevention of reoccurrence. Following percutaneous drainage by pericardiocentesis, up to 60% of cases recur; thus, prolonged catheter drainage is often required.[21] Additionally, pericardial windows and/or sclerosing agents may reduce recurrence.

Cough

Cough is a frequent and distressing symptom in lung cancer patients, present in up to 65% of this population.[22] Cough is more likely to occur in patients with lung tumors originating in the airways.

Medical management may include the following:

- *Cough suppressants*, which include nonopioids and peripherally acting drugs such as benzonatate (Tessalon Perles®)
- *Bronchodilators* may be beneficial if the cough is caused or exacerbated by bronchospasm
- *Opioids* are potent cough suppressants. These agents are reserved for patients with intractable cough resistant to other approaches.
- *Corticosteroids* may be beneficial if the cough is due to radiation therapy.

Hemoptysis

Hemoptysis is a concerning and potentially morbid symptom in lung cancer. For patients whose initial presenting symptom is hemoptysis, surgical resection of the bleeding lobe or lung may be appropriate if the cancer is confined to a hemi-thorax and is amendable to potentially curative surgery. However, most lung cancer patients with clinically significant hemoptysis have advanced disease and are not surgical candidates. Radiation therapy may also be employed to decrease hemoptysis that is not urgently life threatening.

The initial priority in managing major hemoptysis is maintenance of an adequate airway.[23] After determining which lung is bleeding, the patient should be placed on the affected side to limit aspiration into the noninvolved hemithorax and subsequent asphyxiation. Endotracheal intubation may be required; selective right or left mainstem intubation can be performed to protect the nonbleeding lung.

Once a patent airway is established, measures to control bleeding can be undertaken. In most cases, bronchoscopy is required to identify the source of bleeding and to perform one or more of the following therapeutic interventions.

Electrocautery

Electrocautery uses alternating electrical current to produce coagulation and vaporization of endobronchial lesions. It is a relatively inexpensive procedure and can be performed through either a rigid or flexible bronchoscope. Complications include endobronchial fire, inadvertent electrical shock, and hemorrhage.

Argon Plasma Coagulation

Argon plasma coagulation (APC) uses electrically conductive argon plasma as a medium to deliver a high-frequency current to coagulate tissue. Complication rates are low in comparison to other interventions. Additionally, the noncontact feature permits rapid coagulation with minimal manipulation and trauma to the target tissue.

Skeletal Complications

Skeletal metastases are a common manifestation of distant disease spread. Together, lung, breast, and prostate cancer are responsible for approximately 80% of metastatic bone disease.[24] Metastatic bone disease is classified as either osteolytic or osteoblastic, with osteolytic metastases more common in lung cancer. These lesions are characterized by bone disruption due to increased osteoclastic activity. Clinical complications include pain, pathologic fractures, compression of neural structures, hypercalcemia, and bone marrow aplasia, which are collectively referred to as *skeletal-related events*.

The treatment of pain from osseous metastasis involves the use of multiple treatment modalities, including pharmacologic therapy, radiation therapy, surgery, and other invasive techniques. In asymptomatic patients, the use of pharmacologic agents requires careful consideration, as the adverse effects may outweigh any potential benefits. Medications employed for the prevention of skeletal-related events are listed in Table 14.6.

Table 14.6 Medical Prevention of Skeletal-Related Events

Medication	Dosing
Bisphosphonates	
Pamidronate	90 mg IV every 4 weeks
Clodronate	1500 mg IV x 1 every 4 weeks *or*
	300 mg IV daily up to 7 days every 4 weeks *or*
	1600 mg PO x 1 every 4 weeks
Ibandronate	6 mg IV every 4 weeks
Zoledronic acid	4 mg IV every 3–4 weeks
RANKL antagonist	
Denosumab	120 mg SC every 4 weeks

RANKL, receptor activator of nuclear factor kappa-B ligand.

Pharmacologic Therapy

Nonsteroidal Anti-Inflammatory Drugs

Nonsteroidal anti-inflammatory drugs (NSAIDS) are a mainstay of therapy for cancer-induced bone pain. In theory, selective COX-2 inhibitors may be of greater therapeutic potential due to their antitumor and anti-angiogenic properties. Long-term use of NSAIDs conveys risk of gastritis and gastrointestinal ulceration. These agents should be avoided in patients with renal dysfunction.

Opioids

Opioids are a key component of the management of painful osseous metastases. See the section on "Cancer-Associated Pain" and Tables 14.1–14.3 for detailed information and dosing.

Bisphosphonates

Bisphosphonates have been shown to reduce pain and to reduce the incidence of and delay the onset of skeletal-related events (pain, pathologic fractures, compression of neural structures, hypercalcemia, and bone marrow aplasia) in patients with bony metastatic disease. These drugs inhibit bone resorption by interfering with osteoclast function. Preclinical studies have demonstrated direct antitumor properties of bisphosphonates, including induction of tumor cell apoptosis, inhibition of cancer cell invasion, and inhibition of metastatic growth.[25] Among bisphosphonates, zoledronate is considered the most potent in terms of reducing bone resorption and relieving pain.[26]

Bisphosphonate administration requires the following:

- Concurrent administration of supplemental calcium and vitamin D to prevent hypocalcemia (unless hypercalcemia is present)
- Monitoring of renal function and dose reduction in the setting of renal dysfunction
- Avoidance of use around the time of invasive dental procedures and consideration of a baseline dental evaluation to limit the risk of osteonecrosis of the jaw

Additionally, bisphosphonates are highly effective in the treatment of hypercalcemia, which can occur in the setting of skeletal metastases or as a humorally mediated paraneoplastic syndrome. Generally, serum calcium levels will fall within 2–4 days, reach nadir in 4–7 days, and remain suppressed for up to 21 days.

RANK/RANKL Inhibitors

The RANK-RANKL (receptor activator of nuclear factor kappa-B ligand) system, which plays an important role in osteoclast maturation and function, is involved in the development and progression of osseous metastasis. Osteoclast activity is dependent on the binding of receptor activator nuclear factor kappa-β ligand (RANKL), a member of the tumor necrosis factor (TNF) cytokine family expressed on activated T cells and osteoclasts, to RANK.

Denosumab, a fully human monoclonal antibody directed against RANKL, is FDA approved for the prevention of skeletal-related events in patients with osseous metastases from solid tumors. The dose of denosumab is 120 mg subcutaneously every 28 days. No adjustment is required for renal dysfunction. In a phase III randomized controlled trial of denosumab versus zoledronic acid (N = 1776), denosumab was associated with longer overall survival among the 801 patients with lung cancer: median 8.9 versus 7.7 months (HR 0.80; 95% CI, 0.67–0.95; $P = 0.01$).[27]

External Beam Radiation Therapy

Up to 80% of patients receiving palliative radiation therapy for osseous metastasis will experience partial to complete pain relief within 10 to 14 days of initial treatment.[28] The exact mechanism for this analgesic effect is unclear. Radiation therapy has a direct effect on osteoclast formation and tumor cell reduction, but these effects would not account for the early relief many patients experience. Radiation therapy may be administered in multiple modalities based on the extent of osseous disease, functional status of the patient, and dose of radiation therapy needed to treat the disease. Radiotherapy is also used as an adjunct to surgical stabilization to decrease the risk of impending skeletal complications.

Examples of commonly used radiation therapy treatment schedules for painful skeletal metastases are as follows:

- 2000 cGy delivered in 10 fractions of 200 cGy each
- 400 cGy delivered in a single fraction (generally reserved for patients with poor prognosis with life expectancy less than time to onset of late toxicity from high-dose-per-fraction radiation)

Radiopharmaceutical Therapy

Radiopharmaceutical therapy is occasionally used for palliation of diffuse osseous involvement in metastatic disease. Bone targeted isotopes—such as samarium-153 (^{153}Sm), strontium-89 (^{89}Sr), and rhenium-188 (^{188}Re)—are administered intravenously by a trained nuclear medicine physician. This approach is particularly useful for patients with multiple sites of painful metastases. However, these agents carry a risk of potentially permanent myelosuppression and therefore should not be used if further chemotherapy is planned.

Interventional Therapies

Focal Ablation Procedures

Focal ablative therapy, which includes radiofrequency ablation (RFA) or cryotherapy, may provide relief to patients with painful bony metastases.

Appropriate candidates have moderate to severe localized symptoms limited to one or two areas.

Vertebral Augmentation Procedures

Vertebroplasty and kyphoplasty are employed for the treatment of pain, spinal instability, and radiculopathy associated with vertebral compression fractures. Both procedures entail percutanous injection of bone cement into the fractured vertebral body. Kyphoplasty also involves balloon inflation prior to cement injection to restore vertebral height. Notably, a recent large randomized, placebo-controlled trial in patients with osteoporotic vertebral compression fractures showed no difference in pain and pain-related disability between vertebroplasty and a sham procedure.[29] However, the population did not include individuals with acute vertebral fractures, and it is not known whether these findings are generalizable to compression fractures due to malignancy.

Surgery

Up to 30% of patients with bone metastases develop fractures of the long bones requiring surgical intervention, with the femur being the most commonly involved site.[30] Weight-bearing bones are rarely amenable to conservative therapy because of the high degree of weight support and load. Nevertheless, it should be noted that, in general, lung cancer has a shorter survival after development of bone metastases than do prostate or breast cancer. Accordingly, fewer patients may live long enough to develop pathologic fractures.

Prophylactic surgery is often considered for patients with disease involving weight-bearing bones or those with impending fractures. There is no uniformly accepted system for assessing risk and need for surgery. Variables commonly considered[31,32]:

- *Size of lesion*: increased risk if >2.5 cm or greater than two-thirds the diameter of the bone
- *Cortical involvement*: increased risk if >50%
- *Location*: increased risk in weight-bearing bones, especially subtrochanteric region of femur
- *Type*: increased risk if lytic

Surgery entails bone fixation and stabilization with pins, nails, screws, and/or rods. Most patients who undergo surgical stabilization experience an improved quality of life with decreased pain and suffering and reduced complications associated with immobility (e.g., deep venous thrombosis, pressure ulcers).

Neurologic Complications

Brain Metastases

Up to 65% of lung cancer patients will develop brain metastases. Standard treatment options include symptomatic therapy with corticosteroids, whole-brain radiation therapy, stereotactic radiation, and surgical resection.

An algorithm depicting a therapeutic approach to patients with newly diagnosed brain metastases is depicted in Figure 14.1.

Corticosteroids

Corticosteroids decrease edema associated with intracranial metastases. Because it has the most potent anti-inflammatory compared to mineralocorticoid properties, dexamethasone is the preferred agent. A commonly employed regimen is dexmethasone 10 mg bolus, then 4 mg every 6 hours (given orally or intravenously). The dose is tapered as the effects of definitive therapies take effect. In the absence of symptomatic edema, steroids may be withheld and the patient closely observed.

Short-term toxicities of corticosteroids include gastritis and gastrointestinal ulceration, mood changes (including acute psychosis), and hyperglycemia. Over longer treatment courses, patients may experience weight gain, depression, osteoporosis, cataracts, increased intraocular pressure, hypertension, and truncal weight gain. In patients receiving long term (> 1 month) corticosteroids, pneumocystis pneumonia prophylaxis with trimethoprim-sulfamethoxazole should be considered. Dexamethasone is a potent long-acting corticosteroid; an understanding of its dosing equivalency is important for effective clinical use (see Table 14.7).

Surgery

For patients considered surgical candidates, the resection of a single brain metastasis has become a standard option. Clinical factors taken into account include accessibility of the lesion, functional status, and status of extracranial disease.[33] Additionally, selected patients with up to three brain metastases may benefit from resection of the dominant or all lesions.[34] The addition of whole-brain radiation therapy after surgical resection has been shown to prolong survival.[33]

Stereotactic Radiation

Stereotactic radiation capitalizes on advanced tumor localization and patient immobilization technology to deliver high-potency radiation doses in a single fraction or a small number of fractions. The use of stereotactic radiation is generally restricted to lesions <3.5 cm in size and no more than three total lesions. Up to 2400 cGy can be administered in a single fraction. In some instances, whole-brain radiation therapy is administered with stereotactic radiation. This approach decreases neurologic progression but does not improve overall survival.

Table 14.7 Corticosteroid Equivalencies

Name	Equivalent Dose (mg)	Half-Life (hours)
Short-acting		
Hydrocortisone	20	8 to 12
Cortisone	25	8 to 12
Intermediate-acting		
Methylprednisolone	4	12 to 36
Prednisolone	5	12 to 36
Prednisone	5	12 to 36
Triamcinolone	5	12 to 36
Long-acting		
Betamethasone	0.6	36 to 54
Dexamethasone	0.75	36 to 54

Compared to whole-brain radiation therapy alone, stereotactic radiation therapy plus whole-brain radiation therapy results in increased likelihood of performance status improvement or stability. Among patients with single brain metastases or favorable prognosis, overall survival may be improved.[35]

Whole-Brain Radiation Therapy

A commonly used treatment schedule for whole-brain radiation therapy is 300 cGy per fraction x 10 fractions for a total of 3000 cGy. Adverse effects include cortical atrophy, ventriculomegaly and clinical symptoms such as memory loss, frontal gait disorders, and urinary incontinence.[33]

Epidural Spinal Cord Compression

Spinal metastases are among the most debilitating complications of systemic cancer. If untreated, the disease state is relentless and can progress rapidly, leading to worsening pain, sphincter dysfunction, sensory loss, and paralysis.[36]

In lung cancer and other solid tumors, the distribution of metastatic sites resulting in cord compression is as follows:

- Vertebral body, 80%
- Paravertebral, 15%
- Intramedullary, 5%

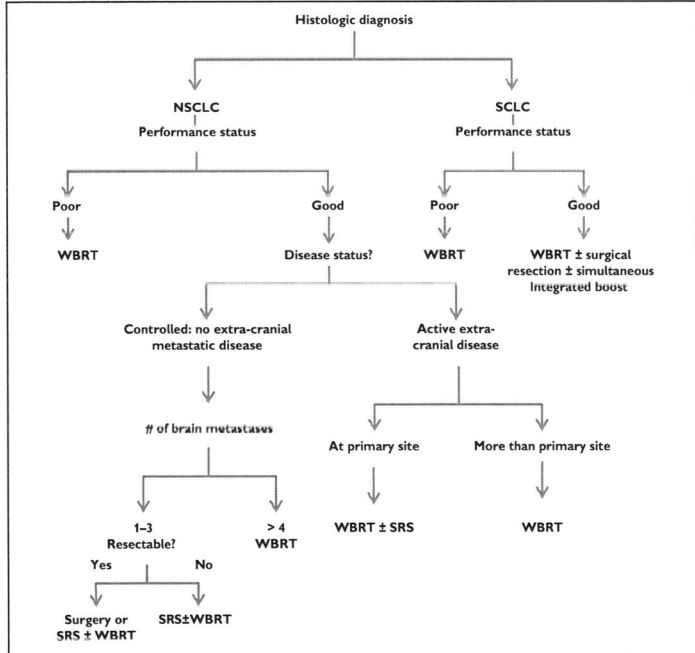

Figure 14.1 Approach to brain metastases in patients with lung cancer.

NSCLC, non-small cell lung cancer; SCLC, small cell lung cancer; SRS, stereotactic radiosurgery; WBRT, whole brain radiation therapy.

Involved spinal levels are as follows:

- Thoracic, 70%
- Lumbar, 20%
- Cervical, 10%

Symptoms of spinal cord compression include the following:

- Back pain (up to 90% of cases)
- Paresthesias
- Weakness
- Sphincter dysfunction

Neurologic status at presentation is highly correlated with functional outcome (see Table 14.8).

Epidural cord compression should be considered in lung cancer patients reporting new-onset back pain. The pain may be local, mechanical, or radicular. Patients describe the pain as being "gnawing" or "aching"; it is often worse when the patient is supine or straining. At the site of tumor involvement there is often tenderness to palpation. Once the tumor mass impinges on nerve roots, radicular pain ensues, which patients describe as "sharp" or "shooting."

If metastatic spinal cord compression is suspected, corticosteroids should be administered immediately prior to any diagnostic testing.[36,37] The reduction in vasogenic edema leads to improved pain control and neurologic function. Magnetic resonance imaging is the most sensitive (>90%) and specific (>90%) imaging test. Definitive treatment is surgical decompression followed by radiation therapy or radiation therapy alone. Surgery should be considered in patients with a good prognosis who are medically operable. Surgical options include laminectomy and circumferential decompression and reconstruction.

Laminectomy

Laminectomy entails removal of spinous processes and adjacent lamina up to the junction of the pedicles, relieving pressure on the compressed spinal cord. The procedure conveys relatively little surgical risk, does not require stabilization hardware, can be performed quickly, and is a widely known surgical technique.

In the majority of cases, however, laminectomy does not address the etiology of the cord compression: metastatic tumor in the vertebral body, which lies anterior to the epidural space. Instead, the removal of posterior vertebral column elements may potentially cause or worsen spinal instability, exacerbating pain and leading to neurologic deterioration.

Table 14.8 Functional Outcomes from Malignant Epidural Spinal Cord Compression	
Pretreatment Neurologic Status	**Likelihood of Ambulation Posttreatment**
Ambulatory	>80%
Paraparetic	<50%
Paraplegic	<10%

Circumferential Decompression and Reconstruction

These surgical methods aim to decompress the spinal cord circumferentially, then reconstruct and stabilize the spine. These aggressive and lengthy operations often require an anterior approach to the affected vertebral body. Depending on spinal level, this may entail a median sternotomy (for high thoracic lesions), a standard thoracotomy (midthoracic), a thoraco-abdominal incision (low thoracic), or a retroperitoneal incision (lumbar). The diseased portion of the vertebral body is resected, and then reconstructed with methylmethacrylate or bone grafting. Internal fixation hardware is then used to stabilize the spine. Radiation therapy is administered postoperatively.

Radiation Therapy

External beam radiation is usually administered as a single, 8–10 cm wide posterior field that encompasses the epidural lesion and a 5 cm (1–2 vertebral bodies) margin above and below the target level. Patients generally receive 3000 cGy delivered in ten 300 cGy fractions.[36,38]

Treatment-Related Complications

Chemotherapy-Associated Complications

Anemia

Symptomatic anemia results in fatigue, dyspnea, depression, and effects on other medical comorbidities leading to increased medical costs, complications, and delays in therapy.[39,40] Treatments for anemia include red blood cell (RBC) transfusions and erythropoiesis-stimulating agents (ESAs).

Transfusions reverse anemia rapidly but have a transient effect. Risks include transfusion associated reactions, transmission of infectious agents, and iron overload.

ESAs, which stimulate the production of red blood cells, can raise hemoglobin levels and reduce transfusion requirements. Recently, substantial concerns regarding ESA-related adverse effects have emerged, including increased risk of thromboembolic events, cerebrovascular events, pulmonary edema, and hypertension. Additionally, a number of studies in cancer patients have suggested an association between ESA use and decreased survival. Nevertheless, a recent meta-analysis of ESAs in lung cancer patients receiving chemotherapy demonstrated no increase in mortality or disease progression.[41] Currently, ESAs are not recommended for patients receiving potentially curative therapy. Other potential causes of anemia, such as dietary deficiencies (check folate, B12), hemolysis (check Coombs, haptoglobin, LDH), and bleeding (check fecal occult blood test, iron studies, reticulocyte count), should be ruled out prior to ESA initiation. Iron deficiency should be corrected before starting an ESA. ESA dosing and titration guidelines are listed in Table 14.9.

Neutropenia

Neutropenia occurs commonly in lung cancer patients receiving myelosuppresive chemotherapy and also in certain patients receiving radiation therapy. Severe neutropenia predisposes patients to infections and may result in treatment delays or dose reductions.

Table 14.9 Erythropoietin Stimulating Agent Dosing and Titration

Initial dosing	Titration If No Response*
Epoetin alfa 150 units/kg SC three times per week	Increase dose to 300 units/kg SC three times per week
Epoetin alfa 40,000 units SC weekly	Increase dose to 60,000 units SC weekly
Darbepoetin alfa 2.25 mcg/kg SC weekly	Increase darbepoetin to up to 4.5 mcg/kg SC weekly
Darbepoetin alfa 500 mcg SC every 3 weeks	

*Typical goal Hb 10–11 g/dL. Week 3: If Hb increased >1 g/dL after 2 weeks of therapy, hold dose until Hb <10 g/dL and resume at reduced dose (decrease dose by 25%). Week 4: If Hb increased <1 g/dL from baseline and Hb <11 g/dL, increase dose. If Hb increased ≥1 g/dL and Hb <11 g/dL, continue current dose. If Hb increased ≥1 g/dL and Hb >11 g/dL, hold dose until Hb <10 g/dL and resume at reduced dose (decrease dose by 25%). Week 8: If Hb increased <1 g/dL from baseline and Hb <11 g/dL, discontinue treatment as patient not responding.

Myeloid growth factors (e.g., granulocyte colony stimulating factor [G-CSF]) are used to prevent and treat neutropenic fever. Commonly employed guidelines for the use of myeloid growth factors in the prevention of neutropenic fever include the following[42]:

- Chemotherapy regimen conveying high risk (>20%) of neutropenic fever: administer
- Chemotherapy regimen conveying intermediate risk (10%–20%) of neutropenic fever: consider
- Chemotherapy regimen conveying low risk (<10%) of neutropenic fever: do not administer
- Prior neutropenic fever or dose-limiting neutropenia: consider administration versus chemotherapy dose reduction

Commonly used guidelines for the use of myeloid growth factors in the treatment of neutropenic fever include the following[42]:

- Continue if already receiving G-CSF
- Administer if risk factors for infection-associated complications:
  - Sepsis syndrome
  - Age >65 years
  - Absolute neutrophil count (ANC) < 100
  - Neutropenia expected to last >10 days
  - Pneumonia
  - Fungal infection
  - Prior neutropenic fever
  - Hospitalized when fever developed

Table 14.10 provides myeloid growth factor dosing. Table 14.11 lists lung cancer chemotherapy regimens considered to be intermediate and high risk for neutropenic fever.[42]

Table 14.10 Myeloid Growth Factor Dosing for Chemotherapy-Induced Neutropenia

Medication	Dosing (Start 24–72 Hours after Completion of Chemotherapy)
Filgrastim (G-CSF, Neupogen)	5 mcg/kg SC daily (round to nearest vial size—300 mcg or 480 mcg) until post-nadir ANC recovery to normal or near-normal levels by laboratory standards
Pegfilgrastim (Neulasta)	6 mg SC once per cycle of treatment
Sargramostim (GM-CSF, Leukine)	250 mcg/m² SC daily (round to nearest vial size—300 mcg or 480 mcg) until post-nadir ANC recovery to normal or near-normal levels by laboratory standards

Table 14.11 Risk of Neutropenic Fever with Lung Cancer Chemotherapy Regimens

High risk (>20%)
— Topotecan
Intermediate risk (10%–20%)
—Cisplatin-paclitaxel
—Cisplatin-vinorelbine
—Cisplatin-docetaxel
—Cisplatin-irinotecan
—Cisplatin-etoposide
—Carboplatin-paclitaxel
—Docetaxel

Gastrointestinal Side Effects

Nausea and Vomiting

Appropriate prevention and treatment of chemotherapy-induced nausea and vomiting are key to the successful administration of medical lung cancer treatments. Table 14.12 lists commonly used drugs and regimens for lung cancer treatment according to emetogenic risk, along with antiemetic recommendations. Table 14.13 provides further information on the dosing and adverse effects of specific antiemetic drugs.

All patients should be given prescriptions for breakthrough antiemetics. Commonly used agents include the following:

- Prochlorperazine 10 mg PO/IV q4–6h prn
- Prochlorperazine 25 mg PR q12h prn
- Haloperidol 0.2 to 2 mg PO/IV q4–6h prn
- Lorazepam 0.5 to 2 mg PO q6h prn
- Metoclopramide 10 to 20 mg PO q6h prn
- Promethazine 12.5 to 25 mg PO/IV q6h prn

Mucositis, Stomatitis, and Esophagitis

Oral mucositis represents a major complication of cytotoxic chemotherapy and radiotherapy. Affected patients may experience pain, dysgeusia, and dysphagia with subsequent dehydration and malnutrition. These symptoms reduce quality

Table 14.12 Emetogenic Risk and Antiemetic Recommendations for Lung Cancer Chemotherapy Regimens

Emetogenic Risk	Lung Cancer Regimens	Antiemetic Recommendations
High (>90%)	Cisplatin >50 mg/m² Cisplatin-docetaxel Cisplatin-etoposide Cisplatin-gemcitabine Cisplatin-irinotecan Cisplatin-paclitaxel Cisplatin-pemetrexed Cisplatin-vinorelbine	Aprepitant PO days 1–3 + 5-HT₃ antagonist IV day 1, then PO days 2–4 + Dexamethasone IV day 1, then PO days 2–4 + Lorazepam IV day 1
Moderate (30%–90%)	Carboplatin-docetaxel Carboplatin-etoposide Carboplatin-gemcitabine Carboplatin-paclitaxel Carboplatin-pemetrexed Carboplatin-vinorelbine Cisplatin <50 mg/m²	5-HT₃ antagonist IV day 1, then PO days 2–4 + Dexamethasone IV day 1, then PO days 2–4 ± Lorazepam IV day 1
Low (10%–30%)	Docetaxel Gemcitabine Pemetrexed	Dexamethasone IV day 1 ± Lorazepam IV day 1 OR Prochlorperazine day 1 ± Lorazepam IV day 1
Minimal (<10%)	Bevacizumab Crizotinib Erlotinib Vinorelbine	None

of life and may lead to treatment delays or dose reductions. Management is directed toward supportive care.

Topical formulations for the treatment of mucositis and esophagitis commonly include various combinations of the following ingredients:
- Lidocaine (local anesthetic)
- Diphenhydramine (antihistamine)
- Antacids
- Nystatin (antifungal)
- Glucocorticoids (anti-inflammatory)
- Sucralfate (coating agent)

In patients with symptoms of gastritis, proton pump inhibitors (PPIs) or sulcrafate may be beneficial. Patients with mild oral candidiasis can be

Table 14.13 Antiemetic Dosing

Drug	IV Dosing	PO Dosing	Side Effects	Comments/Remarks
Serotonin 5HT₃ antagonists				
Dolasetron	100 mg	100 mg	Vascular headaches, constipation, urinary retention, agitation, prolonged QT interval	Avoid if electrolyte abnormalities (hypokalemia or hypomagnesemia) or long QT syndrome
Granisetron	1 mg	2 mg (also available as a 3.1 mg/hour patch)		
Ondansetron	8–24 mg/day	8mg Q8h prn		
Palonosetron	0.5 mg × 1	0.5 mg × 1		
Corticosteroids				
Dexamethasone (pre-chemo)	10–20 mg	10–20 mg	Hyperglycemia, hypertension, irritability, insomnia, edema	Pre-chemo dosing for highly emetogenic therapy
Dexamethasone (delayed emesis)	N/A	4–8 mg bid × 2 days		
Prokinetic agents (dopamine-2, serotonin receptor antagonists)				
Metoclopramide (pre-chemo)	2 mg/kg		Extrapyramidal side effects, flu-like symptoms	Caution with neuroleptics, phenothiazines, or antidopaminergics
Metoclopramide (delayed emesis)	N/A	20–40 mg bid-qid × 3–5 days		
Anti-psychotics (dopamine-2 receptor antagonists)				
Prochlorperazine	10–30 mg	0–20 mg Q4h prn	Constipation, dizziness, dry mouth, nausea, insomnia, restlessness, extrapyramidal side effects, QT prolongation	Caution with concomitant use of other antipsychotics
Haloperidol	1–4 mg	4 mg Q6h prn		

(continued)

Table 14.13 (Continued)

Drug	IV Dosing	PO Dosing	Side Effects	Comments/Remarks
Benzodiazepines				
Lorazepam	1–2 mg	1–4 mg Q6h prn	Sedation, hypotension	
Neurokinin inhibitors				
Aprepitant		125 mg on day 1, then 80 mg daily on days 2 and 3	Neutropenia, bradycardia, fatigue, constipation, urinary retention, QT prolongation	CYP3A4 metabolism and potential drug–drug interactions; dose reduction of concurrently administered corticosteroids recommended
Fosaprepitant	150 mg IV on day 1 only OR 115 mg IV on day 1 followed by aprepitant 80 mg PO daily on days 2 and 3			
Miscellaneous				
Dronabinol		5–20 mg	Dependency, dizziness, cognitive alteration	Caution with concomitant use of other central nervous system depressants

treated with oral nystatin swish and swallow. However, for severe or extensive esophageal candidiasis, treatment with oral fluconazole may be needed. Due to patients' immunocompromised state, the threshold for treating these patients should be low.

Chemotherapy-Induced Peripheral Neuropathy

Peripheral neuropathy may be seen with numerous chemotherapeutic agents. This complication may involve the sensory, motor, and/or autonomic nervous system. Common clinical features include the following:

- *Sensory*: parasthesias, dysesthesias, hypoesthesias, burning, pain
- *Motor*: weakness, atrophy, gait abnormalities
- *Autonomic*: diaphoresis, postural weakness, anhidrosis, orthostasis, constipation, ileus

Chemotherapeutic agents may be associated with isolated sensory or motor neuropathy or combined sensory and motor effects. Commonly used lung cancer treatments associated with peripheral neuropathy include the following[43]:

Sensory
Carboplatin (13%–42%)
Cisplatin (49%–100%)
Etoposide (1%–2%)
Gemcitabine (2%–38%)

Sensory and Motor
Docetaxel (20%–58%)
Paclitaxel (59%–78%)
Vinorelbine (20%–25%)

In about 75% of patients, chemotherapy-induced peripheral neuropathy is reversible with a median time to recovery of 13 weeks after treatment discontinuation. In cases of severe neuropathy, symptoms may improve only partially or not at all.

Currently, no specific agent is routinely recommended for the treatment or prevention of chemotherapy-associated peripheral neuropathy. The standard approach to this clinical entity includes awareness and early detection of neuropathy, along with dose reduction and/or discontinuation of the causative drugs. Several agents have been studied for the prevention of this complication, including nerve growth factor, amifostine, glutathione, glutamine, glutamate, and vitamin B6.[43] Twice daily hand and foot soaks in cold water for 15 minutes have also been reported to mitigate symptoms.

Certain conditions may predispose to the development of chemotherapy-induced peripheral neuropathy:

- Medical conditions (e.g., diabetes, alcohol abuse, impaired renal or hepatic function)
- Advanced age
- Genetic variations in drug metabolism
- Underlying unrelated neuropathy

Table 14.14 lists agents used to treat symptoms of painful sensory peripheral neuropathy.

Table 14.14 Pharmacologic Treatment of Painful Peripheral Neuropathy

Drug	PO Dosing	Advantages	Adverse Effects	Comments/Remarks/Warnings
First-line agents				
Tricyclic antidepressants (TCAs)				
Nortriptyline	Start at 25 mg PO at night. If receiving benefit, titrate up to 50 mg PO at night	Inexpensive, once daily dosing, can treat depression	Anticholinergic effects, hypotension	May prolong QT interval; caution in patients with emotional liability; avoid in patients on SSRIs
Amitriptyline			More sedating than nortriptyline	
Calcium channel alpha 2 delta ligands				
Gabapentin	Start at 300 mg PO three times daily. Titrate slowly to 600 mg PO three times daily, then as tolerated up to 1200 mg PO three times daily	Safe, no significant drug interactions	Somnolence, dizziness, peripheral edema, cognitive impairment, tremors	Caution with renal insufficiency, multiple daily dosing
Pregabalin	Start at 75 mg PO twice daily. If symptoms improved and well tolerated, increase up to 150 mg PO twice daily			Expensive, unknown long-term side effects
Selective serotonin and norepinephrine reuptake inhibitors (SNRIs)				
Duloxetine	60 mg PO daily	Once daily dosing; also have anxiolytic effects	Nausea, dry mouth, constipation, insomnia, dizziness	Slow titration to optimal dosing; when stopping, needs slow taper
Venlafaxine	75 mg PO daily			

Second-line agents

Opioids (see opioid table for dosing); reserved for those who have failed to respond or cannot tolerate first-line treatment

Tramadol	Start at 25 mg PO every 6 hours as needed. If symptoms improved and well tolerated, increase to 50 mg PO every 6 hours as needed	Inexpensive, no significant drug interaction	Cognitive impairment, gait disturbance, lowers seizure threshold	Increased risk for serotonin syndrome

Third-line agents

Antiepileptics

Carbamazepine	Start at 100 mg PO daily. If symptoms improving and tolerated, increase up to 400 mg PO daily	Once daily dosing; can also treat seizures	Aplastic anemia, thrombocytopenia, Stevens-Johnson syndrome, pancreatitis	Caution with drug–drug interactions
Valproic acid	Start at 200 mg PO twice daily. If symptoms improving and tolerated, increase up to 1 g PO twice daily	Inexpensive	Hepatotoxicity, pancreatitis, pancytopenia, teratogenic	Caution with drug–drug interactions

Topical agents—only for localized peripheral neuropathy

Capsaicin	Apply to affect area three times daily	Inexpensive	Temporary relief of symptoms; burning, pain, inflammation	Avoid contact with eyes, mucous membranes and open wounds
Lidocaine (Lidoderm patch)	Apply one patch to area of symptoms for 8–12 hours daily	Expensive, only for localized areas of symptoms	Burning, itching, erythema at the site of application	Caution with patients on antiarrhythmic agents and severe hepatic dysfunction

Toxicities of Epidermal Growth Factor Receptor Inhibitors

Acneiform rash is the most common toxicity of epidermal growth factor receptor (EGFR) inhibitors, occurs with both monoclonal antibodies (mAbs) and tyrosine kinase inhibitors (TKIs), and can be attributed to the expression of EGFR in normal epithelial tissues, such as skin (see Fig. 14.2). Papulopustular lesions develop in up to 75% of patients treated with erlotinib.[44]

The onset of rash is typically 7–10 days after initiation of an EGFR inhibitor. Severity varies over the course of therapy. The rash usually resolves within several weeks after treatment discontinuation. Although termed "acneiform," the rash has an etiology, pathophysiology, and management that is distinct from acne. For severe symptoms, a dermatology referral should be considered.

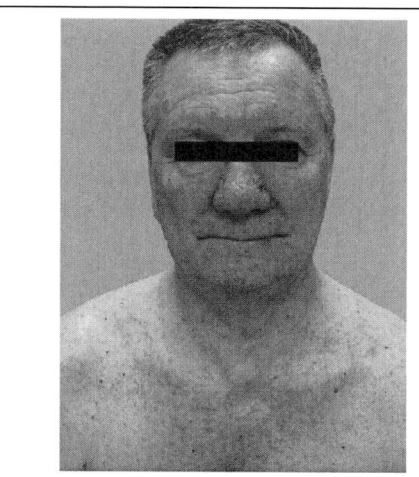

Figure 14.2 Epidermal growth factor receptor (EGFR) inhibitor–associated acneiform rash. (Reprinted from Lacouture ME et al. *Oncology* (Williston Park) 2007;21(11 Suppl 5):17–21, with permission from Elsevier.)

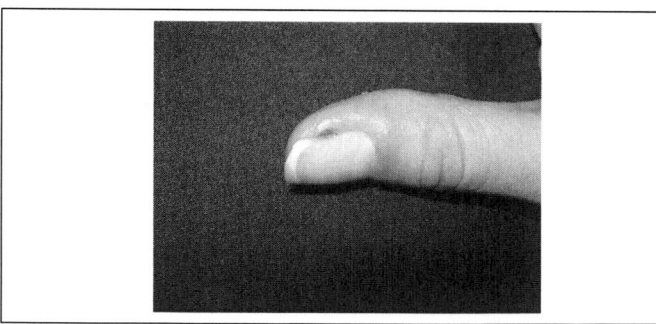

Figure 14.3 Epidermal growth factor receptor (EGFR) inhibitor–associated paronychia. (Reprinted from Lacouture ME, et al. *Clin Lung Cancer.* 2006;8(Suppl 1):S36–42, with permission from Elsevier.)

Other less common dermatologic toxicities include nail, hair, and eye involvement. Paronychia is a painful periungual inflammation and fissuring that affects fingernails and toenails, occuring in up to 15% of patients receiving EGFR inhibitors (Fig. 14.3). For supportive care, the application of petroleum jelly to the periungual area may prevent paronychia. Treatment includes the use of daily soaks with vinegar or bleach.

Up to 5% of patients treated with EGFR inhibitors report hair abnormalities, including scalp and body alopecia, as well as changes in texture (e.g., being more brittle, finer, curlier).[45] Affected areas may revert back to normal after therapy discontinuation.

Table 14.15 Management of Selected Epidermal Growth Factor Receptor (EGFR) Inhibitor–Associated Toxicities

Toxicity	Description	Management
Skin—rash (mild)	• Localized • Minimally symptomatic • No impact on activities of daily living (ADL) • No sign of superinfection	• Continue EGFR inhibitor at current dose and monitor for change in severity • Consider pulsed topical hydrocortisone 1% or 2.5% cream and/or clindamycin 1% gel • Reassess after 2 weeks; if worsens or does not improve, institute "skin rash—moderate" treatment
Skin rash (moderate)	• Generalized • Mild symptoms (e.g., pruritus, tenderness) • Minimal impact on ADL • No sign of superinfection	• Continue EGFR inhibitor at current dose and monitor for change in severity • Pulsed topical hydrocortisone 1% or 2.5% cream and/or clindamycin 1% gel or pimecrolimus 1% cream • Doxycycline 100 mg PO bid or minocycline 100 mg PO bid • Reassess after 2 weeks; if worsens or does not improve, institute "skin rash—severe" treatment
Skin—rash (severe)	• Generalized • Severe symptoms (e.g., pruritus, tenderness) • Significant impact on activities of daily living • Potential for superinfection	• Reduce EGFR inhibitor dose • Pulsed topical hydrocortisone 1% or 2.5% cream and/or clindamycin 1% gel • Doxycycline 100 mg PO bid or minocycline 100 mg PO bid • Methylprednisolone dose pack • Reassess after 2 weeks; if worsens or does not improve, consider dose interruption or discontinuation

(continued)

Table 14.15 (Continued)

Toxicity	Description	Management
Skin—xerosis		• Emollients: zinc oxide (30%), petroleum jelly, or other think emollients (e.g., Aquaphor®, Aveeno®, Cetaphil®, Eucerin®) • Avoid alcohol-based lotions, antibacterial soaps
Skin—pruritus		• Cool compresses • Antihistamines (systemic, topical) • Pulsed topical hydrocortisone 1% or 2.5% cream • Topical menthol lotions
Skin—fissuring		• Monsel's solution (ferric subsulfate), silver nitrate, or zinc oxide (20%–30%) • Protective coverings, cyanoacrylate glue (Krazy Glue, Super Glue)
Skin—desquamation		• Petroleum jelly • Mild (neutral pH) soap
Nails—paronychia	• Periungual pyogenic granuloma-like inflammation, swelling, and fissuring of lateral nail folds and distal finger tufts	• Petroleum jelly • Vinegar or bleach soaks
Eyes—tri chomegaly with eye irritation	• Thickening of lashes	• Avoid contact lens use • Referral to ophthalmologist

Source: Modified in part from *Tarceva Rash Management Guide.* Available at http://prod.bioonc.gene.s3.amazonaws.com/media/20100312/resources/tarceva/tarceva-rash.pdf

Ocular changes—including dry eyes, conjunctivitis, blepharitis, trichomegaly (excessive eyelash growth), and corneal erosions—may occur in up to 30% of patients.[46] Occurrences of any of these symptoms warrant an ophthalmologic evaluation. Treatment is supportive, including warm compresses, eyelash clipping, or short-term course of ophthalmic corticosteroids.

Treatment recommendations for EGFR inhibitor–associated toxicities are listed in Table 14.15.

Radiation Therapy-Associated Toxicities

Thoracic radiation may affect a number of healthy tissues, including the lungs, esophagus, heart, and spinal cord.

Pneumonitis/Fibrosis

While up to 65% of patients receiving thoracic radiation therapy develop posttreatment radiographic changes, only 5%–15% develop clinically manifest radiation-induced lung injury. Consequently, radiation-induced lung injury is a clinical diagnosis, which may be supported by radiographic findings.

The typical time to onset of acute radiation pneumonitis is 4–12 weeks after radiation therapy. For late or fibrotic radiation pneumonitis, typical onset is 6–12 months after radiation therapy. The manifestations of these entities are similar and include cough, dyspnea, chest pain, rales, and hypoxemia. Fever is more common with acute radiation pneumonitis.

Radiographically, volume loss, patchy infiltrates, and a straight-line effect (denoting the radiation therapy port) may be seen. As noted earlier, these findings are not specific to radiation-induced lung injury.

The volume of lung irradiated is the principal predictor of pulmonary complications. It is generally recommended that the V20 (volume of normal lung receiving more than 20 Gy) be no more than 30%–35%.

Corticosteroids are the mainstay of acute treatment of radiation pneumonitis. A common approach is to administer prednisone 30–60 mg PO daily (based on the severity of symptoms) for 2 weeks and then taper gradually. In severe cases, prolonged dosing (up to months in certain patients) may be required. Chronic therapy may include supplemental oxygen, pentoxifylline, and vitamin E.

Esophagitis/Esophageal Strictures

Radiation-induced esophagitis is managed similarly to chemotherapy-associated esophagitis. Esophageal stricture may occur as a late complication and is treated with esophageal dilatation. Esophageal toxicities from radiation therapy are increased if the mean dose to the esophagus exceeds 34 Gy.

Cardiac Toxicity

Via the generation of reactive oxygen species, radiation therapy may lead to inflammatory changes and fibrosis in the cardiovascular system. In general, cardiac toxicities occur years after radiation therapy. Predictors of these complications include the total radiation dose, the dose per fraction, the volume of heart irradiated, the concomitant administration of cardiotoxic systemic agents, and other risk factors such as hypertension and smoking. It is generally recommended to keep the V40 (volume of the heart receiving more than 40 Gy) less than 50%.

Clinical manifestations include coronary artery disease (with the left anterior descending [LAD] and right coronary artery [RCA] most commonly affected), valvular changes, myocardial fibrosis resulting in diastolic dysfunction, pericarditis, and conduction system fibrosis leading to dysrhythmias. Treatment may require coronary stent or pacemaker placement.

Neurologic Toxicity

Radiation delivered to the spinal cord may result in late complications of myelitis, which manifests as both motor and sensory changes. To limit neurologic toxicity, radiation doses to the spinal cord are recommended to be less than 45 Gy. Corticosteroids are the principal treatment.

Palliative and End-of-Life Care

Palliative care, with a focus on symptom management, psychosocial support, and assistance with decision making, has the potential to improve a patient's quality of care and end-of-life care.[47] Recent studies in advanced lung cancer suggest that early initiation of palliative care services not only improves quality of life but also increases overall survival.[48,49]

Table 14.16 Agents Used for the Treatment of Delirium

Medication	Starting Dose (mg)	Dosing Interval	Max Dose per 24 Hours	Formulations	Extrapyramidal Symptoms*	Anticholinergic Symptoms†	Sedation
Haloperidol	0.5–1	0.5–1 mg per hour for urgent symptoms; otherwise Q6 hr	20 mg	Available as oral solution and as injectable product	High	Mild	Moderate
Risperidone	0.25–1	Twice daily or up to Q6 hr prn	6 mg	Available as tablets or as ODT	Moderate	Mild	Mild
Olanzapine	2.5–10	Daily, IM can be given Q2 hr prn up to three doses	20 mg	Available as ODT and IM	Mild	Moderate	Moderate
Quetiapine	12.5–50	Twice daily	800 mg	Oral tablets only	Mild	Moderate	High

*Extrapyramidal symptoms include Parkinsonism (cogwheel rigidity, resting tremor, postural instability), akinesia (inability to initiate movement), akathisia (inability to remain motionless), acute dystonia, tardive dyskinesia (involuntary asymmetric muscle movements).

†Anticholinergic symptoms include ataxia, disorientation, xerostomia, mydriasis (pupil dilation) and resulting photophobia, diplopia, and ileus.

IM, intramuscular; ODT, orally disintegrating tablet.

Secretions

Secretions occur commonly at the end of life and may be distressing for both patients and family members. The mainstay of medical treatment involves the use of anticholinergic medications. Commonly used agents include the following:

- Scopolamine (transdermal disc [1.5 mg]—apply behind the ear every 3 days; or 0.4 mg PO every 4 hours as needed)
- Atropine (0.4 mg sublingual or subcutaneously every 4 hours as needed)
- Glycopyrrolate (0.2–0.4 mg subcutaneously or PO every 4 hours as needed)

Adverse effects include confusion, urinary hesitancy, and constipation. Opioids may also be used to decrease secretions.

Delirium

Delirium is often acute in onset and is precipitated by an inciting event (i.e., infection, iatrogenic [medication, chemotherapy], metabolic). It is important to identify any reversible causes in addition to treating the symptom.

In the interim, for acute symptom management, haloperidol, a first-generation antipsychotic, is the most commonly used agent for controlling delirium. With increased dosing, patients are at risk for extrapyramidal symptoms (e.g., acute dystonia, akinesia [inability to initiate movement], akathisia [inability to remain motionless]) as well as cardiac arrhythmias if given intravenously due to the effect on QT interval. Other antipsychotics have been found to be effective as well. Commonly used agents for the treatment of delirium are listed in Table 14.16.

In cases of severe delirium or uncontrolled pain, where conventional treatment options are not effective, palliative sedation may be the only method to control symptoms. This method requires expert input from a palliative care service.

References

1. Langer C, Hirsh V. Skeletal morbidity in lung cancer patients with bone metastases: demonstrating the need for early diagnosis and treatment with bisphosphonates. Lung Cancer 2010;67:4–11.

2. Yamada K, Ikehara Y, Nakanishi H, Kozawa E, Tatematsu M, Sugiura H. Solitary bone metastasis as the first clinical manifestation in a patient with small bowel adenocarcinoma. J Orthop Sci 2007;12:606–610.

3. Foley KM. Acute and Chronic Cancer Pain Syndromes: Oxford Textbook of Palliative Medicine. 3rd ed. New York: Oxford University Press; 2004.

4. Gatchel RJ, Peng YB, Peters ML, Fuchs PN, Turk DC. The biopsychosocial approach to chronic pain: scientific advances and future directions. Psychol Bull 2007;133:581–624.

5. Cleeland CS, Ryan KM. Pain assessment: global use of the Brief Pain Inventory. Ann Acad Med Singapore 1994;23:129–38.

6. Strouse TB. Pharmacokinetic drug interactions in palliative care: focus on opioids. J Palliative Med 2009;12:1043–50.

7. Trescot AM. Review of the role of opioids in cancer pain. J Natl Comp Cancer Netw 2010;8:1087–94.

8. Argoff CE, Silvershein DI. A comparison of long- and short-acting opioids for the treatment of chronic noncancer pain: tailoring therapy to meet patient needs. Mayo Clinic Proc 2009;84:602–12.

9. Fine PG, Portenoy RK. *A Clinicial Guide to Opioid Analgesia*. 2nd ed. New York: Vendome Group; 2007.

10. Portenoy RK. Treatment of cancer pain. *Lancet* 2011;377:2236–47.

11. Fine PG, Portenoy RK. Establishing "best practices" for opioid rotation: conclusions of an expert panel. *J Pain Symptom Manage* 2009;38:418–25.

12. Katz N, Mazer NA. The impact of opioids on the endocrine system. *Clin J Pain* 2009;25:170–5.

13. Villars P, Dodd M, West C, et al. Differences in the prevalence and severity of side effects based on type of analgesic prescription in patients with chronic cancer pain. *J Pain Symptom Manage* 2007;33:67–77.

14. McNicol E, Horowicz-Mehler N, Fisk RA, et al. Management of opioid side effects in cancer-related and chronic noncancer pain: a systematic review. *J Pain* 2003;4:231–56.

15. Estfan B, Mahmoud F, Shaheen P, et al. Respiratory function during parenteral opioid titration for cancer pain. *Palliative Med* 2007;21:81–6.

16. Kvale PA, Simoff M, Prakash UB. Lung cancer. Palliative care. *Chest* 2003;123:284S–311S.

17. Heffner JE. Management of the patient with a malignant pleural effusion. *Semin Respir Crit Care Med* 2010;31:723–33.

18. Rodriguez-Panadero F, Romero-Romero B. Management of malignant pleural effusions. *Curr Opin Pulm Med* 2011;17:269–73.

19. Chee A, Tremblay A. The use of tunneled pleural catheters in the treatment of pleural effusions. *Curr Opin Pulm Med* 2011;17:237–41.

20. Lestuzzi C, Bearz A, Lafaras C, et al. Neoplastic pericardial disease in lung cancer: impact on outcomes of different treatment strategies. A multicenter study. *Lung Cancer* 2011;72:340–7.

21. Soler-Soler J, Sagrista-Sauleda J, Permanyer-Miralda G. Management of pericardial effusion. *Heart* 2001;86:235–40.

22. Vaaler AK, Forrester JM, Lesar M, Edison M, Venzon D, Johnson BE. Obstructive atelectasis in patients with small cell lung cancer. Incidence and response to treatment. *Chest* 1997;111:115–20.

23. Jean-Baptiste E. Clinical assessment and management of massive hemoptysis. *Crit Care Med* 2000;28:1642–7.

24. Mercadante S. Malignant bone pain: pathophysiology and treatment. *Pain* 1997;69:1–18.

25. Rachner TD, Singh SK, Schoppet M, et al. Zoledronic acid induces apoptosis and changes the TRAIL/OPG ratio in breast cancer cells. *Cancer Lett* 2010;287:109–16.

26. Green JR. Bisphosphonates: preclinical review. *Oncologist* 2004;9(Suppl 4):3–13.

27. Scagliotti G, Hirsch V, Siena S, et al. Overall survival improvement in patients with lung cancer and bone metastases treated with denosumab versus zoledronic acid: subgroup analysis from a randomized phase 3 study. *J Thorac Oncol* 2012;7:1823–9.

28. Poulter CA, Cosmatos D, Rubin P, et al. A report of RTOG 8206: a phase III study of whether the addition of single dose hemibody irradiation to standard fractionated local field irradiation is more effective than local field irradiation alone in the treatment of symptomatic osseous metastases. *Intl J Radiat Oncol Biol Physics* 1992;23:207–14.

29. Kallmes DF, Comstock BA, Heagerty PJ, et al. A randomized trial of vertebroplasty for osteoporotic spinal fractures. *N Engl J Med* 2009;361:569–79.

30. Harrington KD. Impending pathologic fractures from metastatic malignancy: evaluation and management. *Instr Course Lect* 1986;35:357–81.

31. Mirels H. Metastatic disease in long bones. A proposed scoring system for diagnosing impending pathologic fractures. *Clin Orthop Relat Res* 1989;249:256–64.

32. Coleman RE. Clinical features of metastatic bone disease and risk of skeletal morbidity. *Clin Cancer Res* 2006;12:6243s–9s.

33. Soffietti R, Ducati A, Ruda R. Brain metastases. *Handb Clin Neurol* 2012;105:747–55.

34. Kyritsis AP, Markoula S, Levin VA. A systematic approach to the management of patients with brain metastases of known or unknown primary site. *Cancer Chemother Pharmacol* 2012;69:1–13.

35. Andrews DW, Scott CB, Sperduto PW, et al. Whole brain radiation therapy with or without stereotactic radiosurgery boost for patients with one to three brain metastases: phase III results of the RTOG 9508 randomised trial. *Lancet* 2004;363:1665–72.

36. Loblaw DA, Perry J, Chambers A, Laperriere NJ. Systematic review of the diagnosis and management of malignant extradural spinal cord compression: the Cancer Care Ontario Practice Guidelines Initiative's Neuro-Oncology Disease Site Group. *J Clin Oncol* 2005;23:2028–37.

37. Graham PH, Capp A, Delaney G, et al. A pilot randomised comparison of dexamethasone 96 mg vs 16 mg per day for malignant spinal-cord compression treated by radiotherapy: TROG 01.05 Superdex study. *Clin Oncol (R Coll Radiol)* 2006;18:70–6.

38. Taylor JW, Schiff D. Metastatic epidural spinal cord compression. *Sem Neurol* 2010;30:245–53.

39. Houts AC, Loh GA, Fortner BV, Kallich JD. Patient and caregiver time burden associated with anaemia treatment in different patient populations. *Support Care Cancer* 2006;14:1195–204.

40. Groopman JE, Itri LM. Chemotherapy-induced anemia in adults: incidence and treatment. *J Natl Cancer Inst* 1999;91:1616–34.

41. Vansteenkiste J, Glaspy J, Henry D, et al. Benefits and risks of using erythropoiesis-stimulating agents (ESAs) in lung cancer patients: study-level and patient-level meta-analyses. *Lung Cancer* 2012;76(3):478–85.

42. National Comprehensive Cancer Network. *Myeloid Growth Factors* [accessed June 17, 2012]. Available at: http://www.nccn.org/professionals/physician_gls/pdf/myeloid_growth.pdf

43. Hausheer FH, Schilsky RL, Bain S, Berghorn EJ, Lieberman F. Diagnosis, management, and evaluation of chemotherapy-induced peripheral neuropathy. *Sem Oncol* 2006;33:15–49.

44. Shepherd FA, Rodrigues Pereira J, Ciuleanu T, et al. Erlotinib in previously treated non-small-cell lung cancer. *N Engl J Med* 2005;353:123–32.

45. Thatcher N, Nicolson M, Groves RW, et al. Expert consensus on the management of erlotinib-associated cutaneous toxicity in the U.K. *Oncologist* 2009;14:840–7.

46. Zhang G, Basti S, Jampol LM. Acquired trichomegaly and symptomatic external ocular changes in patients receiving epidermal growth factor receptor inhibitors: case reports and a review of literature. *Cornea* 2007;26:858–60.

47. Ferrell B, Koczywas M, Grannis F, Harrington A. Palliative care in lung cancer. *Surg Clin North Am* 2011;91:403–17.

48. Temel JS, Greer JA, Muzikansky A, et al. Early palliative care for patients with metastatic non-small-cell lung cancer. *N Engl J Med* 2010;363:733–42.

49. Borneman T, Koczywas M, Cristea M, Reckamp K, Sun V, Ferrell B. An interdisciplinary care approach for integration of palliative care in lung cancer. *Clin Lung Cancer* 2008;9:352–60.

Index

Page numbers followed by *t* indicate a table and *f* indicate a figure.

237